GASTROINTESTINAL CANCER

The University of Texas System Cancer Center
M. D. Anderson Hospital and Tumor Institute
25th Annual Clinical Conference on Cancer

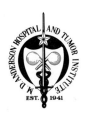

Published for
The University of Texas System Cancer Center
M. D. Anderson Hospital and Tumor Institute
Houston, Texas, by Raven Press, New York

The University of Texas System Cancer Center
M. D. Anderson Hospital and Tumor Institute
25th Annual Clinical Conference on Cancer *(25th :
1980 : M.D. Anderson Hospital
and Tumor Institute)*

Gastrointestinal Cancer

Edited by

John R. Stroehlein, M.D.
and
Marvin M. Romsdahl, M.D., Ph.D.

Departments of Medicine and Surgery
The University of Texas System Cancer Center
M. D. Anderson Hospital and Tumor Institute
Houston, Texas

Raven Press ■ New York

Raven Press, 1140 Avenue of the Americas, New York, New York 10036

Made in the United States of America

Library of Congress Cataloging in Publication Data

Clinical Conference on Cancer (25th : 1980 : M.D.
    Anderson Hospital and Tumor Institute)
    Gastrointestinal cancer.

    Includes index.
    1. Gastrointestinal system—Cancer—Congresses.
2. Digestive organs—Cancer—Congresses. I. Stroehlein,
John R. II. Romsdahl, Marvin M. III. M.D. Anderson
Hospital and Tumor Institute. IV. Title. [DNLM:
1. Gastrointestinal neoplasms—Congresses. W3 C162H 25th
1980g / WI 149 c 641 1980g]
RC280.D5C56 1980   616.99′43   80-5825
ISBN 0-89004-612-3

    This volume is a compilation of the proceedings of The University of Texas System Cancer Center M. D. Anderson Hospital and Tumor Institute 25th Annual Clinical Conference on Cancer, held November 5–7, 1980, in Houston, Texas.
    The material contained in this volume was submitted as previously unpublished material, except in instances in which credit has been given to the source from which some of the illustrative material was derived.
    Great care has been taken to maintain the accuracy of the information contained in the volume. However, the Editorial Staff and The University of Texas System Cancer Center cannot be held responsible for errors or for any consequences arising from the use of the information contained herein.

Preface

This 25th Annual Clinical Conference follows, after 15 years, our previous 1965 conference on Cancer of the Gastrointestinal Tract. Inasmuch as major changes in the incidence of gastrointestinal cancer have not occurred during this time span, the importance of this site in reference to all cancer types is still evident. A slightly downward trend in the percentage of all cancer deaths attributed to gastrointestinal cancer still continues, a statistic influenced greatly by the increased incidence of deaths in both males and females caused by carcinoma of the lung. This trend is affected, to a lesser degree, by the continuing reduced mortality due to stomach cancer. It is of interest that 50% of all cancer deaths in 1900 were attributed to digestive cancer, with this figure dropping to 34% in 1965, and to 26% in 1980. The importance of gastrointestinal cancer is underscored, then, by the realization that approximately one in four of all cancer deaths will result from cancer at this site. It is, therefore, logical to review progress made since our 10th Annual Clinical Conference on this topic in order to assess potential impact on this large number of patients.

In 1965, conference highlights included a relatively new description of the anatomy of the liver, a development which improved the safety and practicality of a surgical approach to neoplasms in this organ. Improved diagnostic techniques, particularly radiographic studies, were emphasized, while radiotherapy and chemotherapy were emerging as serious modalities in a multidisciplinary approach to the management of gastrointestinal cancer.

It is of great interest to view the scope of disciplines now involved in research concerning gastrointestinal cancer, as well as the progress of established methods of treatment. This volume considers developments in epidemiology which point to carcinoma of the colon and rectum and carcinoma of the pancreas as being associated with western world culture. To some extent, this circumstance has served to direct increased attention on carcinogenesis. Consequently, experimental animal models, nutritional and dietary considerations, and an evaluation of the role of microflora and bile have all aroused our interest and curiosity as to their relationship to these important types of cancer in man.

The discovery of a carcinoembryonic antigen (CEA) as a potential marker for colonic and rectal cancer has perhaps been instrumental in expanding other immunological approaches, in the areas of both diagnosis and treatment. Familial polyposis and Gardner's Syndrome have provided a clearly genetic trait distinctly associated with carcinoma of the colon and rectum. Hereditary susceptibility to colorectal cancer in some individuals not afflicted with polyposis has also now been established. Inflammatory diseases of the intestinal tract, because of their association with carcinoma, have prompted pathology studies seeking new information and concepts. We are also witnessing investigations in gastrointestinal cancer that include the basic disciplines of biochemistry and molecular biology. Varied and multidisciplinary research approaches to gastrointestinal cancer have been favorably enhanced by the National Organ Site Program through the National Large Bowel Cancer Project and the National Pancreatic Cancer Project.

These directions in solving problems in gastrointestinal cancer have also been complemented by progress in diagnostic modalities such as endoscopic retrograde cholangiography and pancreatography, colonoscopy, and improved application of air contrast colon examinations, as well as noninvasive techniques such as ultrasonography, computerized axial tomography, and radionuclide scanning of the liver.

From the standpoint of treatment, properly implemented surgery still represents the patient's best, and perhaps only, hope for cure of established cancer of the gastrointestinal tract. Consequently, it is important that specific planning and implementation of the best initial surgical procedure be performed, since second and subsequent operations are often difficult with uncertain outcomes. While systemic chemotherapy and immunotherapy have been extensively investigated as potential adjuvants to surgical treatment, their value in this aspect is still not established. The role of these modalities, particularly chemotherapy, is best applied to patients with unresectable or metastatic disease. Finally, we are hopeful that newly emerging data from both basic and clinical sectors will serve to identify a means for prevention of gastrointestinal cancer in the future.

The problem of gastrointestinal cancer, in its total context, is indeed a challenge. Substantial effort from dedicated individuals, provided with necessary support, will be needed in order to witness further progress. It is rewarding, however, to witness the spectrum of effort and the vitality that is being expended toward this goal.

The Editors

Acknowledgments

We would like to extend our appreciation to all who made the 25th Annual Clinical Conference and the publication of this monograph possible. Our special thanks go to the National Cancer Institute, to the American Cancer Society, Texas Division Incorporated, for cosponsoring the Clinical Conference, and to the Texas Society of Pathology for cosponsoring the Thirteenth Annual Special Pathology Program held in conjunction with the Clinical Conference. We are grateful for support provided for annual clinical and pathology awards and lectureships, including the Heath Award established by former University of Texas Board of Regents chairman William W. Heath and Mavis B. Heath in honor of the former chairman's brothers and the William O. Russell lectureship endowed by Joanne Vandenberge Hill.

For planning and preparation of the conference we wish to thank members of the Program Committees: Howard T. Barkley, Jr., Edward M. Copeland, III, Murray M. Copeland, Gerald D. Dodd, Jr., Emil J Freireich, Herbert A. Fritsche, Jr., Robert C. Hickey, David A. Karlin, Richard G. Martin, Anthony J. Mastromarino, Robert S. Nelson, Marvin M. Romsdahl (Co-chairman), Leslie J. Smith, Jr. (Chairman, Pathology Conference), and John R. Stroehlein (Co-chairman). For arrangements and organizations special thanks to Miss Frances Goff, Staff Assistant to the President, U. T. Cancer Center; Glenn Knotts, Director, Division of Educational Resources; Stephen Stuyck, Head, Department of Public Information and Education; John Bush, Executive Director, University Cancer Foundation; and to The University of Texas System Cancer Center Executive Staff and their associates.

For compiling and editing this volume, we are again grateful to the Department of Scientific Publications, U. T. Cancer Center M. D. Anderson Hospital and Tumor Institute. We especially wish to thank Dorothy Beane, Department Head, and Susan Freitag, Editor, without whose assistance timely publication of this monograph would not have been possible.

Contents

Directions for Future Research

Contributors

William A. Albano
*Departments of Surgery and
  Preventive Medicine
Creighton University School of
  Medicine
Omaha, Nebraska 68178*

H. T. Barkley, Jr.
*Division of Radiotherapy
The University of Texas System Cancer
  Center
M. D. Anderson Hospital and Tumor
  Institute
Houston, Texas 77030*

Oliver H. Beahrs
*Mayo Medical School
Rochester, Minnesota 55901*

Frederick F. Becker
*Department of Pathology
The University of Texas System Cancer
  Center
M. D. Anderson Hospital and Tumor
  Institute
Houston, Texas 77030*

Agop Y. Bedikian
*Department of Developmental
  Therapeutics
The University of Texas System Cancer
  Center
M. D. Anderson Hospital and Tumor
  Institute
Houston, Texas 77030*

Roland W. Bennetts
*Department of Medicine
The University of Texas System Cancer
  Center
M. D. Anderson Hospital and Tumor
  Institute
Houston, Texas 77030*

Michael E. Bernardino
*Department of Diagnostic Radiology
The University of Texas System Cancer
  Center
M. D. Anderson Hospital and Tumor
  Institute
Houston, Texas 77030*

Gerald P. Bodey
*Department of Developmental
  Therapeutics
The University of Texas System Cancer
  Center
M. D. Anderson Hospital and Tumor
  Institute
Houston, Texas 77030*

B. B. Borgelt
*Division of Radiotherapy
The University of Texas System Cancer
  Center
M. D. Anderson Hospital and Tumor
  Institute
Houston, Texas 77030*

Michael A. Burgess
*Department of Developmental
  Therapeutics
The University of Texas System Cancer
  Center
M. D. Anderson Hospital and Tumor
  Institute
Houston, Texas 77030*

Patrick J. Byrne
*Division of Medical Oncology
Vincent T. Lombardi Cancer Research
  Center
Georgetown University School of
  Medicine
Washington, D.C. 20007*

William M. Christopherson
*Department of Pathology
University of Louisville School of
  Medicine
Louisville, Kentucky 40208*

V. P. Chuang
Department of Diagnostic Radiology
The University of Texas System Cancer
   Center
M. D. Anderson Hospital and Tumor
   Institute
Houston, Texas 77030

R. Lee Clark
President Emeritus
The University of Texas System Cancer
   Center
M. D. Anderson Hospital and Tumor
   Institute
Houston, Texas 77030

Edward M. Copeland, III
The University of Texas Medical
   School at Houston and Department
   of Surgery
The University of Texas System Cancer
   Center
M. D. Anderson Hospital and Tumor
   Institute
Houston, Texas 77030

Murray M. Copeland
National Large Bowel Cancer Project
The University of Texas System Cancer
   Center
M. D. Anderson Hospital and Tumor
   Institute
Houston, Texas 77030

Thomas H. Corbett
Chemotherapy Department
Southern Research Institute
Birmingham, Alabama 35202

L. Cuasay
Department of Epidemiology
The University of Texas System Cancer
   Center
M. D. Anderson Hospital and Tumor
   Institute
Houston, Texas 77030

B. Shannon Danes
Department of Medicine
Laboratory for Cell Biology
Cornell University Medical College
New York, New York 10021

Gerald D. Dodd
Department of Diagnostic Radiology
The University of Texas System Cancer
   Center
M. D. Anderson Hospital and Tumor
   Institute
Houston, Texas 77030

O. Howard Frazier
Department of Surgery
The University of Texas System Cancer
   Center
M. D. Anderson Hospital and Tumor
   Institute
Houston, Texas 77030

R. Fuqua
Department of Developmental
   Therapeutics
The University of Texas System Cancer
   Center
M. D. Anderson Hospital and Tumor
   Institute
Houston, Texas 77030

Phil Gold
McGill Cancer Centre
Department of Medicine
Montreal General Hospital
Montreal, Quebec, Canada

David M. Goldenberg
Department of Pathology
University of Kentucky Medical Center
Lexington, Kentucky 40536

Daniel P. Griswold, Jr.
Chemotherapy Department
Southern Research Institute
Birmingham, Alabama 35202

Robert C. Hickey
Executive Vice President
The University of Texas System Cancer
   Center
Director
M. D. Anderson Hospital and Tumor
   Institute
Houston, Texas 77030

D. H. Hussey
Division of Radiotherapy
The University of Texas System Cancer
  Center
M. D. Anderson Hospital and Tumor
  Institute
Houston, Texas 77030

George L. Jordan, Jr.
Cora and Webb Mading
Department of Surgery
Baylor College of Medicine
Houston, Texas 77030

David A. Karlin
Department of Medicine
The University of Texas System Cancer
  Center
M. D. Anderson Hospital and Tumor
  Institute
Houston, Texas 77030

Kamal G. Khalil
Department of Surgery
The University of Texas System Cancer
  Center
M. D. Anderson Hospital and Tumor
  Institute
Houston, Texas 77030

J. Kong
Division of Radiotherapy
The University of Texas System Cancer
  Center
M. D. Anderson Hospital and Tumor
  Institute
Houston, Texas 77030

Josef K. Korinek
Department of Medicine
The University of Texas System Cancer
  Center
M. D. Anderson Hospital and Tumor
  Institute
Houston, Texas 77030

Charles A. LeMaistre
President
The University of Texas System Cancer
  Center
M. D. Anderson Hospital and Tumor
  Institute
Houston, Texas 77030

Martin Lipkin
Gastroenterology Service and
  Diagnostic Unit
Department of Medicine
Memorial Sloan-Kettering Cancer
  Center
New York, New York 10021

Henry T. Lynch
Department of Preventive Medicine/
  Public Health
Creighton University School of
  Medicine
Omaha, Nebraska 68178

Jane Lynch
Department of Preventive Medicine/
  Public Health
Creighton University School of
  Medicine
Omaha, Nebraska 68178

Patrick M. Lynch
Creighton University School of
  Medicine
Omaha, Nebraska 68178

Richard G. Martin
Department of Surgery
The University of Texas System Cancer
  Center
M. D. Anderson Hospital and Tumor
  Institute
Houston, Texas 77030

K. A. Mason
Department of Radiation Oncology
University of California, Los Angeles
Los Angeles, California 90024

G. M. Mavligit
Department of Developmental
  Therapeutics
The University of Texas System Cancer
  Center
M. D. Anderson Hospital and Tumor
  Institute
Houston, Texas 77030

Charles M. McBride
Department of Surgery
The University of Texas System Cancer
  Center
M. D. Anderson Hospital and Tumor
  Institute
Houston, Texas 77030

Eugene M. McKelvey
Department of Developmental
  Therapeutics
The University of Texas System Cancer
  Center
M. D. Anderson Hospital and Tumor
  Institute
Houston, Texas 77030

Marion J. McMurtrey
Department of Surgery
The University of Texas System Cancer
  Center
M. D. Anderson Hospital and Tumor
  Institute
Houston, Texas 77030

A. B. Miller
Faculty of Medicine
University of Toronto
Toronto, Ontario, Canada

A. R. Moossa
Department of Surgery
University of Chicago
Chicago, Illinois 60637

Basil Clifford Morson
St. Mark's Hospital
London, England

Clifton F. Mountain
Department of Surgery
The University of Texas System Cancer
  Center
M. D. Anderson Hospital and Tumor
  Institute
Houston, Texas 77030

Robert S. Nelson
Department of Medicine
The University of Texas System Cancer
  Center
M. D. Anderson Hospital and Tumor
  Institute
Houston, Texas 77030

Garth L. Nicolson
Department of Tumor Biology
The University of Texas System Cancer
  Center
M. D. Anderson Hospital and Tumor
  Institute
Houston, Texas 77030

Yehuda Z. Patt
Department of Developmental
  Therapeutics
The University of Texas System Cancer
  Center
M. D. Anderson Hospital and Tumor
  Institute
Houston, Texas 77030

Matilda Perkins
Department of Surgery
The University of Texas
Health Science Center at San Antonio
San Antonio, Texas 78284

Marvin M. Romsdahl
Department of Surgery
The University of Texas System Cancer
  Center
M. D. Anderson Hospital and Tumor
  Institute
Houston, Texas 77030

Jerrold P. Saxton
Division of Radiotherapy
The University of Texas System Cancer
  Center
M. D. Anderson Hospital and Tumor
  Institute
Houston, Texas 77030

Frank M. Schabel, Jr.
Chemotherapy Department
Southern Research Institute
Birmingham, Alabama 35202

Philip S. Schein
Division of Medical Oncology
Vincent T. Lombardi Cancer Research
    Center
Georgetown University School of
    Medicine
Washington, D.C. 20007

Paul Sherlock
Gastroenterology Service and
    Diagnostic Unit
Department of Medicine
Memorial Sloan-Kettering Cancer
    Center
New York, New York 10021

Frederick P. Smith
Division of Medical Oncology
Vincent T. Lombardi Cancer Research
    Center
Georgetown University School of
    Medicine
Washington, D.C. 20007

J. Leslie Smith, Jr.
Department of Pathology
The University of Texas System Cancer
    Center
M. D. Anderson Hospital and Tumor
    Institute
Houston, Texas 77030

William J. Spanos, Jr.
Division of Radiotherapy
The University of Texas System Cancer
    Center
M. D. Anderson Hospital and Tumor
    Institute
Houston, Texas 77030

John R. Stroehlein
Department of Medicine
The University of Texas System Cancer
    Center
M. D. Anderson Hospital and Tumor
    Institute
Houston, Texas 77030

John L. Thomas
Department of Diagnostic Radiology
The University of Texas System Cancer
    Center
M. D. Anderson Hospital and Tumor
    Institute
Houston, Texas 77030

Manuel Valdivieso
Department of Developmental
    Therapeutics
The University of Texas System Cancer
    Center
M. D. Anderson Hospital and Tumor
    Institute
Houston, Texas 77030

Daniel D. Von Hoff
Department of Medicine
The University of Texas
Health Science Center at San Antonio
San Antonio, Texas 78284

S. Wallace
Department of Diagnostic Radiology
The University of Texas System Cancer
    Center
M. D. Anderson Hospital and Tumor
    Institute
Houston, Texas 77030

Lee W. Wattenberg
Department of Laboratory Medicine
    and Pathology
University of Minnesota
Minneapolis, Minnesota 55455

Sidney J. Winawer
Gastroenterology Service and
    Diagnostic Unit
Department of Medicine
Memorial Sloan-Kettering Cancer
    Center
New York, New York 10021

H. Rodney Withers
Department of Radiation Oncology
University of California, Los Angeles
Los Angeles, California 90024

Paul V. Woolley
Division of Medical Oncology
Vincent T. Lombardi Cancer Research
  Center
Georgetown University School of
  Medicine
Washington, D.C. 20007

Jesus Zornoza
Department of Diagnostic Radiology
The University of Texas System Cancer
  Center
M. D. Anderson Hospital and Tumor
  Institute
Houston, Texas 77030

Introduction

Gastrointestinal Cancer, edited by
John R. Stroehlein and
Marvin M. Romsdahl.
Raven Press, New York © 1981.

Introduction

Charles A. LeMaistre, M.D.

President, The University of Texas System Cancer Center

I am pleased to welcome you to our 25th annual Clinical Conference. Each year, The University of Texas System Cancer Center holds this conference so practicing physicians may have an opportunity to exchange ideas and information about a particular type of cancer.

We hope this year's conference on gastrointestinal cancer will bring new insight to a site of cancer that continues to remain a major health hazard. This fact is true despite efforts undertaken in the last decade which have brought about many improvements in diagnosis and therapy.

Studies conducted in the last 10 years by you and other physicians have improved our understanding of the role of nutrition in gastrointestinal cancer, made clear that changes are taking place in the epidemiology of some GI cancers, enabled the development of promising imaging techniques that have enhanced our diagnostic capabilities, and brought about improvements in treatment.

It now appears, for example, that nutritional support plays a larger part in the treatment of persons with cancer than for persons who have other diseases that involve the same organ system. Not only have we seen that nutritional support measures can lessen the mortality for surgical procedures, but we have found that we can restore immunological competence to patients by using proper nutritional aids. Nutritional research is now being broadened to include studies on anorexia, altered taste perception, and other nutritional and digestive complications that commonly occur in cancers of the gastrointestinal system.

We also are recognizing that changes are taking place in the incidence of some GI cancers. Recent epidemiologic studies have shown that the incidence of gastric cancer is decreasing, while the incidence of pancreatic cancer is on the rise. In addition, we now are seeing fewer rectal lesions and more proximal lesions. We do not yet know what these statistics mean. But we do know that the messages they give us are important, particularly with respect to screening for GI cancers.

Perhaps one of the areas which has made the biggest impact on gastrointestinal cancers is the development of new diagnostic methods. For the first time, we have at our disposal noninvasive methods of viewing the GI system through such diagnostic techniques as cross-sectional imaging and ultra-sound. In addition to allowing us to visualize portions of the gastrointestinal tract that were hidden from view before, these new methods have made feasible the development and safe use of directed-needle biopsies. By combining these new techniques with fiberoptic endoscopy and the air contrast examination, we now are able to better visualize all portions of the gastrointestinal tract. Although there has not yet been an impact on survival, it appears that by using these new diagnostic techniques we are seeing smaller lesions at the time of surgery.

The development of fiberoptic colonoscopy and the use of air contrast barium enemas have had similar positive implications with respect to colon cancer. While the impact of fiberoptic colonoscopy remains uncertain, it has allowed biopsy and removal of polyploid lesions in the colon. Within the next decade, we should be able to tell what the impact of these two diagnostic methods has been and where their future roles in prevention might lie.

While the overall outlook for treatment of gastrointestinal cancers is not as good as we might hope, the five-year survival rates for most localized cancers of the gastrointestinal tract are encouraging. Since the majority of these cancers are not localized at the time of surgery, however, physicians are attempting to minimize recurrence by the use of radiation and chemotherapy and immunotherapy programs. The interest in developing and implementing screening tests for certain cancers recently has been revived, particularly with respect to colorectal lesions. Although the hoped-for serum test specific for colorectal cancer has not been found, physicians again are showing interest in its development and are conducting clinically relevant studies in immunobiology and the use of fecal occult blood testing as a screening modality.

I would like to express my thanks to our partners in this conference—the National Cancer Institute and the Texas Division of the American Cancer Society, which have assisted us in sponsoring this conference for many years. In addition, I would like to add my special thanks to the *National Enquirer* for their gift in support of this conference.

Heath Memorial Award Lecture

Gastrointestinal Cancer, edited by
John R. Stroehlein and
Marvin M. Romsdahl.
Raven Press, New York © 1981.

Introduction of Heath Memorial Award Recipient

Robert C. Hickey, M.D.

*Executive Vice President, The University of Texas System Cancer Center; and
Director, M. D. Anderson Hospital and Tumor Institute*

Dr. Phil Gold, Physician-In-Chief of the Montreal General Hospital and Professor of Medicine and Physiology of the McGill University, is the 1980 recipient of the Heath Memorial Award.

The Heath Award has had a number of distinguished recipients. They are listed in your brochure. The award is given for "outstanding contributions to the better care of the cancer patient by the clinical application of basic science knowledge." Indeed, that is the case today.

Dr. Phil Gold's name is identified with CEA, the carcinoembryonic antigen, discovered and described by him with Dr. S. O. Freedman in 1965. This biological marker has been useful in cancer care, particularly of patients with cancers of the gastrointestinal tract; but mainly, it stimulated an entire field of inquiry about biological markers.

Dr. Gold's career has been intimately tied to McGill University. I have mentioned his faculty status. He earned his bachelor's degree in 1957, then a doctorate of medicine. In 1965 he received a doctorate in physiology and immunology—his thesis being on the carcinoembryonic antigen.

His awards have been many; I shall not enumerate them, but they are listed in the brochure.

The Heath Award was established by the late William W. Heath, former Chairman of the Board of Regents of The University of Texas System, in honor of his brothers. The Award consists of a certificate, a monetary award, and a medallion.

The medallion, which I hold, is depicted in the brochure. On the face are two central figures representing a physician tending his patient. Below the figures is the tree of life. The alpha and omega represent the physician's role in patient care from birth to death. The retort symbolizes the role of research. On the reverse side is the inscription: Dr. Phil Gold, "for outstanding contribution to the care of the patient with cancer."

So ladies and gentlemen, I present to you Dr. Phil Gold of Montreal, the 1980 Heath Awardee. The title of his lecture is Biological Markers in Human Tumors.

Gastrointestinal Cancer, edited by
John R. Stroehlein and
Marvin M. Romsdahl.
Raven Press, New York © 1981.

Biological Markers of Human Tumors

Phil Gold, M.D., Ph.D.

*McGill Cancer Centre and the Department of Medicine of the Montreal General
Hospital, Montreal, Canada*

Cancer represents a complex group of diseases characterized by a common feature: the failure of the malignant cell to respond to the usual homeostatic growth control mechanisms of the host. This results in autonomous cancer cell proliferation that is passed on to all daughter cells by their malignant progenitors. Thus, cancer may well be perceived primarily as a genetic problem. Studies of cancer tissue have, however, involved multiple areas of biological research. Early studies included investigations of the metabolic properties of tumor cells and, subsequently, a search for constituents or properties that might be unique to tumor tissue.

With advances in immunobiology during the first half of the twentieth century, it was inevitable that the concepts and technology of this rapidly expanding field would be applied to studies in cancer research. With the use of antibodies as probes, the putatively unique tumor tissue constituents thus defined gained the common designation of "tumor antigens" and the battle lines were soon drawn between the protagonists of a rapidly unfolding saga. After a number of false starts and somewhat poorly conceived experiments involving outbred animals and tumors of questionable origin, the dogma at mid-century suggested that the concept of tumor-specific antigens was heretical and that the immunological approach to the search for unique constituents of tumor cells should cease (Castro 1978, Richards 1980).

As is so often the case in biology, however, after the final pronouncement had apparently been made, the classic experiments of Foley (1953) provided the first conclusive evidence for the presence of neoantigens in chemically induced tumors of mice. These studies had been made possible by the development of highly inbred, or syngeneic, strains of mice and rats. Foley demonstrated that methylcholanthrene-induced tumors transplanted between syngeneic mice could be rejected under appropriately controlled circumstances. Since the transplantation had been performed between genetically identical animals, the observed rejection reaction could have been precipitated only by an immunological response against a newly developed antigen, on the surface of the tumor cells, that had appeared during the process of neoplastic transformation. The tumor constituents were called "tumor specific transplantation antigens" (TSTA) because tumor rejection had been used as the reaction to detect their presence. Although this observation has been confirmed in numerous virally and chemically induced tumor systems, detection of tumor-specific transplantation antigens in experimental tumors has not always been unequivocal.

In studies that have subsequently been performed, it has been found that the tumor antigens in question are apparently capable of eliciting humoral and/or cell-mediated immune responses on the part of the tumor-bearing host but generally without the functional capacity to destroy the growing tumor. Indeed, some evidence suggests that the host antitumor response may actually stimulate or potentiate tumor cell growth and dissemination (Prehn and Lappe 1971).

ANTITUMOR IMMUNE REACTIONS

The TSTA's noted previously can be detected in both autochthonous and syngeneic hosts immunized against the transplanted tumor cells, by tumor rejection assays, as well as by in vitro assays that measure both cellular and humoral antitumor immune responses (Klein 1966, Old and Boyse 1964, Green et al. 1967). A significant feature of these antigens is that they reflect the antigenically individual characteristics of each tumor type. Thus, each chemically induced neoplasm expresses its own unique tumor-specific antigen, whereas all tumors induced by the same virus share the same TSTA's (Basombrio 1970). Concomitant with antigenic gain, there is sometimes a measurable loss of normal tissue antigens from the cell surface (Ting and Herberman 1971, Haywood and McKhann 1970, Baldwin and Glaves 1972).

Since tumor transplantation studies in man are precluded by ethical considerations, the demonstration of human tumor-specific antigens (TSA's) depends on indirect serologic evidence, provided by such techniques as immunofluorescence, complement fixation tests, cytotoxicity, and a variety of in vitro correlates of cell-mediated immunity (Hellström et al. 1971). By these techniques, tumor antigens and antitumor immunity have been demonstrated for a variety of tumors. In man, the cellular and humoral responses against surface antigens of the tumor appear to be directed principally against antigens shared by all tumors of the same organ and histologic type. This observation is responsible for much of the current optimism concerning the potential usefulness of immunologic manipulation in the control of cancer (Hellström and Hellström 1972). Individually unique tumor antigens may, however, occur but will only be recognized in autologous reaction systems (Lewis et al. 1969).

Cell-mediated immunity has generally been considered primarily responsible for tumor rejection in experimental tumor systems, since resistance to tumor growth can be transferred to histocompatible hosts by means of lymphocytes from tumor-immune or even tumor-bearing hosts. This opinion has, however, been modified because of recent studies that indicate that there is antibody-mediated tumor cell killing through either complement-dependent or antibody-dependent cellular cytotoxic (ADCC) mechanisms.

Table 1. *Assays for Cell-Mediated Immune Response to Tumor Antigen*

Skin tests for delayed hypersensitivity using extracts of tumor cells
Cytotoxicity assays against fresh tumor cells or cultured tumor cell lines
Leukocyte migration inhibition by tumor antigens
Leukocyte adherence inhibition by tumor antigens
Lymphocyte proliferative response to tumor antigens
Macrophage electrophoretic mobility test

Numerous attempts have been made to measure cell-mediated antitumor immunity by in vitro assays in the hope of providing an approach for evaluating the potential role of cell-mediated immunity in the rejection of cancer cells. Moreover, there would be an immediate practical use for such assays if they could be used to diagnose cancer reliably and to monitor the course of cancer growth. The techniques that may be employed in attempts to evaluate cell-mediated antitumor immunity in man are summarized in Table 1.

Although the demonstration of an antitumor immune response, either of the humoral or cell-mediated immune type, has often been taken as evidence suggestive of the presence of tumor-specific antigenicity, such studies have frequently suffered from the fact that autochthonous tumor cells have seldom been used in such work, thus making it difficult to discern whether the immune responses observed in vitro were directed toward a tumor antigen(s) or toward the alloantigens present on the tumor target tissue used in these studies. Furthermore, many of the in vitro procedures that have been, and are being, used are technically difficult and show significant variation in quantitative responses on a day-to-day basis. From the pragmatic standpoint, however, interest in the demonstration of putative human tumor-specific antigens has increased steadily during the past decade, since such substances would have major clinical application as markers in the diagnosis and prognosis of cancer and, perhaps, in the future immunotherapeutic management of the cancer patient.

To date, all the evidence indicates that a given tumor may express a variety of constituents or biological markers that may, semantically at least, be termed "tumor antigens." These tumor markers may be unique to a given tumor, they may be common to all tumors of a given histopathological type, they may represent embryonic and/or transplantation-like antigens, and in addition to the tumor cell surface, they may appear in the cytoplasm, and/or in the nucleus of the cancer cell (Castro 1978, Richards 1980).

HUMAN TUMOR ANTIGENS: BIOLOGICAL MARKERS OF TUMOR GROWTH

Table 2 presents a brief outline of the manner in which human tumor antigens, or markers of human tumor growth, may be classified. It must be noted that the constituents in question may represent quantitative and/or qualitative alterations in normally occurring body components (in which case

Table 2. *Human Tumor Antigens: Biologic Markers of Cancer Growth*

1. Quantitative and/or qualitative changes in synthesis of normal cell products
   Plasma cell disorders
   Endocrine tumors
   Ectopic hormone production (paraneoplastic syndromes)
   Enzymes
2. Oncofetal substances
   Carcinoembryonic antigen
   α_1-Fetoprotein
   Hemoglobin F
   Enzymes
3. Specific tumor antigens

they are tumor antigens only in that they are sought by antibody probes) or that they may be materials that appear de novo during tumor growth (in which case they are true tumor antigens). Examples of quantitative and/or qualitative alterations in normally occurring tissue and serum components include the paraproteins associated with multiple myeloma, Waldenström's macroglobulinemia, light-chain disease, the various heavy-chain disease syndromes, and the hormone- or enzyme-producing tumors (Lokich 1978, Shuster et al. 1980).

ECTOPIC HORMONES AND ENZYMES

Hormones and enzymes comprise two general classes of tumor markers. The interest of the immunologist in these two groups of markers is generally of a methodologic rather than an in vivo mechanistic nature; i.e., the need for high levels of sensitivity and specificity in the detection of these markers has led in several instances to the application of radioimmunological techniques in favor of standard biochemical methods. Hormone production may be associated with endocrine tumors derived from cell types which normally produce these substances. Ectopic hormones, on the other hand, refer to production and secretion from non-endocrine-derived tumors. Two general theories have been proposed to explain this phenomenon. The first suggests that there is derepression or other dysregulation of genetic information leading to expression of an "inappropriate" portion of the genome. The second theory suggests that cells of neuroectodermal crest origin migrate to various body sites during development. These may subsequently undergo malignant transformation and secrete "ectopic" hormones.

A wide variety of tumors has been associated with hormone production, although this occurs most commonly with tumors of the lung (Richardson et al. 1978). Hormone production may be associated with various paraneoplastic syndromes, but in many instances the secreted polypeptide may be only immunologically similar to the normal hormone and biochemically nonfunctional. Furthermore, within the groups of tumors associated with ectopic hormones, the incidence of abnormal serum levels of the hormone may be in the range of 20%-40%. However, in most cases the elevations are minimal, with striking increases occurring in fewer than 5% of cases (Lokich 1978). Another difficulty precluding the widespread diagnostic use of these markers is the lack of a clear-cut relationship between tumor burden and circulating hormone levels, except in the case of human chorionic gonadotrophin secretion from trophoblastic tumors.

Human Chorionic Gonadotrophin (HCG)

HCG represents the best example of the clinical utility of a hormone as a tumor marker. This hormone is normally produced by the human placenta in early pregnancy. The most characteristic pathologic elevations occur in patients with choriocarcinoma. In these cases, the levels of HCG correlate with the "tumor burden," and measurement of the β-subunit by radioimmunoassay allows the detection of circulating HCG when as few as a million tumor cells are present (Ress 1978). Furthermore, circulating HCG levels are a sensitive indicator of therapeutic responses and allow accurate titration of chemotherapeutic agents (Metz et al. 1978).

Although HCG levels are elevated in patients with a large variety of non-trophoblastic tumors, such measurements have not been uniformly useful in diagnosis and management, with the exception of concurrent HCG and α_1-fetoprotein measurements in hepatomas.

Galactosyltransferase Isoenzyme II (GT II)

GT II is an electrophoretically distinct isoenzyme of galactosyltransferase absent from normal serum but found in the sera of 70%-80% of patients with gastrointestinal tract tumors. It is not seen in most cases of nonmalignant disease, the only exceptions being severe alcoholic hepatitis and celiac disease. Preliminary data suggest that GT II levels correlate with the extent of tumor burden and may herald postoperative recurrence of disease.

At present, the assay for GT II is laborious and time-consuming. It requires an electrophoretic purification step followed by a functional assay of galactosyltransferase activity. The development of a radioimmunoassay method for measuring GT II will allow large-scale application and investigation of the utility of this marker (Podolshy et al. 1978).

Placental Alkaline Phosphatase (Regan Isoenzyme)

Alkaline phosphatase isoenzymes exist in a series of different electrophoretic, biochemical, and immunological forms. One of these, the Regan isoenzyme, is a heat-stable variant normally produced by placental tissue and is associated with a variety of malignant neoplasms (Wolf 1978). Raised levels of this isoenzyme were found in 10%-25% of patients with various tumors and in 20%-35% of patients with urogenital neoplasms (Kellen et al. 1976). It is most frequently produced by ovarian tumors, and the incidence of the elevation of the isoenzyme is as high as 75% if one examines the tumor tissue directly (Benham et al. 1978). Tumor excision leads to the disappearance of the enzyme from the circulation.

Terminal Deoxynucleotidyl Transferase (TdT)

TdT is a DNA polymerase that adds deoxyribonucleoside monophosphates to preformed DNA, without a template. The only normal tissues which contain the enzyme are cortical thymus and a subpopulation of bone marrow lymphocytes. As such, it can be considered a marker for prothymocytes (Meyskens and Jones 1978).

The enzyme can be detected in cell extracts by a biochemical assay or in intact cells by immunofluoresence using a specific antiserum. TdT is detectable in almost all cases of untreated acute lymphoblastic leukemia and one third of cases of chronic myelogenous leukemia in blast crisis (Strivastava et al. 1978). Enzyme levels return to normal during disease remissions and rise again with relapse. Of even greater interest has been the finding that 60% of patients with chronic myelogenous leukemia in blast crisis with TdT-positive cells respond to initial therapy, whereas none of the TdT-negative group show such a response (Marks et al. 1978).

The biologic role of this enzyme is not known, but it has shown itself to be useful both in classifying lymphoid tumors and in the clinical management of patients bearing these tumors.

Prostatic Acid Phosphatase

Acid phosphatases are enzymes capable of hydrolyzing phosphate esters in an acidic environment and can be found in many body tissues. Prostatic acid phosphatase is a particular isoenzyme produced by adult prostatic acinar epithelium and its biochemical estimation has been a useful adjunct in the diagnosis and treatment of prostatic cancer (Editorial: Br. Med. J. 1978). Serum acid phosphatase activity is elevated in most (70%-90%) patients with metastatic prostatic cancer but much less frequently (5%-30%) in the early stages of the disease. Furthermore, differentiation of the prostatic enzyme from other acid phosphatases in the serum cannot be accomplished biochemically. The recent developments of fluorescent assays and radioimmunoassays for the isoenzyme have, however, allowed the detection of elevated levels in more than half of patients with Stage A disease and its specific detection in bone marrow aspirates which may permit the detection of clinically imperceptible metastases (Belville et al. 1978).

CARCINOEMBRYONIC ANTIGEN

In 1965, a series of studies was reported concerning the antigenic analysis of adenocarcinoma of the human colon (Gold and Freedman 1965). The results showed that all the colon cancers examined contained an identical tumor antigen which was absent from the comparable normal tissue. It was subsequently shown that all human adenocarcinomas arising from the entodermally derived digestive system epithelium (esophagus, stomach, small bowel, colon, rectum, liver, and pancreas) contained the same tumor-specific antigen (Gold and Freedman 1965). A similar constituent was also found in embryonic and fetal gut, pancreas, and liver during the first two trimesters of gestation. Because this component could not be detected in any other normal, diseased, or neoplastic tissues by the techniques employed at that time, it was named the carcinoembryonic antigen (CEA) of the human digestive system. With the development of sensitive radioimmunoassay systems for the detection of CEA, the question has been raised as to whether this constituent, or other CEA-like components, is present in various normal tissues, nonenteric cancers, and other noncancerous pathologic tissues (Terry et al. 1974, Fuks et al. 1975). At least some of these materials have been shown not to be CEA, but rather CEA-like components that cross-react with CEA if incompletely absorbed anti-CEA antisera are employed in the test system (Mach and Pusztaszeri 1972, Kleist et al. 1972, Gold et al. 1978). The ultimate resolution of this question will require extensive immunochemical and structural analysis of CEA and of other molecules that may bear antigenic similarities to CEA.

Biology of CEA

Employing techniques of cellular agglutination and immunofluorescence, CEA has been localized, at least in part, to the surface of the tumor cell (Gold 1970). The heaviest accumulation of CEA, on both embryonic and cancerous digestive system cells, appears to be on the luminal surface (Burtin and Kleist 1970). Ultrastructurally, CEA has been localized to the glycocalyx of the tumor cell (Gold et al. 1970).

A specific humoral immune response against CEA has been demonstrated in some studies of cancer patients (Gold 1967, Gold et al. 1972, Gold and Gold 1973). The failure to demonstrate such antibodies in other studies (Gerfo et al. 1972, Kleist and Burtin 1966) may be due to differences in the methodology used for antibody detection. Anti-CEA antibodies have been demonstrated in the circulation of pregnant women (Gold 1967). An elegant in vivo demonstration of anti-CEA antibody production has been reported in a patient suffering from carcinoma of the colon and the nephrotic syndrome. Employing immunofluorescent techniques to examine the kidney biopsy from this patient, it was found that CEA, immunoglobulin, and complement had been deposited on the glomerular basement membrane (Costanza et al. 1973). Cell-mediated immunity against antigens common to human colon cancer and fetal gut epithelium was said to have been demonstrated by the colony inhibition technique, and it was suggested that CEA might be the common factor involved (Hellström et al. 1970). However, despite direct attempts to demonstrate the ability of CEA to evoke a cell-mediated response on the part of the tumor-bearing host, no such evidence has ever been obtained (Lejtenyi et al. 1971, Hollinshead et al. 1972).

Studies with tissue-cultured colon cancer cells in vitro (Goldenberg et al. 1972) and xenografted human colon cancer tissue in hamsters (Goldenberg and Hansen 1972) have demonstrated that CEA is produced by tumor cells in situ. In patients who have undergone apparently complete bowel tumor resections, CEA is catabolized rapidly and postoperative serum concentrations frequently fall to undetectable levels within 2-14 days after surgery (Dhar et al. 1972, Holyoke et al. 1972). The site of CEA breakdown in man remains unknown, but the liver appears to be a major site of catabolism for human CEA when injected into animals (Shuster et al. 1973).

Biochemistry and Immunochemistry of CEA

Most procedures for the purification of CEA have utilized perchloric acid extraction and gel infiltration (Terry et al. 1974, Fuks et al. 1975). These procedures may yield "pure" CEA but many other additional steps have been used to achieve final purification. These include block electrophoresis, ion-exchange chromatography, isoelectrofocusing, density gradient centrifugation, lectin affinity chromatography, and immunoaffinity chromatography (Terry et al. 1974, Fuks et al. 1975, Rogers 1976, Ashman and De Young 1977, Krantz et al. in press). Similar products have been obtained by these different methods, but subtle immunochemical differences may result from variations in the purification procedure. Treatment with perchloric acid may cause chemical and/or conformational changes in CEA or select certain molecular subpopulations (Rogers 1976, Kimball and Brattain 1978). CEA prepared by methods that avoid the use of perchloric acid may result in the isolation of a CEA molecule more representative of the native state of the material. Purified CEA yields a single diffuse band by SDS-polyacrylamide gel electrophoresis with an apparent molecular weight of approximately 200,000. The sedimentation coefficient is 7-8 S and a single band in the β-globulin region is obtained on immunoelectrophoresis against anti-CEA antiserum. Ion-exchange chromatography and isoelectrofocusing studies show that CEA is an acidic molecule with considerable charge heterogeneity (Terry et al. 1974, Fuks et al. 1975, Rogers 1976). By electron microscopy, the molecule appears as a morphologically distinctive cruller-shaped, or twisted, rod with dimensions 9 x 40 mm (Slayter and Coligan 1975).

CEA is a glycoprotein with the carbohydrate content varying from about 80% for purified CEA of gastric origin to about 40% for CEA obtained from colon cancer tissue (Terry et al. 1974, Fuks et al. 1975, Banjo et al. 1974). This variation in carbohydrate content, as well as microheterogeneity of inter-mediate and peripheral sugar linkages, probably accounts for a good deal of the heterogeneity which is observed in CEA preparations. Removal of sialic acid residues simplifies the electrophoretic and isoelectrofocusing patterns of CEA (Terry et al. 1974, Fuks et al. 1975, Banjo et al. 1974 a and b, Krupey et al. 1968, Coligan et al. 1972) but does not account for all of the observed hetero-geneity. The amino acid content of CEA suggests that the protein is relatively hydrophilic in nature (Banjo et al. 1974b) and evidence for the presence of 6 intrachain disulphide bridges has been reported (Westwood and Thomas 1975).

Attempts have been made to localize and chemically characterize the tumor-specific antigenic site of the molecule, but results so far have not been conclusive. Glycopeptides have been prepared which exhibited considerable cross-reactivity in the radioimmunoassay for CEA, suggesting that carbohy-drate structure is involved in the tumor-specific site (Banjo et al. 1974a). Chemical cleavage of CEA has produced a glycopeptide fraction, enriched in carbohydrate, that could be visualized on SDS-polyacrylamide gels and that was reactive in the assay for CEA (Leung et al. 1977). Conversely, other studies have shown that most of the carbohydrate may be removed from CEA without affecting its reactivity, and that a number of oligosaccharides of diverse structure are not cross-reactive with CEA (Hammarstrom et al. 1975). Reduced and alkylated CEA had considerably less reactivity, an effect which has been attributed to changes in protein conformation (Westwood and Thomas 1975). Chemical substitution of a number of amino acid residues by appropriately selective reagents affected immunoreactivity only in those cases where gross conformational changes were observed (Westwood et al. 1978).

The CEA molecule has been shown to contain epitopes which are distinct from the tumor antigenic site. Anti-blood group A antiserum is able to bind CEA (Gold and Gold 1973) as well as glycopeptide fragments of CEA (Gold et al. 1973). The CEA molecule may also contain an antigenic grouping which cross-reacts with the fetal sulphoglycoprotein antigen frequently found in the gastric juice of patients with cancer of the stomach (Terry et al. 1974, Fuks et al. 1975).

In the last seven years, names have been given to 12 antigens that cross-react with CEA and which have been identified by the use of incompletely absorbed antisera prepared against purified CEA. (For individual references, see Gold et al. 1978.) Hence, it is clear that true monospecificity of anti-CEA antisera cannot be assured unless exhaustive absorption with normal tissue extracts has been performed. Six of the 12 cross-reacting substances in question appear to be immunologically identical (Terry et al. 1974, Gold et al. 1978) but the relationship of the remaining antigens to these six, and to one another, requires further study. In addition to these already known cross-reacting glycoproteins, still others very likely exist which might interfere with the specificity of the CEA radioimmunoassay. Therefore, the study of cross-reacting substances must become an integral part of CEA research.

In practice, this means that attention must center not only on the analysis of the antigens but most urgently on the specificity of the anti-CEA antisera as well. If an antiserum is used which is directed principally against the common sites of two different macromolecules, one of which is tumor-specific while the other is not, complete identity of the two substances will erroneously be concluded. Furthermore, the apparent detection of the tumor-specific substance in normal tissues or plasma will obscure its tumor specificity. Since antisera of broad specificity are certainly easier to obtain than those directed against a unique site (Tomita et al. 1974), the polyvalent type of antiserum is probably employed more frequently than is generally believed.

The presence of CEA in various normal tissues has been reported (Martin and Martin 1970, Burtin et al. 1972, Gerfo and Herter 1972, Kupchik and Zamcheck 1972). Small amounts of CEA were isolated from normal colonic mucosa by immunoabsorbant chromatography with antibodies against colon carcinoma CEA (Fritsche and Mach 1977). This putative normal CEA showed marked radioimmunological and immunochemical similarities to colon cancer CEA, but no attempt was made to absorb anti-CEA antiserum with this material in order to determine if activity against colon cancer would be completely removed. A purified CEA preparation has also apparently been obtained from the colonic lavage fluid from healthy individuals (Egan et al. 1977b). This material had immunological and biochemical properties similar to those of CEA obtained from bowel cancer, but the interpretation again rests to a great extent on the definition of the antisera employed. Studies employing immunoabsorption with antisera prepared and absorbed in different fashions have failed to confirm the presence of CEA in normal bowel mucosa (our unpublished data), and further work will certainly be needed to resolve these contradictory results.

Radioimmunoassay for CEA

One of the fundamental characteristics of the cell surface of all metabolizing cells is renewal. Components of the cell surface are continuously shed into the surrounding milieu and are replaced by newly synthesized material. Since tumor antigens are found on the surface of neoplastic cells, their shedding and ultimate appearance in the circulation serve as a basis for their measurement in the blood. The potential clinical benefits in the management and diagnosis of malignant disease that might accrue from the measurement of circulating tumor antigens have been the subject of much recent investigation, with the measurement of circulating CEA serving as the prototype model. With regard to CEA, and ultimately all potentially useful tumor antigens, this required the development of sensitive and reproducible radioimmunoassays capable of detecting nanogram quantities of the material.

Because of the sensitivity of the various radioimmunoassay techniques employed in the detection of CEA, compared to the initial studies with CEA that largely employed precipitation reactions in gel, and as noted above, it has been suggested that this molecule is present in very low concentrations in tissues other than gastrointestinal cancers and fetal and embryonic digestive system organs, and that CEA or "CEA-like" substances may be released into the circulation of patients bearing non-enteric cancers and those suffering from other forms of tissue disease. Again, the problem of whether or not the material found in the sera of patients with non-enteric cancers is identical to the CEA isolated from digestive system cancers, or whether it is made up of "CEA-like" substances that may mimic the presence of CEA in sensitive assay systems, remains to be fully elucidated. In any event, the parameters influencing the detection of CEA by radioimmunoassay and the manner in which these factors may be improved are worthy of brief consideration. Although some of the problems have already been noted, their reiteration in the clinical context of the detection of circulation CEA in patients appears warranted.

Antigens used in the various assay systems available are generally purified from the hepatic metastases of colon cancer but the method of purification varies from laboratory to laboratory. There is no universally accepted standard presently available for use as a reference material. Moreover, immunologic and chemical comparisons are available for only a limited number of preparations of purified CEA. Hence, the identity of the antigens used by different investigators has not been clearly demonstrated, and variability in the immunologic activity of the purified standards utilized may well affect the results obtained with any given assay system.

As noted earlier, sufficient evidence has accumulated to indicate that purified CEA preparations manifest a good deal of intermolecular heterogeneity. Recent studies comparing radioimmunoassays for CEA, employing different "standard" CEA preparations and different anti-CEA antisera, demonstrated significant antigenic differences between some of the "standard" CEA materials employed. Furthermore, the serum CEA of one patient and the corresponding tissue CEA obtained from the patient appeared to be antigenically different (Vrba et al. 1975, 1976). Utilizing additional steps beyond those conventionally employed to purify CEA, the heterogeneity of CEA has been further documented. Thus, the CEA of the gastrointestinal tract, as originally defined, is very probably one of a family of "CEA-like" molecules found in a number of pathologic tissues and, in addition to the tumor-specific determinant of the CEA molecule, there are a number of non-tumor-specific determinant groupings on the CEA molecule that are shared with molecular moieties produced by various tissues afflicted with other pathologic conditions (Rogers et al. 1974, Vrba et al. 1976, Edgington et al. 1975).

The problems associated with preparing appropriately specific anti-CEA antiserum, and the difficulties resulting from the use of inadequately specific antiserum, have been considered previously and need no further elaboration here. It may well be that the resolution of this problem awaits the preparation of a monoclonal antiserum directed against the tumor-specific epitope of the CEA molecule.

The Role of the Present Radioimmunoassays for CEA in Clinical Medicine

The potential clinical uses for human tumor markers, in general, are outlined in Table 3. The ideal immunodiagnostic assay for cancer should distinguish accurately between those patients with cancer and those with benign conditions or with no disease whatever. The tests should be sensitive, so that there is a low or negligible incidence of false-negative assays, and should have high specificity, so that there is a low incidence of false-positive assays. In addition, when possible the tests should be organ-specific and allow for the localization of the tumor mass. Applying these criteria to the presently available radioimmunoassays for CEA, it is immediately obvious that the current assays deviate from the ideal in several respects. Although sensitive and reproducible, the tests currently employed suffer primarily from a lack of specificity, since a variety of benign disorders are associated with elevated levels of CEA—albeit the titers are usually pesistently low (Egan et al. 1977a, b). Similarly, the current tests do not demonstrate absolute organ specificity, since a number of different tumors are associated with circulating CEA values of high and/or rising titers (Egan et al. 1977a, b, Hansen et al. 1974, Lawrence et al. 1972). Resolution of the difficulties described, in terms of antigen and antiserum preparations, should allow the radioimmunoassays for CEA to approach the ideal situation more closely. At the present time, however, the radioimmunoassays for CEA should not be employed indiscriminately as a tool for cancer screening of apparently healthy individuals in the population, in that negative results may be obtained in subjects with early cancerous lesions, while positive results do not always indicate the presence of malignant growth. Again, it should be noted that many of the nonmalignant conditions associated with positive assays, even at the present time, usually show transient and/or low elevations of CEA rather than persistent, rising levels of CEA, and are distinguishable from cancerous growth on this basis. The clinical experience with serial CEA measurement in patients with established colorectal cancer is shown in Figures 1–3. Several types of CEA profiles have been observed in patients where the CEA levels were elevated preoperatively

Table 3. *Potential Uses for Human Tumor Markers*

1. Population screening
2. Adjunct in the diagnosis of cancer
3. Preoperative indicator of tumor burden
4. Indicator of therapeutic success
5. Evidence of postoperative recurrence
6. Use in tumor localization

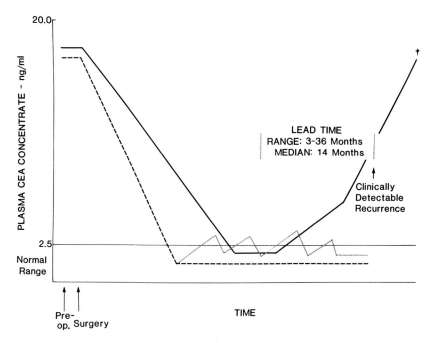

FIG. 1. Patterns observed in colorectal cancers when CEA levels are measured serially in patients in whom CEA is elevated preoperatively and potentially curative surgery is subsequently performed.

(Figures 1 and 2). Postoperatively, resection of the primary tumor may result in a fall of serum CEA values to the normal range within 30 days of surgery, indicating potentially curative resection of the tumor (Figure 1). If the CEA level remains within the normal range subsequently, it strongly indicates the absence of either local or metastatic recurrence. Occasionally, however, small spikes in circulating CEA are seen during serial studies of a patient. Although the explanation for this phenomenon is unclear, no tumor recurrence has been observed in most instances. However, if two consecutive CEA determinations, performed 4–6 weeks apart, show progressive elevation in circulating CEA levels after having returned to normal in the postoperative period, a recurrence of the tumor must be strongly suspected. It is possible that early and aggressive second-look surgery based upon rising CEA values may reveal locally resectable, rather than the disseminated metastatic, recurrence of the tumor. The value of such a procedure has not as yet been demonstrated with any degree of clarity.

One of the most interesting findings of serial postoperative determinations of circulating CEA levels is that CEA elevations can herald the onset of tumor regrowth from 3 to 36 months prior to any evidence of clinical recurrence. It is to be hoped that in the future, the advent of more effective chemotherapeutic

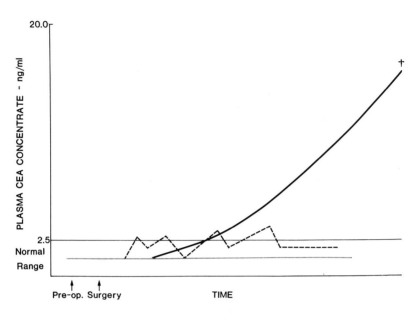

FIG. 2. As Figure 1 but with negative preoperative circulating CEA values.

and immunotherapeutic agents will allow us to take advantage of this lead time so that treatment can be initiated early, when the tumor load is small and a significant therapeutic effect may be more readily achieved.

In many instances, the CEA levels do not return to normal but remain elevated or only fall slightly in the postoperative period (Figure 3). This pattern reflects a significant residual tumor mass that has not been surgically resected and, thus, a poor prognosis. In approximately 15% of patients with established colon cancer, CEA is not elevated in the preoperative period, even though the patient may have a Dukes' Stage D lesion, and despite the fact that the tumor tissue may contain large quantities of extractable CEA. In such cases, the CEA level usually remains within the normal range throughout the patient's clinical course, but may, occasionally, become slightly increased as a preterminal event. In some cases, elevated CEA levels show a preterminal decrease for as yet undetermined reasons.

Another area requiring further investigation has been suggested by studies showing that CEA levels correlate well with regression or progression of cancer growth during chemotherapy of cancers of the gastrointestinal tract, lung, and breast, and the serial CEA determinations may be useful in monitoring the effectiveness of such treatment. Early evidence indicates that the radioimmunoassay for CEA may well be of value in monitoring the management of cancer patients receiving radiotherapy.

While recognizing the theoretical and practical limitations presently associated with the radioimmunoassay for CEA vis-à-vis its clinical applications,

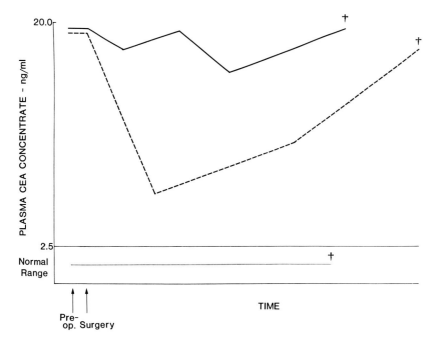

FIG. 3. Serial CEA levels in the plasmas of patients with metastatic disease demonstrated at the time of surgery.

being guided by these restrictions, and using the test in every case in association with clinical acumen and the usually employed ancillary diagnostic tests for cancer, there seems little doubt that the radioimmunoassay for CEA has a definite role to play in the diagnosis and management of the cancer patient. It is not too optimistic to expect that the further definition of the physiochemical and immunochemical properties of CEA and related materials, and the advent of more specific anti-CEA antisera, will result in more specific, and perhaps more sensitive, tests for the detection of minimal tumor growth.

In like fashion, the levels of CEA in body secretions and excretions, such as pleural fluid, ascites fluid, amniotic fluid, gastrointestinal secretions, cerebrospinal fluid, and urine, in addition to the levels of CEA in the circulation, may provide important information concerning the status of any given cancer patient.

Radioimmunolocalization of Tumors Employing ^{131}I-Anti-CEA

During the past two or three years, a new dimension has been added to the use of the CEA system in cancer diagnosis. This has occurred through the advent of the technique of radioimmunolocalization of tumors employing radiolabeled anti-CEA antibodies. Injecting the ^{131}I-anti-CEA antiserum intravenously in patients bearing CEA-producing tumors, and utilizing appropriate computerized subtractive methods to overcome the problem of radioactivity in the intravascular space, it has been possible to obtain excellent scintigram imaging of the tumor mass. The First International Symposium dealing with this new technology (Cancer Res. 40:2973-2976, 1980) has recently been held and there is every indication that this type of procedure will eventually provide the physician with a very powerful probe in localization of tumor tissue.

ACKNOWLEDGMENTS

Portions of this manuscript have been published previously in the following volumes:

Shuster J., D. Thomson, and P. Gold. 1978. Immunodiagnosis, *in* Immunological Aspects of Cancer, J. E. Castro, ed. MTP Press Ltd., Lancaster, England, pp. 283–312.

Gold, P., S. O. Freedman, and J. Shuster. 1979. Carcinoembryonic antigen. Historical perspective, experimental data, *in* Immunodiagnosis of Cancer, Part I, R. B. Herberman and K. R. McIntire, eds. Marcel Dekker, Inc., New York and Basel, pp. 147–164.

Fuks, A., J. Shuster, and P. Gold. 1980. Theoretical and practical considerations of the utility of the radioimmunoassay for carcinoembryonic antigen (CEA) in clinical medicine, *in* Cancer Markers, S. Sell, ed. The Humana Press, Clifton, New Jersey, pp. 315–327.

Gold, P., and J. Shuster. 1980. Historical development and potential uses of tumor antigens as markers of human cancer growth. *Cancer Res.* 40:2973–2976.

REFERENCES

Ashman, L. K., and N. J. De Young. 1977. Immunoadsorbent purification of the carcinoembryonic antigen. Immunochemistry 14:329–336.

Baldwin, R. W. 1970. Tumor specific antigens associated with chemically induced tumors. Rev. Eur. Etud. Clin. Biol. 15:593–598.

Baldwin, R. W., and D. Glaves. 1972. Deletion of liver-cell surface membrane components from aminoazo-dye-induced rat hepatomas. Int. J. Cancer 9:76–85.

Banjo, C., P. Gold, C. W. Gehrke, S. O. Freedman, and J. Krupey. 1974a. Preparation and isolation of immunologically active glycopeptides from carcinoembryonic antigen (CEA). Int. J. Cancer 13:151–163.

Banjo, C., J. Shuster, and P. Gold. 1974b. Intermolecular heterogeneity of the carcinoembryonic antigen. Cancer Res. 34:2114–2121.

Basombrio, M. A. 1970. Search for common antigenicities among twenty-five sarcomas induced by methylcholanthrene. Cancer Res. 30:2458–2462.

Belville, W. D., H. D. Cox, D. E. Mahan, J. P. Olmert, B. T. Mittemeyer, and A. W. Bruce. 1978. Bone marrow acid phosphatase by radioimmunoassay. Cancer 41:2286–2291.

Benham, F. J., M. S. Povey, and H. Harris. 1978. Placenta-like alkaline phosphatase in malignant and benign ovarian tumors. Clin. Chim. Acta 86:201–215.

Burtin, P., and S. von Kleist. 1970. Immunochemical studies on human colonic tumors, *in* Carcinoma of the Colon and Antecedent Epithelium, W. J. Burdette, ed. Charles C Thomas, Springfield, pp. 150–157.

Burtin, P., E. Martin, M. C. Sabine, and S. von Kleist. 1972. Immunological study of polyps of the colon. J. Natl. Cancer Inst. 48:25–32.

Castro, J. E. 1978. An overview of tumor immunology and immunotherapy, in Immunological Aspects of Cancer, J. E. Castro ed. Lancaster, England, MTP Press Ltd., pp. 1–14.

Coligan, J. E., J. T. Lautenschleger, M. L. Egan, and C. W. Todd. 1972. Isolation and characterization of carcinoembryonic antigen. Immunochemistry 9:377–386.

Costanza, M. E., V. Pinn, R. S. Schwartz, and L. Nathanson. 1973. Carcinoembryonic antigen-antibody complexes in a patient with colonic carcinoma and nephrotic syndrome. N. Engl. J. Med. 289:520–522.

Dhar, P., T. Moore, N. Zamcheck, and H. Z. Kupchik. 1972. Carcinoembryonic antigen (CEA) in colonic cancer. J. Am. Med. Assoc. 221:31–35.

Edgington, T. S., R. W. Astarita, and E. F. Plow. 1975. Association of an isomeric species of carcinoembryonic antigen with neoplasia of the gastrointestinal tract. N. Engl. J. Med. 293:103.

Editorial. 1978. Radioimmunoassay of serum prostatic acid phosphatase in prostatic cancer. Br. Med. J. ii:719–720.

Egan, M. L., D. G. Pritchard, J. E. Shively, and V. L. W. Go. 1977a. CEA-like substance in normal colon washings. Proc. Am. Assoc. Cancer Res. 18:40.

Egan, M. L., D. G. Pritchard, C. W. Todd, and V. L. W. Go. 1977b. Isolation and immunochemical and chemical characterization of carcinoembryonic antigen-like substances in colon lavages of healthy individuals. Cancer Res. 37:2638–2643.

Foley, E. J. 1953. Antigen properties of methylcholanthrene-induced tumors in mice of strain of origin. Cancer Res. 13:835.

Fritsche, R., and J. P. Mach. 1977. Isolation and characterization of carcinoembryonic antigen (CEA) extracted from normal human colon mucosa. Immunochemistry 14:199–227.

Fuks, A., C. Banjo, J. Shuster, S. O. Freedman, and P. Gold. 1975. Carcinoembryonic antigen (CEA): Molecular biology and clinical significance. Biochim. Biophys. Acta 417:123–152.

Gerfo, P. Lo, and F. J. Herter. 1972. Demonstration of tumor-associated antigen in normal colon and lung. J. Surg. Oncol. 4:1–7.

Gerfo, P. Lo, F. P. Herter, and S. J. Bennett. 1972. Absence of circulating antibodies to carcinoembryonic antigen in patients with gastrointestinal malignancies. Int. J. Cancer 9:344–348.

Gold, J. M., C. Banjo, S. O. Freedman, and P. Gold. 1973. Immunochemical studies of the intramolecular heterogeneity of the carcinoembryonic antigen (CEA) of the human digestive system. J. Immunol. 111:1872–1879.

Gold, J. M., S. O. Freedman, and P. Gold. 1972. Human anti-CEA antibodies detected by radioimmunoelectrophoresis. Nature New Biol. 230:60–62.

Gold, J. M., and P. Gold. 1973. The blood group. H-like site on the carcinoembryonic antigen. Cancer Res. 33:2821–2824.

Gold, P. 1967. Circulating antibodies against carcinoembryonic antigens of the human digestive system. Cancer 20:1663–1667.

Gold, P. 1970. The model of colonic cancer in the study of human tumor-specific antigens, in Carcinoma of the Colon and Antecedent Epithelium, W. J. Burdette, ed. Charles C Thomas, Springfield, pp. 131–142.

Gold, P., P. Burtin, T. M. Chu, S. G. Hammerstrom, H. J. Hanson, B. G. Johansson, S. von Kleist, J.-P. Mach, A. M. Neville, J. E. Shively, P. Stroebel, N. Zamcheck, D. Goldenberg, and J. Westwood. 1978. CEA Group Report, International Research Group for Carcinoembryonic Proteins. Meeting, Copenhagen 1977. Scand. J. Immunol. suppl. 8:27–38.

Gold, P., and S. O. Freedman. 1965a. Demonstration of tumor-specific antigens in human colonic carcinomata by immunological tolerance and absorption techniques. J. Exp. Med. 121:439–462.

Gold, P., and S. O. Freedman. 1965b. Specific carcinoembryonic antigens of the human digestive system. J. Exp. Med. 122:467–481.

Gold, P., J. Krupey, and H. Ansari. 1970. Position of the carcinoembryonic antigen of the human digestive system in ultrastructure of tumor cell surface. J. Natl. Cancer Inst. 45:219–222.

Goldenberg, D. M., and H. J. Hansen. 1972. Carcinoembryonic antigen present in human colonic neoplasms serially propagated in hamsters. Science 175:1117–1118.

Goldenberg, D. M., R. A. Pavia, H. J. Hansen, and J. P. Vandevoorde. 1972. Synthesis of carcinoembryonic antigen in vitro. Nature, Lond. 239:189–190.

Green, H. N., H. M. Anthony, R. W. Baldwin, and J. W. Westrop. 1967. Antigen modifications in malignancy, *in* An Immunological Approach to Cancer. Butterworth, London, pp. 165–198.

Hammarstrom, S., E. Engvall, B. G. Johansson, S. Svensson, G. Sundblad, and I. J. Goldstein. 1975. Nature of the tumor-associated determinant(s) of carcinoembryonic antigen. Proc. Natl. Acad. Sci. USA 72:1528–1532.

Hansen, J. H., J. J. Snyder, E. Miller, J. P. Vandervoorde, O. Neal Miller, L. R. Hines, and J. J. Burns. 1974. Carcinoembryonic antigen (CEA) assay. Human Pathol. 5:139.

Haywood, G. R., and C. F. McKhann. 1970. Relationship between tumor-specific and H-2 antigens on mouse sarcomas. Fed. Proc. 29:371.

Hellström, I., and K. E. Hellström. 1972. Some aspects of human tumor immunity and their possible implications for tumor prevention and therapy, *in* Frontiers in Radiation Therapy and Oncology, Vol. 7. S. Karger, Basel, pp. 3–15.

Hellström, I., K. E. Hellström, and T. H. Shepard. 1970. Cell-mediated immunity against antigens common to human colonic carcinoma and fetal gut epithelium. Int. J. Cancer 6:346–351.

Hellström, I., K. E. Hellström, H. O. Sjogren, and G. A. Warner. 1971. Demonstration of cell-mediated immunity to human neoplasms of various histological types. Int. J. Cancer 7:1–16.

Hollinshead, A. C., C. G. McWright, T. C. Alford, D. H. Glew, P. Gold, and R. B. Herberman. 1972. Separation of skin reactive intestinal cancer antigen from carcinoembryonic antigen of gold. Science 177:887–889.

Holyoke, D., G. Reynoso, and T. N. Chu. 1972. Carcinoembryonic antigen (CEA) in patients with carcinoma of the digestive tract. Ann. Surg. 176:559–564.

Kellen, J. A., R. S. Bush, and A. Malkin. 1976. Placenta-like alkaline phosphatase in gynecological cancers. Cancer Res. 36:269–271.

Kimball, P. M., and M. G. Brattain. 1978. A comparison of methods for the isolation of carcinoembryonic antigen. Cancer Res. 38:619–623.

Klein, G. 1966. Tumor antigens. Annu. Rev. Microbiol. 20:223–252.

Kleist, S. von, and P. Burtin. 1966. On the specificity of autoantibodies present in colon cancer patients. Immunology 10:507–515.

Kleist, S. von, G. Chavanel, and P. Burtin. 1972. Identification of an antigen from normal human tissue that cross-reacts with the carcinoembryonic antigen. Proc. Natl. Acad. Sci. USA 69:2492–2494.

Krantz, M. J., S. Laferte, and N. Ariel. 1980. Radioimmunoassay of carcinoembryonic antigen. Methods in Enzymology (in press).

Krupey, J., P. Gold, and S. O. Freedman. 1968. Physicochemical studies of the carcinoembryonic antigens of the human digestive system. J. Exp. Med. 128:387–398.

Kupchik, H. Z., and N. Zamcheck. 1972. Carcinoembryonic antigen(s) in liver disease. II. Isolation from human cirrhotic liver and serum and from normal liver. Gastroenterol. 63:95–102.

Lawrence, D. J. R., V. Stevens, R. Bettelheim, D. Darcy, C. Leese, C. Tuberville, P. Alexander, E. W. Johns, and A. M. Neville. 1972. Role of plasma carcinoembryonic antigen in diagnosis of gastrointestinal mammary and bronchial carcinoma. Br. Med. J. 3:605.

Lejtenyi, M. C., S. O. Freedman, and P. Gold. 1971. Response to lymphocytes from patients with gastrointestinal cancer to the carcinoembryonic antigen of the human digestive system. Cancer 28:115–120.

Leung, J. P., Y. Eshdat, and V. T. Marchesi. 1977. Colonic tumor membrane-associated glycoprotein: Isolation of antigenically active peptides after chemical cleavage. J. Immunol. 119:664–670.

Lewis, M. C., R. L. Ikonopisov, R. C. Narin, T. M. Phillips, F. G. Hamilton, D. C. Bodenham, and P. Alexander. 1969. Tumor-specific antibodies in human malignant melanoma and their relationship to the extent of the disease. Br. Med. J. iii:547–552.

Lokich, J. J. 1978. Tumor markers: Hormones, antigens, and enzymes in malignant disease. Oncology 35:54–57.

Mach, J. P., and G. Pusztaszeri. 1972. Carcinoembryonic antigen (CEA): Demonstration of a partial identity between CEA and a normal glycoprotein. Immunochemistry 9:1031–1034.

Marks, S. M., D. Baltimore, and R. McCaffrey. 1978. Terminal transferase as a predictor of initial responsiveness to vincristine and prednisone in blastic chronic myelogenous leukemia. (A co-operative study.) New Engl. J. Med. 298:812–814.

Martin, F., and M. S. Martin. 1970. Demonstration of antigens related to colonic cancer in the human digestive system. Int. J. Cancer 6:352–360.

Metz, S. A., B. Weintrub, S. W. Rose, J. Singer, and R. P. Robertson. 1978. Ectopic secretion of chorionic gonadotropin by a lung carcinoma. Pituitary gonadatropin and subunit secretion and prolonged chemotherapeutic remission. Am. J. Med. 65:325–333.

Meyskens, F. L., and S. E. Jones. 1978. Terminal transferase: Its evolving role. New Engl. J. Med. 298:845–846.

Old, L. J., and E. A. Boyse. 1964. Immunology of experimental tumors. Annu. Rev. Med. 15:167–186.

Plow, E. F., and T. S. Edgington. 1975. Isolation and characterization of a homogeneous isomeric species of a carcinoembryonic antigen: CEA-S. Int. J. Cancer 15:748.

Podolshy, D. K., M. M. Weister, K. J. Isselbacher, and A. M. Cohen. 1978. A cancer-associated galactosyltransferase isoenzyme. New Engl. J. Med. 299:703–705.

Prehn, R. T. 1968. Tumor-specific antigens of putatively non-viral tumors. Cancer Res. 28:1326–1330.

Prehn, R. T., and M. A. Lappe. 1971. An immunostimulation theory of tumor development. Transplant. Rev. 7:26–54.

Ress, L. H. 1978. Hormone production by tumors. Antibiotics Chemother. 22:161–165.

Richards, V. 1980. Cancer immunology—an overview. Prog. Exp. Tumor Res. 25:1–60.

Richardson, R. L., F. A. Greco, R. K. Oldham, and G. W. Liddle. 1978. Tumor products and potential markers in small cell lung cancer. Sem. Oncol. 5:253–262.

Rogers, G. T. 1976. Heterogeneity of carcinoembryonic antigen. Implications on its role as a tumor marker substance. Biochim. Biophys. Acta 458:355–373.

Rogers, G. T., F. Searle, and K. D. Bagshawe. 1974. Heterogeneity of carcinoembryonic antigen and its fractionation by con A affinity chromatography. Nature 251:519.

Shuster, J., M. Seilverman, and P. Gold. 1973. Metabolism of human carcinoembryonic antigen in xenogeneic animals. Cancer Res. 33:65–68.

Shuster, J., D. M. P. Thomson, A. Fuks, and P. Gold. 1980. Immunologic approaches to diagnosis of malignancy. Prog. Exp. Tumor Res. 25:89–139.

Slayter, H. S., and J. E. Coligan. 1975. Electron microscopy and physical characterization of the carcinoembryonic antigen. Biochemistry 14:2323–2330.

Strivastava, B. I. S., S. A. Kahn, J. Minowada, and A. Freeman. 1978. High terminal deoxy-nucleotidyl transferase activity in pediatric patients with acute lymphocytic and acute mylocytic leukemias. Int. J. Cancer 22:4–9.

Terry, W. D., P. A. Henkart, J. E. Coligan, and C. W. Todd. 1974. Carcinoembryonic antigen: Characterization and clinical applications. Transplant Rev. 20:100–129.

Ting, C. C., and R. B. Herberman. 1971. Inverse relationship of polyoma tumor specific cell surface antigen to H-2 histocompatibility antigens. Nature, Lond. 232:118–120.

Tomita, J. T., J. W. Safford, and A. A. Hirata. 1974. Antibody responses to different determinants on carcinoembryonic antigen CEA. Immunology 26:291–298.

Vrba, R., E. Alpert, and K. J. Isselbacher. 1975. Carcinoembryonic antigen: Evidence for multiple antigenic determinants and isoantigens. Proc. Natl. Acad. Sci. USA, 72:4602.

Vrba, R., E. Alpert, and K. J. Isselbacher. 1976. Immunological heterogeneity of serum carcinoembryonic antigen (CEA). Immunochemistry 13:87.

Westwood, J. H., and P. Thomas. 1975. Studies on the structure and immunological activity of carcinoembryonic antigen—the role of disulphide bonds. Br. J. Cancer 32:708–719.

Westwood, J. H., P. Thomas, R. G. Edwards, P. M. Scopes, and M. W. Barrett. 1978. Chemical modifications of the protein of carcinoembryonic antigen: Associated changes in immunological activity and conformation. Br. J. Cancer 37:183–189.

Wolf, P. L. 1978. Clinical significance of an increased or decreased serum alkaline phosphatase level. Arch. Path. 102:497–501.

Current Concepts

Gastrointestinal Cancer, edited by
John R. Stroehlein and
Marvin M. Romsdahl.
Raven Press, New York © 1981.

Epidemiology of Gastrointestinal Cancer

A. B. Miller, M.B.

NCIC Epidemiology Unit, McMurrich Building, Faculty of Medicine, University of Toronto, Toronto, Ontario, Canada

INTRODUCTION

One of the most fruitful sources of data on the descriptive epidemiology of gastrointestinal cancers are cancer registries throughout the world (Waterhouse et al. 1976). The latest volume (Volume 3) is similar to its predecessors in that it shows a substantial variation in incidence of different cancers in different parts of the world. In Table 1 the range of incidence of the cancers being considered in this symposium is given, together with the sex ratio. The latter is derived by the ratio of the means of the age standardized incidence rates, derived from the 77 different populations with data in Volume 3. Some of these populations come from the same registry. Thus, considerable information can be obtained by contrasting different racial groups, as for example in the cancer registries of Israel, Singapore, Hawaii, and a number of the U.S. registries.

The table indicates that the range of incidence is greatest for esophageal and liver cancer, followed by gallbladder, colon, stomach, rectal, and pancreatic cancer. Substantial ranges of incidence are found where there are registries reporting very low incidence. This is particularly so for esophageal and liver

Table 1. *Range of Incidence and Sex Ratio for Gastrointestinal Cancers*

Site	Range of incidence*		Sex ratio
	Males	Females	
Esophagus	130	50	3.2
Stomach	12	20	2.0
Colon	23	20	1.0
Rectum	16	9	1.5
Liver	130	85	2.1
Gallbladder	44	22	0.6
Pancreas	10	13	1.6

*Source: Waterhouse et al. (1976). Range of incidence in rates standardized to world population.
Ratio of mean of rates standardized to world population, derived from Waterhouse et al. (1976).

cancer, since a low incidence is found in the Caucasian populations of North America and Europe. A low incidence of stomach cancer is of course now found in North America; in contrast, a high incidence of stomach cancer is found in Japan, while there is a low incidence of colon and rectal cancer. The sex ratios indicate a similarity in incidence for the two sexes only for colon cancer, with a moderate male excess for cancer of the stomach, rectum, and pancreas and a substantial male excess for esophageal and liver cancer. Only for gallbladder cancer is there an excess in females.

Table 2 indicates the extent to which there is a correlation between the incidence of various cancers from the same data source (Waterhouse et al. 1976). It is of interest from this table that the lowest correlation between the incidence in males and females in the same registry is for esophageal cancer and the highest is for colon cancer. Significant positive correlations within the same sex only occur for colon and rectal cancer and for colon and rectal cancer with pancreatic cancer. There are significant negative correlations for colon and stomach cancer. However, in men, esophageal cancer is positively correlated with liver cancer, and in women liver cancer is negatively correlated with colon and rectal cancer.

The table also indicates the extent to which colon and, to a lesser extent, rectal and pancreatic cancer are correlated with breast, endometrial, and ovarian cancer in women.

It was Burkitt (1971) who pointed out that when one sees similarities in frequency of occurrence for the different diseases, then one should look for common factors in etiology. This table suggests that there may be different etiological factors in esophageal cancer in males and in females. However, similar factors may operate in the etiology of colon, rectal, and pancreatic

Table 2. *Correlation between Incidence of Various Cancers Based on Data Standardized to the World Population*

FEMALES				MALES			
	Esophagus	Stomach	Colon	Rectum	Liver	Gallbladder	Pancreas
Esophagus	0.38*	0.05	−0.03	−0.19	0.80	−0.22	0.20
Stomach	0.11	0.94*	−0.40	−0.24	−0.04	0.20	−0.17
Colon	−0.12	−0.40	0.95*	0.85	−0.15	−0.24	0.60
Rectum	−0.08	−0.18	0.67	0.76*	−0.22	−0.14	0.41
Liver	0.05	0.06	−0.33	−0.39	0.89*	−0.14	0.05
Gallbladder	−0.28	0.13	−0.27	−0.01	−0.08	0.74*	−0.07
Pancreas	−0.14	−0.23	0.54	0.44	−0.23	0.17	0.77*
Breast	−0.17	−0.46	0.84	0.72	−0.39	−0.15	0.63
Cervix uteri	0.06	0.09	−0.12	−0.14	0.20	0.14	0.13
Endometrium	−0.29	−0.28	0.69	0.45	−0.15	−0.16	0.49
Ovary	−0.25	−0.40	0.63	0.51	−0.26	0.04	0.60

*Correlation between same site in males and females. All coefficients above and to the right refer to males, all below and to the left to females.
A coefficient greater than 0.22 is statistically significant (P≤0.05)
(Data derived from Waterhouse et al., 1976)

cancer in both sexes, with liver and esophageal cancer in men, and with breast, endometrial, and ovarian cancer in women. The inverse correlation of colon with stomach cancer could have been forecast from the reverse frequencies found in different countries, but this again suggests that one is looking for entirely different etiological factors.

Epidemiology contributes greatly to the elucidation of etiology, especially when exposure can be clearly identified and when strong associations are found with dose response and correct temporal relationships compatible with biological knowledge, suggesting that the factor is important in causation. These types of factors have not been prominent in the epidemiology of gastrointestinal cancers, but nevertheless substantial leads are beginning to accumulate which suggest etiological hypotheses. Many of these, as might be anticipated, relate to factors in our diet.

Because of the substantial differences in the occurrence of gastrointestinal cancers internationally, and thus the dissimilarities in the etiology that one can suspect, in the remainder of this presentation I shall review what is known about the epidemiology and etiology of the various gastrointestinal cancers in general. Wherever appropriate, however, I shall point to similarities in possible causation with other cancer sites, both within and outside of the gastrointestinal tract.

EPIDEMIOLOGY OF INDIVIDUAL SITES

Esophageal Cancer

Esophageal cancer shows substantial variation in incidence, with some of the lowest rates in white Caucasians (Hirayama et al. 1980). Within the United States, however, there is a significant difference in incidence between blacks and whites, especially in males. Internationally there is a high incidence belt running from the Caspian littoral to North China. The high incidence area in Northern Iran which shows some substantial differences between geographically adjacent areas has been subject to a great deal of investigation, particularly by the International Agency for Research on Cancer. So far, however, no specific carcinogen has been identified (Joint Iran-International Agency for Research on Cancer Study Group, 1977).

However, a number of environmental factors have been associated with high incidence. Incidence is higher in people of low socioeconomic status, and there are undoubted effects of both tobacco and alcohol which appear to act synergistically in increasing risk (Tuyns et al. 1979). The strong correlation in men of alcohol consumption with liver cancer and the marked sex differential in most geographic areas supports the theory of some carcinogen in alcoholic beverages, possibly a nitrosamine. Dietary deficiency, especially of iron in some groups, has been suspected as an important cause, but there is now a strong suspicion that some major dietary deficiency as yet unidentified may be associated with the increased risk in Northern Iran. In this area, risk seems to be as high in women as in men, and alcohol and tobacco do not appear to be responsible. One hypothesis yet to be excluded is that dietary deficiency accompanied by exposure to opium is important.

Stomach Cancer

As is well recognized, stomach cancer occurs with high frequency in Japan and other parts of Asia and South America, but with low and decreasing frequency in North America and Europe (Hirayama et al. 1980). Among the etiologic factors recognized as potentially important are a number of host factors. Thus, some individuals seem to be genetically predisposed to stomach cancer, especially those of blood type A. Various precancerous lesions have also been identified, especially atrophic gastritis and intestinal metaplasia (Correa et al. 1970, Haenszel et al. 1976). The study of these changes in surveys in Colombia has shown that even within this high-incidence country there is substantial variation in incidence between different areas (Cuello et al. 1976), and this variation is well correlated with different levels of nitrate in the diet and drinking water (Correa et al. 1976, Tannenbaum et al. 1979). Another host factor associated with increased risk is pernicious anemia.

A number of environmental factors have also been identified. Tobacco has so far been supported as a risk factor only by the prospective study of Hirayama in Japan, where the risk ratio is approximately 1.6 (Hirayama 1977). Asbestos has been recognized, however, as likely to increase the risk of gastric and, for that matter, esophageal, colon, and rectal cancer in a number of studies. The risk ratios are approximately 3 (Miller 1978).

However, it is to dietary factors that we turn for what are expected to be the most important causes of stomach cancer. Factors which are suspected of being carcinogenic include those associated with the pickling or smoking of food for preservation; benzpyrene derived from processes of cooking, particularly broiling and barbecuing; and nitrosamines or nitrosamides derived from an interaction between high nitrate-containing food and water and dietary amines in the stomach, in the presence of achlorhydria (Mirvish 1971, Weisburger et al. 1980a). Agents suspected of being protective against stomach cancer include milk, particularly in Japan (Hirayama 1977), refrigeration, and exposure to reducing agents such as ascorbic acid, which may interfere with the nitrate/nitrite dietary amine nitrosamide production reaction (Weisburger et al. 1980b).

Although data have been obtained from experimental animals (Weisburger et al. 1980b) that support the protective effect of vitamin C against the production of nitrosamines, there is some doubt as to the possible effect in man because the total amount of vitamin C in the U.S. diet has changed little in the periods preceding and accompanying the fall of gastric cancer incidence (Page and Friend 1978). There has admittedly been a switch in food consumption patterns whereby the main source of vitamin C in the past, potatoes, has been replaced more recently by green vegetables, salads, and fruits. Nevertheless, the available data do not support a substantial deficiency of vitamin C in the past that would coincide with a relatively simple effect of this substance acting as a protective agent only recently.

One possible factor that deserves further investigation is that butylated hydroxytoluene and similar agents may be largely responsible for the reduction in gastric cancer incidence, since these substances, among others, have been found to exert a protective effect against chemical carcinogens (Wattenberg 1975).

Case-control studies have not been particularly rewarding in defining more specifically the role of diet and other factors in the etiology of stomach cancer. A study in Hawaiian Japanese showed an excess consumption by stomach cancer patients of salted/dried fish or salt-pickled vegetables (Haenszel et al. 1972). However, a study in Japan did not reproduce these findings, although it did show a higher risk in farmers and a lower risk for lettuce and celery users (Haenszel et al. 1976b). A study in Israel showed a higher consumption of starches among gastric cancer patients than in three matched control groups (Modan et al. 1974). A study in the United States suggested that a low risk of gastric cancer was associated with eating lettuce and other uncooked vegetables (Graham et al. 1972). Further studies, using more refined methodology, are required to resolve these discrepancies.

Colon and Rectal Cancer

A number of factors have been associated with cancer of the colon and rectum. These include adenomatous polyps, believed by many to be the precancerous lesion for some if not all such cancers (Haenszel and Correa 1971, Morson 1974). (This topic is discussed further by Dr. Morson, 1981, see pages 99 to 115, this volume.)

A substantially increased risk is well-recognized for individuals with familial polyposis and long-standing ulcerative colitis (Hirayama et al. 1980). Associations have been noted between breast cancer and urban living, rectal cancer and beer (Enstrom 1977). Biochemical studies have identified an association with high excretion of fecal bile acids and steroids (Hill 1975), and a number of dietary variables have been implicated in etiology.

The most important association with increased risk of cancer of the colon and rectum (and for that matter, those cancers in women with which colon cancer is most highly correlated—breast, endometrial, and ovarian cancer) is a high intake of total fat (Armstrong and Doll 1975).

Although some studies have suggested that the variable might be animal protein (Hirayama 1977, Haenszel et al. 1973), it seems more likely that fat is the important variable because of the higher correlations internationally (Armstrong and Doll 1975). This also fits in with the biochemical mechanisms postulated and, to some extent, established in animal experimental studies. There is, however, no unanimity even from correlation type studies. Thus,

Enig et al. (1978) have suggested that animal fat is, if anything, negatively correlated with colon and rectal cancer incidence in the United States.

A high intake of dietary fiber has been particularly associated with protection from colon cancer (IARC Microecology Group 1977, Reddy et al. 1978), although it is not clear whether all components of dietary fiber are equally protective. Wattenberg has pointed to the effect of dietary constituents on the metabolism of chemical carcinogens by the microsomal mixed function oxidase system (Wattenberg 1975). Naturally occurring inducers of increased activity in this system are found in cruciferous vegetables such as brussels sprouts, cabbage, and cauliflower. Graham et al. (1978) found a possible protective effect of such vegetables against colon cancer.

Case control studies of colon and rectal cancer have not produced consistent findings. A study in Hawaiian Japanese pointed to the importance of Western-type meals and especially beef intake (Haenszel et al. 1973), but these findings were not replicated in Japan (Haenszel et al. 1980), although a negative association with consumption of cabbage was found in the latter study. A study in Israel suggested the importance of foods low in fiber in the etiology of colon but not rectal cancer (Modan et al. 1975). However, a study in Canada has shown an association of both colon and rectal cancer with saturated fat intake but not with estimated consumption of crude fiber (Jain et al. 1980).

Rectal cancer has been associated with beer consumption in some (Enstrom 1977, Dean et al. 1979) but not all studies (Jensen 1979). It has also been pointed out that there is a greater correlation between rectal cancer mortality and beer consumption than between rectal cancer and saturated fat (McMichael et al. 1979).

Gallbladder Cancer

There is a high incidence of gallbladder cancer in Latin America, Japan, and Southeast Asia and, as already noted, in females to a greater extent than in males (Hirayama et al. 1980). Although relatively uncommon in the United States, it has been associated with gallstones, obesity, and type 4 hyperlipoproteinemia. Dietary risk factors postulated include both high caloric and high fat diets. As yet, these associations of postulated risk factors must remain hypothetical, but they probably justify further investigation. However, the uniformly poor correlation of gallbladder cancer with the other cancers suggested as being associated with a high fat diet (Table 2) appears to mitigate against high fat diets being relevant.

Liver Cancer

Liver cancer is found in high incidence in sub-Sahara Africa and in Southeast Asia (Hirayama et al. 1980). It is, of course, low in incidence in North America. It has been associated with a number of precancerous lesions, particularly with cirrhosis, hemochromatosis, and chronic hepatitis. Among environmental factors associated with the disease are alcohol, aflatoxin, vinyl chloride, and hepatitis B virus. Studies in China suggest a strong association with polluted water, probably because of exposure to hepatitis B virus (Su 1979). Although liver cell adenomas have been shown to be associated with oral contraceptive use (Christopherson and Mays 1977), no clear association has been identified with primary liver cell cancers.

Because this is a cancer from which we seem to be largely protected, there has not been a great deal of investigation of its etiology. It is, however, perhaps relevant that the most favored etiological factor in Africa is exposure to aflatoxin (Linsell and Peers 1977). Our own food storage and inspection policies, particularly of peanuts and foods made from them, may well be protecting us from what is a most important condition in Africa, one which is proving difficult to control.

Pancreatic Cancer

Pancreatic cancer is found in high incidence in Western industrial countries and in some racial groups, particularly the Maoris of New Zealand, native Hawaiians, and black Americans (Fraumeni 1975, Hirayama et al. 1980). The only recognized host factor is diabetes; so far there are no clear associations with environmental factors, although the disease has been associated with lower socioeconomic status, with exposure to tobacco (Fraumeni 1975), and with a high fat diet (Armstrong and Doll 1975, Miller 1980, Wynder 1975). The high correlation between pancreatic cancer and other cancers suspected of being associated with a high fat diet (Table 2) supports this latter hypothesis.

The disease has been increasing in Western countries, although in the last few years this increase may have come to an end. By use of mathematical modeling approaches, Moolgavkar (personal communication, 1980) has postulated that a substantial proportion of pancreatic cancer may be attributable to cigarette consumption. A number of studies are on-going of the current etiology of pancreatic cancer, especially under the aegis of the National Pancreatic Cancer Project. It is possible that we will learn more about the etiology of this cancer, which is so difficult to diagnose and treat, in the next few years.

CONCLUSION

It is apparent from this review that it is difficult to derive a common thread for the etiology of all gastrointestinal tumors. One possible encouraging feature is that factors which protect against one cancer are different from those which appear to be carcinogenic for others. Thus the fears that some have expressed that control of colon cancer may be achieved only at the cost of an increase in the incidence of gastric cancer are likely to prove groundless.

It seems likely that future studies will identify substantial interactions between factors and will further specify the extent to which factors are responsible in different areas. Thus, the apparent differing importance of fiber and fat in different investigations of the etiology of colon cancer may be only partially due to differences in the methodology of dietary studies. It is indeed possible that in order to achieve full protection from colon cancer, one needs to combine a high fiber with a low fat diet (Miller 1980). The vegetable/cereal manufacturers are helping us with the former, but so far there has been very little incentive to reduce the total amount of fat in our diet. I believe this is one of the most important preventive measures that we should urge upon our population. We have possibly been successful in reducing cardiovascular disease by a combination of reduction of cigarette smoking in adults and a partial substitution of saturated fat with polyunsaturated fat. However, trends in fat consumption indicate that although there has been a transfer in the consumption of fat from animal to vegetable sources, the total amount of fat in our diet has increased (Page and Friend 1978). I believe we now have to supplement the substitution with a reduction in total fat intake, preferably achieving no greater than a 30% contribution of fat to our total calorie consumption.

REFERENCES

Armstrong, B., and R. Doll. 1975. Environmental factors and cancer incidence and mortality in different countries, with special reference to dietary practices. Int. J. Cancer 15:617–631.

Burkitt, D. P. 1971. Guest editorial: Some neglected leads to cancer causation. J. Natl. Cancer Inst. 47:913–919.

Christopherson, W. M., and E. T. Mays. 1977. Liver tumors and contraceptive steroids: Experience with the first one hundred registry patients. J. Natl. Cancer Inst. 58:167–171.

Correa, P., C. Cuello, and E. Duque. 1970. Carcinoma and intestinal metaplasia in Colombian migrants. J. Natl. Cancer Inst. 44:297–306.

Correa, P., C. Cuello, E. Duque, L. C. Burbano, F. T. Garcia, O. Bolanos, C. Brown, and W. Haenszel. 1976. Gastric cancer in Colombia III. Natural history of precursor lesions. J. Natl. Cancer Inst. 57:1027–1035.

Cuello, C., P. Correa, W. Haenszel, G. Gordillo, C. Brown, M. Archer, and S. Tannenbaum. 1976. Gastric cancer in Colombia I. Cancer risk and suspect environmental agents. J. Natl. Cancer Inst. 57:1015–1020.

Dean, G., R. Maclennan, H. McLoughlin, and E. Shelley. 1979. The causes of death of blue-collar workers at a Dublin brewery, 1954–1974. Br. J. Cancer 40:581–589.

Enig, M. G., R. J. Munn, and M. Keeney. 1978. Dietary fat and cancer trends—a critique. Fed. Proc. 37:2215–2220.

Enstrom, J. E. 1977. Colorectal cancer and beer drinking. Brit. J. Cancer 35:674–683.

Fraumeni, J. F. 1975. Cancers of the pancreas and biliary tract. Epidemiological considerations. Cancer Res. 35:3437–3446.

Graham, S., H. Dayal, M. Swanson, A. Mittleman, and G. Wilkinson. 1978. Diet in the epidemiology of cancer of the colon and rectum. J. Natl. Cancer Inst. 61:709–714.

Graham, S., W. Schotz, and P. Martino. 1972. Alimentary factors in the epidemiology of gastric cancer. Cancer 30:927–928.

Haenszel, W., J. W. Berg, M. Segi, M. Kurihara, and F. B. Locke. 1973. Large bowel cancer in Hawaiian Japanese. J. Natl. Cancer Inst. 51:1765–1779.

Haenszel, W., and P. Correa. 1971. Cancer of the colon and rectum and adenomatous polyps. A review of epidemiologic findings. Cancer 28:14–24.

Haenszel, W., P. Correa, C. Cuello, N. Guzman, L. C. Burbano, H. Lores, and J. Munoz. 1976a. Gastric cancer in Colombia II. Case-control study of precursor lesions. J. Natl. Cancer Inst. 57:1021-1026.

Haenszel, W., M. Kurihara, F. B. Locke, K. Shimuzu, and M. Segi. 1976b. Stomach cancer in Japan. J. Natl. Cancer Inst. 56:265-274.

Haenszel, W., M. Kurihara, M. Segi, and R. K. C. Lee. 1972. Stomach cancer among Japanese in Hawaii. J. Natl. Cancer Inst. 49:969-988.

Haenszel, W., F. B. Locke, and M. Segi. 1980. A case-control study of large bowel cancer in Japan. J. Natl. Cancer Inst. 64:17-22.

Hill, M. J. 1975. Metabolic epidemiology of dietary factors in large bowel cancer. Cancer Res. 35:3398-3402.

Hirayama, T. 1977. Changing patterns of cancer in Japan with special reference to the decrease in stomach cancer mortality, *in* Origins of Human Cancer. Cold Spring Harbor Laboratory, Cold Spring Harbor, New York, pp. 55-75.

Hirayama, T., J. A. H. Waterhouse, and J. F. Fraumeni, eds. 1980. Cancer risks by site. UICC Technical Report Series Vol. 41. International Union Against Cancer, Geneva.

IARC Microecology Group. 1977. Dietary fibre, transit-time, faecal bacteria, steroids and colon cancer in two Scandinavian populations. Lancet 2:207-211.

Jain, M., G. M. Cook, F. G. Davis, M. C. Grace, G. R. Howe, and A. B. Miller. 1980. A case-control study of diet and colo-rectal cancer. Int. J. Cancer 26:757-768.

Jensen, O. M. 1979. Cancer morbidity and causes of death among Danish brewery workers. Int. J. Cancer 23:454-463.

Joint Iran-International Agency for Research on Cancer Study Group. 1977. Esophageal cancer studies in the Caspian littoral of Iran: Results of population studies—a prodrome. J. Natl. Cancer Inst. 59:1127-1138.

Linsell, C. A., and F. G. Peers. 1977. Aflatoxin and liver cell cancer. Trans. R. Soc. Trop. Med. Hyg. 71:471-473.

McMichael, A. J., J. D. Potter, and B. S. Hetzel. 1979. Time trends in colo-rectal cancer mortality in relation to food and alcohol consumption. United States, United Kingdom, Australia and New Zealand. Int. J. Epidemiol. 8:295-303.

Miller, A. B. 1978. Asbestos fibre dust and gastro-intestinal malignancies. Review of literature with regard to a cause-effect relationship. J. Chron. Dis. 31:23-33.

Miller, A. B., G. B. Gori, S. Graham, T. Hirayama, M. Kunze, B. S. Reddy, and J. H. Weisburger. 1980. Nutrition and Cancer. Preventive Medicine 9:189-196.

Mirvish, S. S. 1971. Kinetics of nitrosamide formation from alkylureas, n-alkylurethans, and alkylguanidines: Possible implications for the etiology of human gastric cancer. J. Natl. Cancer Inst. 46:1183-1193.

Modan, B., V. Barell, F. Lubin, M. Modan, R. A. Greenberg, and S. Graham. 1975. Low-fiber intake as an etiologic factor in cancer of the colon. J. Natl. Cancer Inst. 55:15-18.

Modan, B., F. Lubin, V. Barell, R. A. Greenberg, M. Modan, and S. Graham. 1974. The role of starches in the etiology of gastric cancer. Cancer 34:2087-2092.

Morson, B. C. 1974. Evolution of cancer of the colon and rectum. Cancer 34:845-849.

Page, L., and B. Friend. 1978. The changing United States diet. Bioscience 28:192-197.

Reddy, B. S., A. R. Hedges, K. Laakso, and E. L. Wynder. 1978. Metabolic epidemiology of large bowel cancer. Fecal bulk and constituents of high-risk North American and low-risk Finnish population. Cancer 42:2832-2838.

Su Delong. 1979. Drinking water and liver cell cancer. An epidemiologic approach to the etiology of this disease in China. Chin. Med. J. 92:748-756.

Tannenbaum, S. R., D. Moran, W. Rand, C. Cuello, and P. Correa. 1979. Gastric cancer in Colombia IV. Nitrite and other ions in gastric contents of residents from a high risk region. J. Natl. Cancer Inst. 62:9-12.

Tuyns, A. J., G. Pequignot, and J. S. Abbatucci. 1979. Oesophageal cancer and alcohol consumption. Importance of type of beverage. Int. J. Cancer 23:443-447.

Waterhouse, J., C. Muir, P. Correa, and J. Powell, eds. 1976. Cancer incidence in five continents Volume III. IARC Scientific Publication No. 15. International Agency for Research on Cancer, Lyon.

Wattenberg, L. W. 1975. Effects of dietary constituents on the metabolism of chemical carcinogens. Cancer Res. 35:3326-3331.

Weisburger, J. H., H. Marquardt, N. Hirota, H. Mori, and G. Williams. 1980a. Induction of glandular stomach cancer in rats with an extract of nitrite-treated fish. J. Natl. Cancer Inst. 64:163–167.

Weisburger, J. H., H. Marquardt, H. F. Mower, N. Hirota, H. Mori, and G. Williams. 1980b. Inhibition of carcinogenesis: Vitamin C and the prevention of gastric cancer. Preventive Medicine 9:352–361.

Wynder, E. L. 1975. An epidemiological evaluation of the causes of cancer of the pancreas. Cancer Res. 35:2228–2232.

Gastrointestinal Cancer, edited by
John R. Stroehlein and
Marvin M. Romsdahl.
Raven Press, New York © 1981.

Intravenous Hyperalimentation and Cancer: An Update

Edward M. Copeland, III, M.D.

The University of Texas Medical School at Houston, and
The University of Texas System Cancer Center
M. D. Anderson Hospital and Tumor Institute, Houston, Texas

Recently, intravenous hyperalimentation (IVH) has been demonstrated to result in nutritional repletion of patients with cancer both before, during, and after antineoplastic therapy. Cancer, per se, does not appear to significantly increase energy requirements; however, surgery, chemotherapy, and radiation therapy do limit nutritional intake for varying periods of time, and sequential therapy can eventually lead to inanition and malnutrition. In an already undernourished patient, the increased risk of complications secondary to malnutrition can limit the dose of chemotherapy or radiation therapy, and the patient may no longer be classified as a reasonable treatment candidate, even though he has a potentially responsive lesion. The margin of safety between the therapeutic dose and lethal dose of many chemotherapeutic agents is much smaller in a malnourished patient than in a well-nourished one.

No doubt, a growing neoplasm extracts nutrients from the host and can result in host catabolism, particularly if the patient does not ingest nutrients in quantities sufficient to supply the demands of the neoplasm and the patient. The metabolic interactions between cancer and the host are not fully understood. It does appear, however, that once cancer disseminates, there is a relationship between the volume of cancer and the magnitude of weight loss. As Holland and her group (Plumb and Holland 1977) have indicated, much of the depression and hopelessness encountered in cancer patients can be a reactive state associated with the diagnosis of cancer, with the effects of treatment, or with the stage of disease. Such a depressive response alone can reduce the normal amount of food intake. Also important in the early diagnosis of anorexia and weight loss is the observation that depression can occur in response to the anticipated threat of a symptom or sign that the individual perceives as evidence of a potential malignant process. Since symptoms of a malignant disease often antedate diagnosis by as long as six months, it is not unusual to find that patients have lost 6% of their usual body weight prior to diagnosis and are not malnourished. Nevertheless, patients with certain cancers, such as oat cell carcinoma of the lung, can have extreme weight loss prior to diagnosis of their disease and, yet when diagnosed, the volume of tumor is relatively small. Theologides (1979) has postulated that anorexia and weight loss are secondary to certain peptides, oligonucleotides, and other metabolites produced by the cancer. Others, including myself, believe that much of the malnutrition seen in cancer patients is iatrogenic and the result of inadequate nutritional intake during and after treatment with antineoplastic agents.

Absorption of nutrients via a functional gastrointestinal tract is the best means of maintaining adequate nutrition; however, delivery of nutrients to the gastrointestinal tract does not always result in nutritional restoration of the malnourished patient because the syndrome of malnutrition may include malabsorption. In the severely malnourished individual, gastrointestinal columnar mucosal cells become cuboidal and the brush border is reduced in height. Decreased production of mucosal cells and decreased migration from the intestinal crypts occur, gastrointestinal motility diminishes, and overgrowth of facultative and anaerobic bacteria results. All of these environmental, morphological, and absorptive abnormalities are reversible after protein-calorie replenishment. The process is slow, however, because adequate enteral nutriments are initially partially malabsorbed, and the uncomfortable symptoms of diarrhea, nausea, bloating, and abdominal pain limit the patient's desire to eat or obtain nutriments via nasogastric, gastrostomy, or jejunostomy feedings. Unfortunately, nutritional supplementation via the gastrointestinal tract can thus be time-consuming, or the gastrointestinal tract may be unavailable for nutrient administration. Under these circumstances, the use of intravenous hyperalimentation has been indicated. IVH has interrupted the vicious cycle created by malnutrition because adequate nutrients can be provided to the patient as adjunctive support during oncologic therapy. Similarly, if the primary disease is of the gastrointestinal tract, this organ may be rested during IVH because absorption and assimilation of foodstuffs across the gastrointestinal mucosa is not necessary. The concept of "bowel rest" has been an extension of nutritional therapy since the introduction of IVH.

MANAGEMENT OF MALNUTRITION

Nutritional depletion is defined by our team as a recent, unintentional loss of 10% or more of body weight, a serum albumin concentration of less than 3.4 g/dl, and/or a negative reaction to a battery of recall skin test antigens. Patients who satisfy two of these three criteria and who have a reasonable chance of responding to appropriate antineoplastic therapy are candidates for IVH. Similarly, patients who are incapable of adequate enteral nutrition because of the malnutrition imposed by previous oncologic therapy are candidates for nutritional rehabilitation with IVH. Also suited for IVH are nutritionally healthy patients whose treatment plan requires multiple courses of chemotherapy, possibly combined with surgery or radiation therapy. IVH is employed in these patients if maintenance of optimum nutrition during therapy is considered important to maximize the chances for response to treatment, to reduce complications of oncologic therapy, or to improve the quality of life. We like our simplified definition of malnutrition, although there are many more complex tests for evaluating nutritional status, most of which can be correlated with somatic compartments. The fat compartment can be evaluated by measuring the triceps' skin fold thickness, the visceral protein compartment by measuring serum albumin concentration and also by skin testing for delayed hypersensitivity, and the skeletal muscle compartment by measuring upper arm circumference and creatinine-height index. Although our team uses all available tests, and each test is an important one, the practicing physician without the aid of an organized nutritional support service cannot always perform all available tests. Percent weight loss, serum albumin level, and reactivity to skin tests will serve to identify most patients requiring aggressive nutritional rehabilitation.

The patient's initial nutritional status, the effect of the planned oncologic therapy on nutritional intake, the anticipated systemic reaction to the planned antineoplastic therapy, and the need for rapid nutritional recovery after the completion of oncologic therapy will indicate whether maintenance or anabolic levels of calories and protein are required prior to, during, and/or after cancer treatment. A simple way to calculate calorie and protein needs is to supply calories at 35 kcal/kg/day, if maintenance levels are necessary, or 45 kcal/kg/day, if anabolism needs to be promoted. Nitrogen (protein in grams divided by 6.25) should be given in the ratio of about 1 gram per 150 nonprotein calories.

As a single test, nitrogen balance cannot assess the nutritional status of the patient. Nitrogen balance studies determine the need for additional protein and calorie intake to offset body protein losses and to meet energy demands during the time period in which the nitrogen balance studies are determined. Since amino acids are distinguished from other nutrients by the presence of nitrogen, nitrogen balance is commonly used as a nutritional index. When cumulative nitrogen output exceeds nitrogen input for several days, the patient may become protein-calorie malnourished; conversely, when cumulative nitrogen intake combined with the proper amount of calories as both fat and carbohydrate exceeds nitrogen output for several days, anabolism will usually ensue.

PARENTERAL NUTRITION

Solutions for intravenous hyperalimentation generally contain 3.5%-5% amino acids and 20%-30% dextrose. The osmolarity of this solution is between 1,800-2,400 mOsm, necessitating infusion via a large bore central vein rather than through a peripheral vein. Usually, the subclavian vein is catheterized percutaneously via the infraclavicular approach, so that the tip of the feeding catheter can be placed in the middle of the superior vena cava. Accurate positioning of the catheter tip is verified by obtaining a chest roentgenogram prior to beginning the hypertonic IVH solutions. Improper positioning of the catheter in a smaller vessel, such as the jugular vein, will result in thrombophlebitis, often within 48 hours of initiating the infusion. A constant rate of administration is necessary to promote proper utilization of the infused glucose, amino acids, minerals, and vitamins. Initially, 1,000 ml is delivered in 24 hours to confirm the patient's ability to effectively metabolize the administered glucose. In the absence of hyperglycemia and glycosuria, the flow rate is increased to 1,000 ml every 12 hours. The islet cells of the pancreas will again need the opportunity to adapt with an increase in insulin output in response to the increased glucose infusion. Extremely wasted patients may tolerate only 2,000 ml per day until partial nutritional rehabilitation has been obtained. Usually, however, the average adult requiring IVH will tolerate a daily ration of 3,000 ml within the first 3-5 days of beginning therapy. An expected initial 3-4 pound weight gain is anticipated secondary to rehydration, but then the patient should gain lean body mass at a rate of about one-half pound per day. Body weight gain greater than one pound per day should be considered fluid retention, and the IVH delivery rate should be slowed or a diuretic given. The abrupt cessation of IVH may lead to insulin shock or reactive hypoglycemia. Therefore, IVH should be tapered off during the 24- to 48-hour period prior to completely discontinuing it.

Metabolic status should be reviewed routinely in order to detect any need to alter the flow rate or composition of the nutrient solution. On a regular basis, the following factors should be evaluated: fractional urine sugar concentration every six hours; daily intake and output; daily weight; serum electrolytes, blood urea nitrogen, and blood sugar levels three times a week; serum levels of albumin, magnesium, phosphorous, calcium, and creatinine once a week; liver function tests, coagulation parameters, and complete blood count once a week; and patient reevaluation for any temperature elevation. IVH team members should change the patient's catheter dressing and IVH delivery tubing three times a week, each time repreparing the skin with ether or acetone and an antiseptic solution. An antimicrobial ointment and a sterile dressing are reapplied to cover the catheter-skin entrance site. Proper technique must be utilized always; when it is, a single feeding catheter can remain in place for prolonged periods of time without complications.

Intravenous fat solutions are now available for parenteral use in the United States. Although they are isotonic, 290 mOsm per liter, and can be infused via a peripheral vein without fear of inducing thrombophlebitis, their primary role in intravenous nutritional therapy for cancer patients, to date, is to provide the essential fatty acid, linoleic acid. The fatty acid fraction of the commercially available fat preparations is approximately 54% linoleic acid, adequate quantities of which can be delivered by the thrice weekly administration of one 500 ml bottle of the fatty acid solution. The fat should be infused through a peripheral vein and should not be mixed with the IVH solution. Delivery of the fatty acid solution via the Y-connector of the IVH delivery system has proven safe; nevertheless, peripheral administration remains our current recommendation.

Stimulation of tumor growth from the nutritional repletion of malnourished human beings has not been identified; nevertheless, results from rat experiments do suggest that this possibility exists in the mammalian species and that appropriate antineoplastic therapy should be instituted early during nutritional rehabilitation (Steiger et al. 1980, Daly et al. 1980). Data in rats, however, cannot be applied directly to malnourished cancer patients, since doubling times of human malignant tumors are measured in days or weeks, and the cancer may not kill the patient until several years after the initial clone of malignant cells has developed. The doubling time of animal tumors often can be measured in hours, and this relatively rapid growth can result in death of the animal within five to seven weeks after initial tumor inoculation. Dietary protein repletion or depletion would be expected to have a more obvious and measurable effect on a tumor such as a Walker-256 carcinosarcoma because of its rapid growth characteristics. Because of this rapidity of tumor growth during nutritional repletion in protein-depleted rats, cell-cycle-specific chemotherapeutic drugs have been shown to have a greater effect on some tumors in rodents during nutritional repletion when compared to the effect on similar tumors in animals remaining in a protein-depleted state (Reynolds et al. 1980). Unfortunately, tumors in cachectic human beings during nutritional therapy have not been noted to be more responsive to DNA-specific chemotherapeutic drugs.

CLINICAL MATERIAL

At our institution, over 1,500 patients have received IVH as nutritional support for oncologic therapy during the last eight years. In 1976, our group evaluated the results of IVH in the treatment of 406 consecutive cancer patients suffering from a wide variety of malignant diseases (Copeland and Dudrick 1976). At that time, this was the largest series of cancer patients reported who had received IVH. The majority of these patients were considered to be poor candidates for oncologic therapy because of the significant degree of malnutrition identified prior to embarking upon a course of antineoplastic therapy that might provide major palliation or cure. Subsequent to this 1976 report, several retrospective and prospective randomized studies have been reported. Studies currently sponsored by the Diet, Nutrition, and Cancer Programs of the National Cancer Institute are nearing completion and, at present, neither response rates nor survival has been improved in patients receiving IVH. In many of these studies, patients with only minimal degrees of malnutrition were entered into the randomization process, or if malnourished patients were within the studies, little data on the nutritional efficacy of IVH are given to allow an evaluation of the capacity of the nutrient solutions to result in nutritional repletion. That malnutrition is a poor prognostic indicator for response to chemotherapy is an established fact. Whether or not nutritional repletion, either by parenteral or enteral means, can reverse malnutrition and convert a predictably poor responder into a good responder via nutritional repletion remains unknown. Unfortunately, many of the randomized prospective trials reported today do not equate response of the tumor to chemotherapeutic drugs with the host response to the attempts at nutritional repletion. In fact, host weight gain in these studies is often composed predominantly of an increase in total body water and fat mass with very little documentation of an increase in lean body tissue. Obviously, it is important to know if a previously malnourished patient who has been nutritionally replenished with IVH is a better candidate for response to oncologic therapy than is his malnourished counterpart. The answer to such a question will not be known until a study is done combining the following necessary elements: (1) good definition of malnutrition; (2) randomization of malnourished patients between IVH and standard nutritional maintenance; (3) control group of well-nourished patients on standard nutritional maintenance; (4) drugs with moderate gastrointestinal toxicity; (5) cancer that is moderately responsive to drugs; and (6) nutritional response to therapy correlated with tumor response to therapy. Although the answer to the proposed question from the chemotherapeutic standpoint is unknown at this time, the remainder of this manuscript will present clinical data relevant to the use of intravenous hyperalimentation in the cancer patient population.

Surgery

The benefits of nutritional rehabilitation in the preoperative period for the malnourished surgical patient needs little further documentation. Comparison of parenterally supported patients with esophageal carcinoma to conventionally treated patients has shown better maintenance of weight and nitrogen balance and far fewer complications in the patients supported by parenteral nutrition (Moghissi et al. 1977). A randomized trial of preoperative intravenous nutrition versus conventional treatment in patients with gastric cancer revealed significantly less infection and weight loss and slightly less mortality in those patients supported by parenteral nutrition (William et al. 1976). Seniukov et al. (1978) reported an evaluation of the efficacy of IVH used postoperatively in malnourished patients with carcinoma of the larynx. Seventy patients received IVH, and 90 patients were fed via a nasogastric feeding tube. The two groups of patients were carefully selected to be matched for stage of disease and dose of preoperative radiation therapy. Primary wound healing occurred in 75% of the parenterally fed group versus 40% of the enterally fed group. From this study, it would appear that patients who were given their nutrient mixture by vein, and thereby guaranteed a certain caloric intake, had significantly better postoperative wound healing than did a similar group of patients who were fed by the gastrointestinal tract and who, no doubt, malabsorbed a portion of the administered nutrients. Dionigi and co-workers (1979) compared 98 patients with surgically resectable gastrointestinal cancers treated with IVH pre- and postoperatively to 94 surgical patients with similar gastrointestinal tumors treated with conventional fluid therapy. The IVH group was in better nitrogen balance, weight gain was significantly greater, wound healing was better, and their general well-being was improved; and the average hospital stay for the IVH group was 18 days compared to 25 days for those in the conventionally treated group.

In our series, 100 patients received IVH as nutritional support for a general or thoracic surgical procedure. Although this group of patients was reported retrospectively, in our opinion, without IVH, recovery from the magnitude of the surgical procedure would have been questionable in each patient. Fifty-two patients underwent curative resections, which included esophagectomies, gastrectomies, and abdominal-perineal resections. The overall operative mortality rate was only 4%. In those patients who received IVH pre- and postoperatively, weight gain and a rise in the serum albumin concentration were obtained almost entirely during the preoperative period. Body weight and serum albumin concentration were maintained during the postoperative period, but no increase in either occurred. Those patients who received IVH only postoperatively, usually had developed one of the complications of prolonged malnutrition, such as wound dehiscence, paralytic ileus, intra-abdominal abscess, or wound infection, before IVH was begun. Weight gain was difficult to attain in these patients, probably because of increased energy expenditures secondary to the surgical complications. In contrast, those patients who received IVH preoperatively had virtually no postoperative complications and were often eating within five days after bowel resection. Based on comparative data such as that of Seniukov and Dionigi and the retrospective data from our group, we recommend that a malnourished patient be nutritionally replenished preoperatively rather than waiting for some catastrophic postoperative complication to occur before thinking of nutritional repletion with IVH.

Radiation Therapy

Little has been published on the use of IVH as an adjunct to the use of radiation therapy. In a prospective randomized study of 20 adult patients receiving radiotherapy to the pelvis and the abdomen, IVH allowed weight gain and a slight improvement in visceral protein status of patients receiving it compared to patients treated with conventional nutritional regimens (Valeno et al. 1978). In our series, 39 malnourished patients required treatment with IVH in order to complete a planned course of radiation therapy. IVH was utilized for an average period of 37.6 days, and the average weight gain was 7.8 pounds. Anorexia, nausea, and vomiting disappeared during IVH unless the patient attempted to eat, in which case all symptoms recurred. Fifty-four percent of the patients responded with a greater than 50% reduction in tumor size. Responding patients gained an average of 13.0 ± 6.4 pounds during IVH (average 36.2 days) and radiation therapy (average 3,832 r), whereas nonresponding patients gained only 4.9 ± 8.8 pounds ($p < 0.001$) during IVH (average 42.8 days) and radiation therapy (average 3,819 r). Similarly, a significant rise in serum albumin concentration occurred only in those patients whose tumors responded to radiation therapy. Ninety-five percent of the patients completed their planned course of radiation therapy and improved symptomatically. IVH allowed a planned course of radiation therapy to be delivered to a group of poor-risk, malnourished cancer patients, a positive correlation between tumor response and nutritional status was identified, and symptoms of radiation enteritis were reduced as long as patients were not allowed oral intake.

Chemotherapy

In our series, 175 patients received IVH and chemotherapy. IVH was utilized for an average period of 22.8 days and resulted in an average weight gain of 5.6 pounds. Gastrointestinal symptoms of nausea, vomiting, and diarrhea were reduced or better tolerated if IVH was used with chemotherapy; also, patients were not required to eat in order to maintain body composition. A 50% or greater reduction in measurable tumor mass was obtained in 27.8% of patients. This response rate is actually rather low, because many of these 175 patients had relapsed after initial response to chemotherapy and were being treated with a different drug regimen that was known to have limited effectiveness. Responding patients survived for an average period of 8.2 months, whereas nonresponding patients survived an average of 1.9 months. Depression of the leukocyte count below 2,500 cells/mm³ occurred in 51.5% of patients and lasted for an average duration of 7.7 days; nevertheless, only four pathogenic organisms were grown on cultures from 212 consecutive subclavian vein catheters. Three patients had simultaneous positive blood and catheter cultures, for an incidence of catheter-related sepsis of only 1.4%.

The concept of increased tolerance for 5-fluorouracil (5-FU) during "bowel rest" and nutritional maintenance with IVH was documented initially in animals (Souchon et al. 1975). This experience was extrapolated to human beings suffering from malnutrition and metastatic colon cancer. Sixteen patients were placed on IVH for seven days prior to beginning treatment with 5-FU (15 mg/kg/day diluted in 50 ml of 5% dextrose in water and delivered intravenously during a one-hour period). Ten malnourished patients with metastatic colon cancer who did not receive IVH during 5-FU administration served as controls. In the IVH group, five patients (31%) responded with a greater than 50% reduction in measurable tumor volume and received a total dose of 7.4 g of 5-FU over an average period of 8.6 days. One control patient (10%) responded to an average total dose of 3.8 g of 5-FU given over an average period of only 4.4 days. The control group lost an average weight of 4.2 pounds during the study, whereas the IVH group gained weight. These data are similar to those of Moertel et al. (1974) who had reported previously that patients who have gastrointestinal cancer and a good performance status have a better response to 5-FU than do patients with similar disease processes but a poor performance status. Whether the increased response in nutritionally replenished patients was secondary to a better nutritional status or to the tolerance of a larger dose of 5-FU remains to be evaluated. Another explanation for the poor results of chemotherapy with 5-FU in malnourished patients may be related to folate-deficient states commonly found in cachectic cancer patients (Bertino 1979).

In a prospective, randomized trial utilizing patients with non-oat cell carcinoma of the lung, Issell et al. (1978) reported that patients who received IVH ten days prior to chemotherapy and continued it for 31 days throughout the first course of chemotherapy experienced less nausea and vomiting and had a significant improvement in measured nutritional parameters when compared to the group treated by conventional nutritional methods. A response to chemotherapy was identified in four patients in the IVH group and in only one patient in the non-IVH group. These data are preliminary, but would indicate that nutritionally replenished, malnourished patients have a response advantage over those patients not treated by aggressive nutritional methods. Also, Issell's group has done sequential nutritional assessment indicating that patients who responded to aggressive nutritional therapy were more likely to be responders to chemotherapeutic drugs. Such results support retrospective data previously reported by Copeland, Lanzotti, and their co-workers (1975).

Valdivieso et al. (in press), utilizing both radiation therapy and chemotherapy to treat patients with oat cell carcinoma of the lung, noted an 85% complete response rate for patients randomized to IVH, versus a 59% complete response rate for patients randomized to nutritional support by conventional mechanisms. Also, 90% of the IVH patients maintained ambulatory status during treatment, versus 57% of the conventional therapy group. Similarly, those patients treated with IVH during oncologic therapy had a significantly greater rate of conversion of skin test reactions to positive (38%→67%) than did the conventional therapy group (36%→46%) ($p = 0.03$).

In preliminary reports by Nixon et al. (in press), Popp et al. (in press), Jordan et al. (in press), and Samuels et al. (in press), however, no such advantage for the IVH patient with metastatic colon cancer, lymphoma, adenocarcinoma of the lungs, or metastatic testicular cancer could be identified. In fact, in Nixon's study, colon cancer patients randomized to receive IVH and treated with 5-FU had a significantly shorter survival time than similarly treated patients not nutritionally supported with IVH. Unfortunately, the number of patients in the study is small; distribution of metastatic sites was 1.95 per patient for the IVH group and only 1.2 per patient for the control group; and the median duration of disease was 11.5 months for the IVH group and 15 months for the control group. Thus, the IVH group had more metastatic sites and a shorter duration of disease, indicating a more rapidly progressive metastatic process. The response to 5-FU was poor in both groups, 15% versus 12%, respectively. Therefore, the study of Nixon and co-workers indicates that IVH has no effect on altering rapidly progressive malignant disease, particularly if response to antineoplastic therapy is poor, and does not indicate that IVH is necessarily dangerous to this patient population, as was concluded by Nixon's group. Death occurred promptly in the IVH group, yet there was no evidence of tumor growth acceleration from the administration of IVH. Nevertheless, the authors indicate that the IVH patients died quite rapidly from disease progression. The actual causes of death and the evidence that disease progression was attributed to IVH is not presented in their data.

In the study of Popp et al. (in press), patients with lymphoma were randomized to receive IVH versus the usual outpatient diet. In both the IVH and the non-IVH groups, well-nourished patients had a response advantage over malnourished patients (92% versus 45%). Therefore, response correlated to initial nutritional status and not to the method of nutritional replenishment. The nutritional status of the control and IVH groups was initially the same, no nutritional values are given for the post-IVH period, and the nutritional intake of patients receiving outpatient chemotherapy is unknown. Popp and his co-workers have compared patients with similar initial nutritional states and probably the same nutritional intake and, as expected, have found no differences in the groups. In a subsequent publication (in preparation), these co-workers have indicated that weight gain in the IVH group was primarily as an increase in total body water and fat content. Yet, the capacity to increase protein synthesis over catabolism in malnourished cancer patients and the ability to increase lean body mass during IVH has been well-documented by this group (Brennan and Bert, in press) studying patients with esophageal carcinoma and testicular carcinoma in the past. Why protein anabolism could not be accomplished in the lymphoma patient is not addressed in their data.

Jordan et al. (in press) found the response of extensive adenocarcinoma of the lung to a multiple chemotherapeutic regimen unchanged by the use of IVH. Again, the response advantage was for those patients who were well-nourished at the initiation of chemotherapy, regardless of the method of nutritional supplementation. Of the responding patients, 95% were initially fully ambulatory, and 87% had lost less than 6% of their usual body weight. Although some patients were randomized to receive IVH, no data on sequential nutritional assessment are available, and IVH patients may not have had a protein anabolic response to the infused nutrient solutions.

Samuels et al. (in press) investigated IVH as an adjunct to the treatment of healthy, young, adult male patients with metastatic testicular carcinoma treated with vinblastine and bleomycin. Samuels' group concluded that response rate was unchanged by the use of IVH adjunctively in patients who were nutritionally intact at the outset of chemotherapy, that granulocyte depression and nadirs were the same in the IVH and non-IVH groups, that there was some protection afforded the platelets by the use of IVH, that weight loss was prevented by IVH, but that more infections (not catheter-related) occurred in the IVH group. Samuels' final comments were that IVH should be reserved for those patients who present with significant weight loss or who fail to regain lost weight during rest periods between chemotherapy courses.

A series of well-controlled studies done by van Eys et al. (1980a, b) utilizing children with metastatic, pediatric neoplasms either to or from bone have shown the safety of the technique in the pediatric age group and have shown that infectious complications correlate significantly with the initial nutritional status of the patient, with IVH being only a secondary factor. His group concluded that IVH may be used to rehabilitate pediatric patients nutritionally, even during intensive chemotherapy, and that the ability to deliver chemotherapy may be improved by IVH, particularly in malnourished patients in the late stages of disease. Chemotherapy dose reductions were more often necessary in the control group patients than in the IVH group, and catheter-related sepsis was only 3%.

Rickard et al. (1979) have made interesting observations with the use of IVH in the treatment of children with advanced neoplastic diseases. They did sequential nutritional assessment and found that a period of 9–14 days of IVH was often not adequate to result in an increase in synthesis of either visceral or skeletal proteins, whereas 28 days of IVH would result in such anabolic changes. Similarly, a short course of IVH frequently did not result in a conversion of previously negative skin test reactions to positive, whereas 28 days of IVH did result in the conversion to positive of seven of nine previously negative reactors. The implication from these data is important to grasp, for it implies that just because the physician chooses to use IVH, the patient will not necessarily become nutritionally replenished. The induction of anabolism depends upon the content, time, and method of administration of the IVH solutions and the initial and continuing catabolic responses of the patient, as well as the degree of initial malnutrition, the energy expenditure of the patient required during oncologic therapy, and, last but not least, the expertise of the physician in the utilization of IVH. Those clinical studies that fail to include sequential nutritional assessment in order to identify the effect of IVH on net protein synthesis cannot justifiably state that "nutritional repletion" of the host has no effect on the response of a particular tumor to a chemotherapeutic drug regimen.

CONCLUSION

For the moment, as a treatment modality for the cancer patient, IVH remains in the supportive category. It should be used only when enteral nutritional rehabilitation and maintenance have failed and nutritional rehabilitation is necessary for proper delivery of adequate antineoplastic treatment programs. There are some exciting avenues of research open to the investigator utilizing IVH in the treatment of the cancer patient. The investigator has total control over the nutritional intake of the patient, and nutritional solutions might be tailored to meet the nutritional requirements of the host while at the same time depriving the tumor of an essential nutrient for its growth. For example, the depletion of the amino acid, asparagine, by treatment with asparaginase has been useful in the treatment of acute lymphoblastic leukemia in man. The possibility of synchronizing tumor cell replication during nutritional repletion also exists and is being investigated. For the moment, however, the indication for the use of IVH in the cancer patient population is to allow specific oncologic therapy to be administered to a group of malnourished patients who might otherwise not be acceptable candidates for intensive antineoplastic therapy. In this group, IVH has been safe, efficacious, and possibly life-saving. Nutritional repletion has resulted in an apparent reduction in sepsis, proper wound healing, a return of skin test reactivity, and possibly an increase in tumor response to chemotherapy.

REFERENCES

Bertino, J. R. 1979. Nutrients, vitamins, and minerals as therapy. Cancer 43:2137–2141.

Brennan, M. F., and M. E. Burt. 1981. Nitrogen metabolism in cancer patients. Cancer Treat. Rep. (in press).

Copeland, E. M., and S. J. Dudrick. 1976. Nutritional aspects of cancer, *in* Current Problems in Cancer, R. C. Hickey, ed. Year Book Medical Publishers, Inc., Chicago, pp. 1–51.

Copeland, E. M., B. V. MacFadyen, Jr., V. Lanzotti, and S. J. Dudrick. 1975. Intravenous hyperalimentation as an adjunct to cancer chemotherapy. Am. J. Surg. 129:167–173.

Daly, J. M., H. M. Reynolds, B. J. Rowlands, S. J. Dudrick, and E. M. Copeland. 1980. Tumor growth in experimental animals: Nutritional manipulation and chemotherapeutic response. Ann. Surg. 191:316–322.

Dionigi, R., R. Guaglio, A. Bonera, M. Cerri, R. Rondanelli, and M. Campani. 1979. Clinical-pharmacological aspects, application and effectiveness of total parenteral nutrition in surgical patients. Int. J. Clin. Pharmacol. Biopharm. 17:107–118.

Issell, B. F., M. Valdivieso, H. A. Zaren, S. J. Dudrick, E. J Freireich, E. M. Copeland, and G. P. Bodey. 1978. Protection against chemotherapy toxicity by IV hyperalimentation. Cancer Treat. Rep. 62:1139–1143.

Jordan, W. M., M. Valdivieso, C. Frankmann, M. Gillespie, B. F. Issell, G. P. Bodey, and E. J Freireich. 1981. Treatment of advanced adenocarcinoma of the lung with ftorafur, Adriamycin, cyclophosphamide, and platinum (FACP) and intensive intravenous hyperalimentation (IVH). Cancer Treat. Rep. (in press).

Lanzotti, V. C., E. M. Copeland, S. L. Goerge, S. J. Dudrick, and M. L. Samuels. 1975. Cancer chemotherapeutic response and intravenous hyperalimentation. Cancer Chemother. Rep. 59:437–439.

Moertel, C. G., A. J. Schutt, R. G. Hahn, and R. J. Reitemeier. 1974. Effects of patient selection on results of phase II chemotherapy trials in gastrointestinal cancer. Cancer Chemother. Rep. 58:257–260.

Moghissi, K., J. Hornshaw, P. R. Teasdale, and E. A. Dawes. 1977. Parenteral nutrition in carcinoma of the oesophagus treated by surgery: Nitrogen balance and clinical studies. Br. J. Surg. 64:125–128.

Nixon, D. W., S. Moffitt, D. H. Lawson, J. Ansley, M. J. Lynn, M. H. Kutner, S. B. Heymsfield, M. Wesley, R. Chawla, and D. Rudman. Total parenteral nutrition as an adjunct to chemotherapy of metastatic colorectal cancer. Cancer Treat. Rep. (in press).

Plumb, M. J., and J. Holland. 1977. Comparative studies of psychological function in patients with advanced cancer: I. Self-related, depressive symptoms. Psychosom. Med. 39:264–276.

Popp, M. B., R. I. Fisher, R. M. Simon, and M. F. Brennan. 1981. A prospective randomized study of adjuvant parenteral nutrition in the treatment of diffuse lymphoma. I. Effect on drug tolerance. Cancer Treat. Rep. (in press).

Reynolds, H. M., J. M. Daly, B. J. Rowlands, S. J. Dudrick, and E. M. Copeland. 1980. Effects of nutritional repletion on host and tumor response to chemotherapy. Cancer 45:3069–3074.

Rickard, K. A., J. L. Grosfeld, A. Kirksey, T. V. N. Ballantine, and R. L. Baehner. 1979. Reversal of protein-energy malnutrition in children during treatment of advanced neoplastic disease. Ann. Surg. 190:771–781.

Samuels, M. L., D. E. Selig, S. Ogden, C. Grant, and B. Brown. 1981. Intravenous hyperalimentation and chemotherapy in stage III testicular cancer: A randomized study. Cancer Treat. Rep. (in press).

Seniukov, M. V., I. M. Khmelevskii, O. G. Zubov, V. I. Sloventantor, and N. A. Kaplan. 1978. Parenteral feeding of patients with cancer of the larynx undergoing combination therapy. Vestn. Otorinolaringol. 2:66–72.

Souchon, E. A., E. M. Copeland, P. Watson, and S. J. Dudrick. 1975. Intravenous hyperalimentation as an adjunct to cancer chemotherapy with 5-fluorouracil. J. Surg. Res. 18:451–454.

Steiger, E., J. Oram-Smith, E. Miller, L. Kuo, and H. N. Voss. 1975. Effects of nutrition on tumor growth and tolerance to chemotherapy. J. Surg. Res. 18:455–461.

Theoligides, A. 1979. Cancer cachexia. Cancer 43:2004–2012.

Valdivieso, M., G. Bodey, R. Benjamin, H. Barkley, M. Freeman, M. Ertel, T. Smith, and C. Mountain. 1981. Role of intravenous hyperalimentation as an adjunct to intensive chemotherapy for small bronchogenic carcinoma. Cancer Treat. Rep. (in press).

Valeno, D., L. Overt, A. Malcolm, and G. L. Blackburn. 1978. Nutritional support for cancer patients receiving abdominal and pelvic radiotherapy: A randomized-prospective clinical experiment of intravenous versus oral feeding. Surg. Forum 29:145–148.

van Eys, J., E. M. Copeland, A. Cangir, G. Taylor, B. Cohen-Teitell, P. Carter, and C. Ortiz. 1980a. A clinical trial of hyperalimentation in children with metastatic malignancies. Med. Pediatr. Oncol. 8:63–73.

van Eys, J., E. M. Copeland, G. Taylor, A. Cangir, P. Carter, B. Cohen-Teitell, and C. O. Ortiz. 1980b. Supportive therapy with curative intent, *in* Status of the Curability of Childhood Cancers, J. van Eys and M. Sullivan, eds. Raven Press, New York, pp. 33–46.

William, R. H. P., R. V. Heatley, M. H. Lewis, and L. E. Hughes. 1976. A randomized controlled trial of preoperative intravenous nutrition in patients with stomach cancer. Br. J. Surg. 63:667.

Gastrointestinal Cancer, edited by
John R. Stroehlein and
Marvin M. Romsdahl.
Raven Press, New York © 1981.

Carcinogenesis and Experimental Models

Frederick F. Becker, M.D.

*Department of Pathology, The University of Texas System Cancer Center
M. D. Anderson Hospital and Tumor Institute, Houston, Texas*

The major goals of experimental animal models of carcinogenesis are to give us a greater understanding of the genesis of tumors in man and, where applicable, an opportunity to manipulate the various sequences and contributory factors for a more salutatory termination. For the following reasons, this has been particularly true of animal models of chemical carcinogenesis:

(1) Many of the morphologic, biologic, and biochemical aspects of this process bear striking similarities to those assumed to be the result of chemical exposure in man;

(2) Agents which have been proven to be carcinogenic in man have generally resulted in similar alterations in animals;

(3) Although the tumors that result in animals may occasionally differ in morphology or biologic function from comparable tumors in man (such as those of the breast), in the main they are sufficiently similar in these characteristics to be useful as models;

(4) The results derived from the study of different target tissues resemble each other in important and fundamental characteristics. Similarly, these alterations are often common to a variety of agents of differing chemical classes; and

(5) Many of the crucial alterations induced by chemical carcinogens and many factors shown to influence their development have been shown to play a role in carcinogenesis that results from physical or viral agents; in those instances where the etiology is unknown, these alterations are often present (NCI 1976).

The vastness of the field and the complexity of its components will permit only a broad overview. In this presentation, therefore, the emphasis is placed on currently accepted principles, or major questions, which seem to apply to many systems.

If many of the alterations that result from exposure to chemicals are similar to each other, then certainly some of the problems are also common to the overall process (Table 1) (Berenblum 1978).

Until recently, relatively high doses of chemical carcinogens were used in most carcinogenic regimens. The aim of that approach was to deliver a

Table 1. *Problems in Analyzing Components of Chemical Carcinogenesis*

1. Carcinogenic versus noncarcinogenic alterations.
2. Population at risk for malignancy; "premalignant."
3. Time of irrevocable alteration(s); multiphasic sequence.
4. Primary malignancy, as early as possible.

maximum exposure in a limited time period commensurate with the short life span of the target species. The total dose would be comparable to that which might be accumulated by a human over a much longer time. The major problem resulting from the exposure of tissues to high levels of carcinogens, whether administered chronically or in a single large dose, is to differentiate between carcinogenic and noncarcinogenic alterations. These agents are primarily toxic and induce a spectrum of alterations which parallel, but are probably unrelated to, those which eventuate in a malignant event. Support for this hypothesis can be derived from the extent of interaction of these agents, complexing as they do with almost every macromolecule of the target cell. Further, the overt cell injury, morphologic changes, and other measures of toxicity which are often evident are absent at lower but effective doses of these agents when used in regimens such as those which take advantage of the heightened sensitivity of the replicating cell.

The identification of a population of cells or lesions at risk, and subsequently focusing one's analytic techniques upon these cells, is also of considerable importance. It is becoming increasingly certain that the actual number of cells at risk in a given tissue is relatively small, often no more than 1×10^{-6}. It is evident, therefore, that subsequent to the administration of a carcinogen, the analysis of a specific function or cellular component of an entire target organ would be skewed toward those alterations which occur in cells which will not become malignant.

Further, as will be discussed later, the process is often a multiphasic one, with frequent overlap of phases of differing importance (Farber 1976, 1980, Pitot and Sirica 1980). Therefore, it would be extremely valuable to identify points of crucial and irrevocable change, such that the results of analysis of focal tissues obtained at this time would have more meaning.

And lastly, we must be aware that the entire process of malignant evolution, before and after the appearance of a cancer, is a progressive one (Emmelot and Scherer 1980). To utilize tumors which have been repeatedly transplanted, or explanted and cultured, is to make one vulnerable to the possibility that the characteristics under analysis are related more to those manipulations than to the original ability of the malignant cell to escape the control mechanisms of the host.

Some years ago, Dr. George W. Teebor and I reported a model for the analysis for these problems in a liver carcinogenic system (Teebor and Becker 1971, Becker and Klein 1971, Becker et al. 1971). To increase the likelihood that we might identify discrete alterations, we developed an intermittent regimen during which we fed the carcinogen N-2-acetylaminofluorene (AAF) to rats for three-week periods, interrupted by a week of normal diet. After one cycle, small islands of cells appeared that were proliferative and possibly clonal in origin. Under the continued influence of the carcinogen, these foci grew, began to compress the surrounding liver, and eventually appeared as grossly evident nodules. Despite a considerable accumulated exposure to AAF, if the dietary exposure was terminated following the third feeding cycle, the majority of these nodules disappeared and few if any carcinomas resulted. However, if we administered one additional cycle of AAF, a remarkable functional alteration then occurred. A population of nodules could be identified that were somewhat larger and differed slightly in appearance. However, these contained cells quite similar in morphology to those resulting from three cycles. When carcinogen was now terminated, these nodules persisted and often eventuated as carcinomas. Later, the origin of primary hepatocellular carcinomas (PHC) was often evident entirely within the confines of these nodular lesions when serial sacrifices and histologic examination were performed. It should be pointed out, however, that other PHC may have a use in non-nodular tissues. Thus, persistence of these nodules signaled the acquisition of autonomy in the sense of no longer requiring the stimulus or momentum imparted by the carcinogenic agent. One of the characteristics which appeared to be contributory to persistence was the presence of an elevated rate of cell division within these lesions (Becker and Klein 1971). The cells which form these nodules have been examined extensively and present with a plethora of alterations consisting of a return to partial fetal expression, alteration of normal morphology and function, etc. (Becker and Shurgin 1975, Farber 1976, Stout and Becker 1978, 1979, Chan and Becker 1979, Lapeyre and Becker 1979, Emmelot and Scherer 1980). To date, however, no single characteristic or aggregate of these characteristics is sufficient to explain their predilection for malignant transformation. Of considerable interest, another feature of these nodular, persistent lesions was their heterogeneity. Thus, analysis of their component cell population by enzyme histochemistry, immunofluorescent staining for various fetal antigens, and tests of metabolic activity gave evidence for heterogeneity. And, analysis of their staining for various fetal antigens and by tests of metabolic activity gave evidence for heterogeneity of populations within their component structure.

The examination of this carcinogenic regimen has given rise to a concept which I have termed the *Three S's* of chemical carcinogenesis, i.e., Sequentiality, Subpopulations, and Stochastic progression (Becker 1979). The first is that this is a sequential process in which one cellular alteration gives rise to others in an irrevocable and obligate manner. The second is that the process is characterized by subpopulations; subpopulations of gross lesions, of cells comprising these lesions, and, evidently, of macromolecules within these lesions. And finally, that the process is stochastic in the sense that a large number of primarily affected cells give rise to lesser numbers of (significant) lesions and often eventuate in a single carcinoma. It is my hypothesis that these three components apply equally well to other carcinogenic systems induced by chemical agents such as those characteristically seen in bladder, lung, and skin, as well as to sequences induced by other carcinogenic agents and in those situations where the etiologic agent is as yet unknown. Typical of the latter would be carcinoma of the breast in the human patient.

In addition to the three S's as described, which were conceptually developed from an analysis of the above regimen, the examination of the persistent nodules resulted in my overall concept of the "premalignant lesions" or, as I prefer to refer to them, lesions at high risk for malignancy (Table 2) (Becker 1975, 1979). As mentioned previously, the cells of these nodules demonstrate a persistent mitotic activity, well above that seen in the normal or non-nodular tissues which surround them.

In addition, the component cells demonstrate a lack of normal maturation. For example, it has been demonstrated that these cells remain predominantly diploid, while normal hepatocytes demonstrate an increasing tetraploidy in age-matched rats (Becker et al. 1971). Similarly the cell may demonstrate the presence of fetal antigens or, more impressively, enzymatic activities normally associated with fetal life. This has been particularly striking in the demonstration of enzyme γ-glutamyl transpeptidase, one of the earliest markers for the presence of such cells after chemical exposure (Fiala and Fiala 1973). They often demonstrate cytologic atypia, particularly at the level of high resolution microscopy. Here, aberrations of their mitochondria, and even more impressively of their component membrane systems, are striking. Most notably, the architecture or polarity of these cells is atypical whether in the relationship of cell to like cell; to supporting cell elements; the distance to vascular spaces; or the overall arrangement of suborgan structure. The aggregate of these altered cells is a tumor, whether a nodule, papilloma, or polyp. These changes which are seen in the hepatic nodule of the rat, papillomas induced by chemical agents in the bladder or breast, the papillomas of skin that arise from the classic initiation-promotion sequence, the polyps of familial colonic disease, or the neurofibromas of von Recklinghausen's disease are evidence for the commonality of alterations in premalignant lesions. The

Table 2. *Lesions at High Risk for Malignancy*

Persistent mitotic activity
Loss of maturation—arrest of ploidy
                            fetal proteins
Cytological atypia—negative/positive
Abnormal architecture—cell to cell
                              cell to vasculature
                              cell to stroma
Accumulation of cells—"tumor"

similarity of these systems could not be better demonstrated than those of the papilloma of the mouse induced by carcinogens, with subsequent application of the promoting agents (to be described) and those seen in familial polyposis. Indeed, I have previously speculated (perhaps facetiously) that the lesions induced in mice skin by a series of chemical agents would appear to be the experimental equivalent of an everted colon or the latter, an inverted mouse.

However, despite the consistency of these alterations from system to system, none as yet has permitted us to identify that crucial factor which, during the lag period before the appearance of malignancy, predisposes these cells to progression. Several speculative proposals may be offered which are applicable to *all* high risk lesions and might explain the expression and progression to malignancy prevalent within them. Pierce and others have emphasized the influence of the microenvironment on the expression of the malignant cell and its dormancy (Pierce 1974). Riccardi has stressed the modification of expression of the altered function of mutated cells by adjoining nonmutated cells (Riccardi 1977). It is possible, therefore, that progression to malignancy by cells of the high risk lesions may be strongly influenced by the alterations in normal architectural relationships of these cells.

A final aspect of the cellular composition of these nodules which may be applicable to other lesions considered to be premalignant is the possibility that, although they express phenotypic differences in the form of subpopulations of component cells, the lesions as a whole may be clonally derived (Emmelot and Scherer 1980). Evidence offered from our own studies and those of others has strongly indicated that progression from the original "initiated," early cell clusters to the nodular lesions is one of a progressive growth of a single population of cells, i.e., clonal growth. The phenotypic heterogeneity of the component cells may result from normal maturation processes as seen in hepatocytes, perhaps related to their architectural localization. Recently, Pretlow has presented evidence that the villous adenoma of the colon may represent such a clonal population (Adolfphson et al. 1980).

For many years, tumor induction in mouse skin represented the archetypal model for the two-component concept of carcinogenic evolution, initiation, and promotion (Berenblum 1978). Initiation has been defined as the initial, irreversible alteration induced by chemical agents in a small subpopulation of cells, which prepares them for eventual evolution to malignancy (Emmelot and Scherer 1980). It is generally believed that these alterations occur in the genetic apparatus, DNA. By definition they are considered to be mutational since mutation is now defined by many as any aberration of DNA, regardless of whether or not a mensurable function becomes manifest or is lost (Knudson 1977). Although by earlier definition or concept initiation was invariably the result of exposure to a carcinogen, circumstances can now be identified in which chemical agents not usually carcinogenic for that particular organ can induce this obligate, preliminary, irrevocable alteration. For example, when methylnitrosourea is administered during the regenerative response subsequent to 70% hepatectomy, it becomes a liver carcinogen (Craddock 1976). It is now considered possible that the action of several viral oncogens may be as initiators and, similarly, that a genetically determined alteration may serve a similar function. It is becoming increasingly certain that the process of initiation is much more complicated than previously understood. For example, it is generally accepted that the interaction of the carcinogen with DNA is but the first stage of initiation. However, it must also be pointed out that several classic carcinogens have not been shown to have any interaction with DNA.

Regardless of these exceptions to the DNA-rule, subsequent to the bonding of the activated metabolite of carcinogens to DNA, at least one wave of cell division is required to "imprint" the aberration. In some instances the cell division can occur at a considerable time after exposure (Farber 1976, 1980, Emmelot and Scherer 1980).

Promotion is a form of cocarcinogenesis or enhancement. In its purest form it is the result of exposure to a noncarcinogenic agent, subsequent to completion of a noncarcinogenic initiation; that is, one in which no progression to malignancy would normally occur (Berenblum 1978). In addition to the non-carcinogenic nature of the promoter, a degree of reversibility exists during its chronic application, until an irrevocable, probably malignant, alteration is induced (Weinstein et al. 1979). In the classic instance of mouse skin, promotion has been uniquely the result of derivatives of croton oil and in particular phorbol esters (Berenblum 1978). More recently, it has been demonstrated that phenobarbital can have a similar effect when administered to rats which have been appropriately prepared (Peraino et al. 1978). Despite many years of analysis of promotion in the mouse skin, the basis for this process remains unknown. Similarly, no insights have yet been achieved by examination of phenobarbital's actions. However, it is obvious that a general "feeling" exists that promotion may be related to a proliferative stimulus of the initiated cells (Pitot and Sirica 1980, Weinstein et al. 1979, Marks et al. 1978). The possibility that the potentially promoting effects of hormones in target tissues or dietary constituents (such as fat in the intestinal tract and elsewhere) bear similarities to other processes has intensified efforts to understand them (Winder et al. 1978, Higginson 1979, Weisburger 1979). Other stimuli to the intensity of this effort are two current concepts:

(1) That whereas the initiating "factors" of life such as predisposing mutation or a minimal-required exposure to a chemical carcinogen may be difficult to eliminate and impossible to reverse, an attack on the promotional stage may be feasible. Thus, agents such as retinoids act after initiation (Sporn et al. 1979).

(2) Several investigators have suggested that the majority of human tumors do not result from any known exposure to a carcinogen. Thus, they point out that possibly the "promotional" effect of components of our lifestyle may be more influential and more vulnerable to attack (Winder et al. 1978, Higginson 1976).

However, the complexity of this sequence is exemplified by an experiment performed in my laboratory some years ago (Becker 1975). When rats received three cycles of AAF, those demonstrating reversible lesions which would not eventuate as carcinomas were challenged with a subcarcinogenic dose of a second agent, dimethylnitrosamine, and the liver of every rat demonstrated multiple carcinomas in a relatively short period of time. Thus, although these nodules were morphologically reversible, it is likely that the genetic lesion(s) was not reversible. The second challenge with a known carcinogen (mutagen) may have occurred in a population of cells derived from the clonal proliferation of the original, initiated population. Thus a sequence of initiation → promotion → "initiation" might be possible. Although a number of instances exist in gastrointestinal cancer where the initiation-promotion sequence could be effective, none is so evident as in familial polyposis. Here, the genetic tendency which is evident exists only for a mutational event which predisposes to the formation of polyps. Thus a proliferative-control or maturation-control defect might result. Then, the promotional or promotional-initiation activity of the fecal content would account for subsequent evolution to malignancy at a rate no different from that for polyps in a normal liver (Knudson 1977).

In the liver, and possibly in other organs, particularly the gastrointestinal tract, malignant disease may result from a variety of carcinogenic "regimens." We have been able to induce carcinoma in the liver by a single necrotizing dose of the potent carcinogen diethylnitrosamine, by the application of a smaller dose of diethylnitrosamine when given in combination with partial hepatectomy, and by even smaller doses of diethylnitrosamine in combination with partial hepatectomy with subsequent exposure to phenobarbital. Our ability to manipulate these carcinogenic systems, our understanding of the complexity of the cells and lesions which result from these regimens, and a better ability to correlate these with more finite measures of cell function and macromolecular composition may make possible an eventual understanding of the carcinogenic process and, with that, an increased possibility of reversing or preventing this sequence.

REFERENCES

Adolfphson, C., J. Prchal, T. Pretlow, H. Colcher, and B. Hirschowitz. 1980. The clonal origin of a clonal villous adenoma. Proc. Am. Assoc. Cancer Res. 21:51.

Becker, F. F. 1975. Alteration of hepatocytes by subcarcinogenic exposure to N-2-fluorenylacetamide. Cancer Res. 35:1734–1736.

Becker, F. F. 1979. Evolution chemical carcinogenesis and mortality: the cycle of life, *in* Carcinogens: Identification and Mechanisms of Action, A. C. Griffin and C. R. Shaw, eds. Raven Press, New York, pp. 5–17.

Becker, F. F., R. A. Fox, J. M. Klein, and S. R. Wolman. 1971. Chromosome patterns in rat hepatocytes during N-2-fluorenylacetamide carcinogenesis. J. Natl. Cancer Inst. 46:1261–1269.

Becker, F. F., and K. M. Klein. 1971. The effect of L-asparaginase on mitotic activity during Nfluorenylacetamide hepatocarcinogenesis: Subpopulations of nodule cells. Cancer Res. 31:169–173.

Becker, F. F., and A. Shurgin. 1975. Concanavalin A agglutination of cell from primary hepatocellular carcinomas and hepatic nodules induced by N-2-fluorenylacetamide. Cancer Res. 35:2879–2883.

Berenblum, I. 1978. Historical perspective, *in* Mechanisms of Tumor Promotion and Cocarcinogenesis, T. J. Slaga, A. Sivak, and R. K. Boutwell, eds. Vol. 2, Raven Press, New York, pp. 1–10.

Chan, J. Y. H., and F. F. Becker. 1979. Decreased fidelity of DNA polymerase activity during N-2-fluorenylacetamide hepatocarcinogenesis. Proc. Natl. Acad. Sci. U.S.A. 76:816–818.

Craddock, V. M. 1976. Cell proliferation and experimental liver cancer, *in* Liver Cell Cancer, H. M. Cameron, D. A. Linsell, and G. P. Warwick, eds. Elsevier Scientific Publishing Co., Oxford, pp. 153–202.

Emmelot, P., and E. Scherer. 1980. The first relevant cell stage in rat liver carcinogenesis. The quantitative approach. Biochim. Biophys. Acta 605:247–304.

Farber, E. 1976. The pathology of experimental liver cell cancer, *in* Liver Cell Cancer, H. M. Cameron, D. A. Linsell, and G. P. Warwick, eds. Elsevier Scientific Publishing Co., Oxford, pp. 243–278.

Farber, E. 1980. The sequential analysis of liver cancer induction. Biochim. Biophys. Acta 605:149–166.

Fiala, S., and E. S. Fiala. 1973. Effect of prolonged chemical carcinogenesis of γ-glutamyl transpeptidase in rat and mouse livers. J. Natl. Cancer Inst. 51:151–158.

Higginson, J. 1979. Environmental carcinogenesis: a global perspective, *in* Environmental Carcinogenesis, P. Emmelot and E. Kriek, eds. Elsevier Press, Amsterdam, pp. 9–24.

Knudson, A. G., Jr. 1977. Genetic and environmental interactions in the origin of human cancer, *in* Genetics of Human Cancer, J. J. Mulvihill, R. W. Miller, and J. F. Fraumeni, Jr., eds. Raven Press, New York, pp. 391–397.

Lapeyre, J. N., and F. F. Becker. 1979. S-methylcytosine content of nuclear DNA during chemical hepatocarcinogenesis and in carcinogenesis which results. Biochem. Biophys. Res. Commun. 87:698–705.

Marks, F., S. Bertsch, W. Grimm, and J. Schweizer. 1978. Hyperplastic transformation and tumor promotion in mouse epidermis: possible consequences of endogenous mechanisms controlling proliferation and differentiation, *in* Mechanisms of Tumor Promotion and Cocarcinogenesis, T. J. Slaga, A. Sivak, and R. K. Boutwell, eds. Vol. 2, Raven Press, New York, pp. 97–116.

National Cancer Institute Carcinogenesis Program, Division of Cancer Cause and Prevention. 1976. Symposium on Early Lesions and the Development of Epithelial Cancer. October 21 to 23, 1975. Bethesda, Md., Cancer Res. 36(7 pt 2).

Peraino, C., J. M. Fry, and D. Z. Grube. 1978. Drug induced enhancement of hepatic tumorigenesis, *in* Mechanisms of Tumor Promotion and Cocarcinogenesis, T. J. Slaga, A. Sivak, and R. K. Boutwell, eds. Vol. 2, Raven Press, New York, pp. 421–432.

Pierce, G. B. 1974. The benign cells of malignant tumors, *in* 32nd Symposium of the Society for Developmental Biology: Developmental Aspects of Carcinogenesis and Immunity, T. J. King, ed. Academic Press, Inc., New York, pp. 3–22.

Pitot, H. C., and A. E. Sirica. 1980. The stages of initiation and promotion in hepatic carcinogenesis. Biochim. Biophys. Acta 605:191–216.

Riccardi, V. M. 1977. Cellular interactions as a limiting factor in the expressions of oncogenic mutations: a hypothesis, *in* Genetics of Human Cancer, J. J. Mulvihill, R. W. Miller, and J. F. Fraumeni, Jr., eds. Raven Press, New York, pp. 383–385.

Sporn, M. D., D. L. Newton, J. M. Smith, N. Aeton, A. E. Jacobson, and A. Brossi. 1979. Retinoids and coprevention: the importance of the terminal group of the retinoid molecule in modifying activity and toxicity, *in* Identification and Mechanisms of Action. A. C. Griffin and C. Shaw, eds. Raven Press, New York, pp. 441–453.

Stout, D. L., and F. F. Becker. 1978. Alteration of the ability of liver microsomes to activate N-2-fluorenylacetamide to a mutagen of *Salmonella typhimurium* during hepatocarcinogenesis. Cancer Res. 38:2274–2278.

Stout, D. L., and F. F. Becker. 1979. Metabolism of 2-aminofluorene and 2-acetylaminofluorene to mutagens by rat hepatocyte nuclei. Cancer Res. 39:1168–1173.

Teebor, G. W., and F. F. Becker. 1971. Regression and persistence of hyperplastic hepatic nodules induced by N-2-fluorenylacetamide and their relationship to hepatocarcinogenesis. Cancer Res. 31:1-3.

Weinstein, I. B., L. S. Lee, P. D. Fisher, A. Mufson, and H. Yamasaki. 1979. Environmental carcinogenesis. The mechanism of action of tumor promoters and a molecular model of two stage carcinogenesis, *in* Environmental Carcinogenesis, P. Emmelot and E. Kriek, eds. Elsevier Press, Amsterdam, pp. 265-286.

Weisburger, J. H. 1979. On the etiology of gastro-intestinal tract cancers, with emphasis on dietary factors, *in* Environmental Carcinogenesis, P. Emmelot and E. Kriek, eds. Elsevier Press, Amsterdam, pp. 215-240.

Winder, E. L., D. Hoffmann, D. McCoy, L. Cohen, and B. Reddy. 1978. Tumor promotion and cocarcinogenesis are related to man and his environment, *in* Mechanisms of Tumor Promotion and Cocarcinogenesis, T. J. Slaga, A. Sivak, and R. K. Boutwell, eds. Vol. 2, Raven Press, New York, pp. 59-78.

Gastrointestinal Cancer, edited by
John R. Stroehlein and
Marvin M. Romsdahl.
Raven Press, New York © 1981.

Immunobiology and Biochemical Markers of Gastrointestinal Cancer

David M. Goldenberg, Sc.D., M.D.

Division of Experimental Pathology, Department of Pathology, University of Kentucky Medical Center, Lexington, Kentucky

INTRODUCTION

During the past decade or more, there has been considerable interest in the identification and exploitation of human tumor antigens. This is based upon the view that such substances could serve as tumor "markers" in the diagnosis and monitoring of cancer. Tumor markers can be unique to the individual tumor, restricted to tumors of a specific organ or tumor type, or common to a larger group of tumors or to all cancer types. They might share characteristics with embryonic or fetal cells, with blood-group antigens, or with a variety of tissue antigens occurring in man under normal or nonmalignant conditions. These markers may be secretory products, or constituents of the cell surface, of the cytoplasm, or even of the cell nucleus. Indeed, examples of all of these possibilities exist in the literature (Gold and Goldenberg 1980). Unfortunately, however, if a truly qualitatively tumor-distinct marker exists, it has remained elusive. As the detection method becomes more sensitive for putatively tumor-specific substances, the number of qualitatively distinct tumor markers shrinks (Goldenberg 1976, Gold and Goldenberg 1980). The advent of the hybridoma monoclonal antibody technology (Köhler and Milstein 1975), however, encourages us to continue in the pursuit of cancer-distinct markers and molecules, and this has indeed been reported recently for colorectal carcinoma (Herlyn et al. 1979).

Some antigens associated with tumors appear to have a relatively narrow distribution among normal tissues and organs, thus being broadly categorized as organ- or tissue-specific antigens. Indeed, this was a subject of interest at the beginning of tumor immunology, in the work of Hirszfeld et al. (1929) and of Witebsky (1930, Witebsky et al. 1956). Since malignant tumors very frequently contain morphological and functional characteristics of the cell and tissue types from which they arise, the retention and expression of organ-specific antigens by neoplasms is not surprising. And yet, this has been a relatively neglected area of tumor immunology.

The gastrointestinal system has been the area of greatest attention in efforts to define tumor-distinct and organ-specific antigens. This paper will review the current status of some clinical applications of tumor-associated markers in gastrointestinal cancer. Of course, not all substances reported to be elevated in gastrointestinal tumors will be described. Instead, a selection of those which have been initially extracted and defined in gastrointestinal tumors, and that are of current clinical interest, will be reviewed. In addition to their role as blood markers, some consideration will be given to the use of tumor-associated substances as molecular targets for tumor-localizing radioactive antibodies, both in terms of detection and therapy.

GASTROINTESTINAL MARKERS

Listing

Table 1 presents a list of the more prominent markers known for gastrointestinal tissues and tumors, excluding more recent observations made with hybridoma antibodies. This list contains a few substances which have been studied well by numerous investigators over a long period of time, such as AFP and CEA, and others about which we have relatively little information, such as TennaGen. Still, since some of the antigens appear to be restricted to gastrointestinal tissues, while others have been evaluated clinically in pa-

Table 1. *Tumor-Associated Markers in Gastrointestinal Cancer*

Antigen	Year	Investigator	Organ-Specific	Cancer-Specific
1. AFP, α-fetoprotein	1963	Abelev et al.	No	No
2. CEA, carcinoembryonic antigen	1965	Gold and Freedman	No	No
3. FSA, fetal sulfo-glycoprotein	1968	Häkkinen et al.	Perhaps	No
4. IMG, intestinal mucosa specific glycoprotein	1971	Kawasaki et al.	Cell-specific	No
5. CMA, colonic mucoprotein antigen	1974	Gold and Miller	Cell-specific	No
6. CSAs, colon-specific antigens	1976	Goldenberg et al.	Cell-specific	No
7. SGA, sulfated glyco-peptidic antigen	1978	Bara et al.	Cell-specific	No
8. GOA, goblet cell antigen	1979	Rapp et al.	Cell-specific	No
9. ZGM, zinc glycinate marker	1976	Pusztaszeri et al.	No	No
10. CSAp, colon-specific antigen-p	1977	Pant et al.	Cell-specific	No
11. BFP, basic fetoprotein	1977	Ishii	No	No
12. GT-II, galactosyltrans-ferase-isoenzyme	1978	Podolsky et al.	No	No
13. POA, pancreatic oncofetal antigen	1978	Gelder et al.	No	No
14. TennaGen	1979	Potter et al.	No	No

tients with gastrointestinal tumors, they will be summarized briefly in terms of organ- or cancer-specificity.

AFP is a serum protein occurring during gestation and again expressed by certain neoplasms, particularly primary liver cancer and teratocarcinomas of the testis and ovary (Abelev 1971). It can also be elevated in patients with benign liver diseases, particularly viral hepatitis and when liver necrosis and regeneration are present (Smith 1971, Silver et al. 1974, Hirai et al. 1972). Thus, AFP is neither organ- nor cancer-specific.

CEA was originally described as a gastrointestinal-restricted, cancer-specific, oncofetal antigen (Gold and Freedman 1965), but it has since been shown that the radioimmunoassay for CEA detects elevated amounts in the blood of patients with diverse cancers and also in a number of benign disease states (reviewed in Hansen et al. 1974, Goldenberg 1976). Again, this antigen is neither organ- nor cancer-specific.

The FSA described in the gastric juice of patients with gastric cancer and other pathological conditions may be related to cellular atypia and cancer (Häkkinen 1979). However, no information on its tissue distribution has been published. IMG, CMA, CSAs, SGA, and GOA are probably related gastrointestinal mucoproteins selectively distributed in goblet cells and in signet-ring tumor cells, and are present in normal, diseased, and malignant colonic tissues (Kawasaki et al. 1971, Gold and Miller 1974, Goldenberg et al. 1976a, Bara et al. 1978, Rapp et al. 1979, Gold 1979, Gold and Goldenberg 1980). They may have antigenic cross-reactivity, but this has not been investigated yet. ZGM is neither organ- nor cancer-specific (Saravis et al. 1978), as is also the case for BFP (Ishii 1979) and for TennaGen (Potter et al. 1979). CSAp, however, is similar to some of the other antigens mentioned as being restricted to goblet cells and signet-ring tumor cells, while showing a quantitative increase in certain tumors, particularly colorectal carcinomas (Pant et al. 1977, Pant et al. 1978, Goldenberg 1978a, Pant and Goldenberg 1979). It is very likely distinct from the other cell-specific glycoprotein markers listed in the table because of a number of immunochemical and physicochemical differences (Shochat et al. 1981). Obviously, it would be of significant convenience to investigators in this field if a central reference laboratory for evaluating the immunological identity and relationship of these and other forthcoming antigens were in operation.

The final two markers of interest are GT-II and POA. The galactosyltransferase isoenzyme is elevated in the serum of patients with a number of different cancer types, and although it was not elevated in normal individuals tested, it did show increases in individuals with alcoholic hepatitis and celiac disease (Podolsky et al. 1978). Therefore, it too does not appear to be either organ-specific or cancer-specific. Likewise, POA is elevated in the serum of patients with diverse cancers, as well as in individuals with benign diseases of various organ systems (Gelder et al. 1978, Hunter et al. 1979), and thus cannot be considered either organ- or cancer-specific.

Table 2. *Selected Blood Markers for Gastrointestinal Cancer*

Diagnosis	AFP	CEA	GT-II	POA	BFP	TnGn	CSAp
			Percent Elevated				
Stomach cancer	18	61	75	25	31	74	0
Colorectal cancer	5	72	73	14	26	89	52
Pancreatic cancer	23	91	83	48	NA*	92	20
Primary liver cancer	70	NA	100	0	NA	NA	NA
Benign GI disease	35[†]	37	0	18	3	36	10
Normals	1	11	0	3	0	7	8

*NA, not available.
[†]Hepatitis for AFP cases.

Clinical Results

A summary of the clinical results of some of these markers used in patients with gastrointestinal tumors is presented in Table 2. It emphasizes many of the points already mentioned, but on a comparative basis. AFP is elevated to the greatest percentage in patients with primary liver cancer, as well as transiently in patients with viral hepatitis. A number of tumors derived from the embryonic foregut also have elevated AFP values (Waldmann and McIntire 1974, McIntire et al. 1975), as represented here by stomach and pancreatic cancers. AFP is of less value for the diagnosis of liver cancer than for monitoring disease activity (Purves et al. 1973, Olweny et al. 1975, McIntire et al. 1976).

Table 3 indicates that CEA levels are elevated most in patients with gastrointestinal cancers, ranging from 61% in gastric cancer to 91% in pancreatic cancer. However, the relatively high percentage of patients with benign gastrointestinal diseases showing CEA elevations precludes its use, by itself, for diagnosis (Goldenberg 1979). In colorectal cancer, preoperative CEA values appear to have some prognostic significance, where high levels indicate a higher probability of more advanced disease (Herrera et al. 1976, Wanebo et al. 1978). The most accepted application of the CEA test is in monitoring disease activity in colorectal cancer patients (Holyoke et al. 1975, Mayer et al. 1978, Mach et al. 1978, Sugarbaker et al. 1976). Prospective studies of CEA used alone as an indication for second-look surgery have indicated that a high rate of localized tumor can be found (Martin et al. 1979). This 65% rate of localized tumor found at second-look surgery is apparently much higher than the earlier published results found by second-look surgery before CEA became available (Gilbertsen and Wangensteen 1962). It should be emphasized that it is never a single CEA value that is used to assess clinical status, but always the pattern of changes in circulating CEA.

The galactosyltransferase isoenzyme-II is an interesting new marker which is elevated in a number of gastrointestinal as well as other tumor types, including leukemia, lymphomas, breast cancer, lung cancer, and so on (Table 4). Although normal individuals tested appeared not to have elevations of this isoenzyme, a considerable percentage of patients with celiac disease and with alcoholic hepatitis had abnormal serum values (Podolsky et al. 1978). As is true for CEA, GT-II levels increase with advanced stage of disease in colorectal cancer (Podolsky et al. 1978). Thus, this enzyme marker may also play an important role, perhaps in combination with CEA, in monitoring tumor recurrence and response in colorectal cancer patients.

The results with POA, or pancreatic oncofetal antigen, are less impressive when compared to GT-II (Table 5). The percent positivity among different cancer types appears to be less than with GT-II and, moreover, there are elevations in a number of benign disease states which preclude the use of this new antigen for diagnostic purposes, unless it is used in conjunction with other modalities. There is, indeed, an indication that POA in combination with CEA and diagnostic ultrasound is of potential value in patients with high clinical suspicion of pancreatic cancer (Hunter et al. 1979). Furthermore, POA

Table 3. *Circulating CEA Levels in Various Conditions* *

Clinical Status	% Elevated CEA
Malignant diseases	
Colorectum, all stages	72-81
Dukes' A	38-44
Dukes' B	60-76
Dukes' C	60-75
Metastasized	80-89
Stomach	61
Pancreas	91
Breast	47
Lung	76
Prostate	40
Bladder	42
Gynecologic	65
Lymphomas	35
Acute and chronic leukemias	37
Nonmalignant diseases	
Alcoholic cirrhosis of liver	70
Alcohol addiction	65
Pulmonary emphysema	57
Kidney transplant	56
Pancreatitis	53
Granulomatous colitis	47
Pneumonia	46
Gastric ulcer	45
Ulcerative colitis	31
Normals	
Healthy, unselected	11
Healthy, nonsmokers	3
Healthy, smokers	19
Healthy, pregnant	3

*Adapted from Goldenberg 1976.

Table 4. *Results of Serum Galactosyltransferase Isoenzyme (GT-II) Tests* *

Diagnosis	No. Positive/Total	% Positive
Colorectal cancer	85/117	73
Inflammatory bowel	0/20	0
Pancreatic cancer	15/18	83
Pancreatitis	0/15	0
Stomach cancer	12/16	75
Esophageal (squamous) cancer	4/9	44
Gallbladder and biliary cancer	2/4	50
Cholelithiasis and biliary cirrhosis	0/6	0
Hepatoma	2/2	100
Alcoholic hepatitis	3/15	20
Celiac disease	18/20	90
Breast cancer	18/23	78
Bronchogenic cancer	13/20	65
Prostatic cancer	4/4	100
Renal cancer	1/2	50
Hodgkin's lymphoma	4/8	50
Chronic lymphocytic leukemia	2/2	100
Melanoma	0/2	0
Osteosarcoma	0/1	0
Unknown primary	3/4	75
Normals	0/85	0

*Adapted from Podolsky et al. 1978.

appears to be of some use for serial monitoring of patients with pancreatic cancer if the initial values are elevated (Gelder et al. 1978, Hunter et al. 1979).

Basic fetoprotein, or BFP, was found in human fetal serum as well as in fetal gut and brain tissues (Ishii 1977, Ishii and Hattori 1976). BFP appears to be

Table 5. *Serum POA Results* *

Diagnosis	No. Positive/Total	% Positive
Pancreatic cancer	38/80	48
Pancreatitis	3/24	13
Biliary cancer	5/14	36
Benign biliary	3/11	27
Hepatoma	0/4	0
Colorectal cancer	6/42	14
Inflammatory bowel	1/11	9
Gastric cancer	4/16	25
Gastric ulcer	3/10	33
Lung cancer	18/90	20
Benign lung disease	1/12	8
Smokers	1/37	3
Breast cancer	3/23	13
Benign breast disease	2/27	7
Other malignant tumors	1/56	2
Pregnancy	11/87	13
Normals	3/102	3

*Adapted from Gelder et al. 1978.

Table 6. *Results of BFP Assay**

Diagnosis	No. Tested	% Positive
Stomach cancer	105	31
Colorectal cancer	50	26
Benign GI disease	152	3
Lung cancer	55	31
Benign lung disease	32	9
Breast cancer	78	22
Benign breast disease	3	0
Miscellaneous cancer	140	47
Hepatitis	58	43
Cirrhosis of liver	27	33
Aplastic anemia	12	50
Other benign diseases	58	10
Normals	105	0

*Adapted from Ishii 1979.

associated with a number of different cancer types (Table 6). Unfortunately, it too cannot help discriminate between cancer and benign disease, particularly benign liver disease. It appears that BFP values correlate well with stage of disease and with tumor burden, particularly in gastrointestinal cancer patients (Ishii 1979).

TennaGen, or Tennessee Antigen, is a glycoprotein produced by a number of cancer types, having the highest incidence in adenocarcinomas of the gastrointestinal tract (Potter et al. 1978). Clinical studies have shown that TennaGen is increased in the blood of patients with diverse kinds of cancer, but it is also elevated in patients with benign gastrointestinal disease and benign pulmonary disease (Table 7). This limits its value as a diagnostic marker. In contrast to almost all the other tumor markers discussed, TennaGen appears to be elevated in a high percentage of patients with early colorectal cancer, having levels of over 90% positivity in patients with Dukes' A and B lesions (Potter et al. 1978). Moreover, changes in the level of the

Table 7. *Results of TennaGen Test**

Diagnosis	No. Positive/Total	% Positive
Colorectal cancer	170/192	89
Benign GI disease	197/548	36
Stomach cancer	28/38	74
Pancreatic cancer	23/25	92
Lung cancer	68/86	79
Benign lung disease	46/139	33
Breast cancer	60/133	45
Other malignant tumors	100/183	55
Normals-smokers	41/590	7
Normals-nonsmokers	19/282	7

*Adapted from Potter et al. 1979.

Table 8. *CSAp Radioassay Results*

Diagnosis	No. +/Total	% Positive
Gastric cancer	0/10	0
Colorectal cancer	16/31	52
Pancreatic cancer	3/15	20
Ovarian cancer	0/24	0
Brochogenic cancer	2/29	7
Cervical cancer	1/19	5
Benign GI disease	1/10	10
Normals	2/25	8

antigen in the serum appear to reflect disease activity following therapy (Potter et al. 1978).

The final marker to be discussed is our CSAp, or colon-specific antigen-p (Goldenberg et al. 1976b, Pant et al. 1977, 1978, Pant and Goldenberg 1979). We have recently isolated a tryptic fragment from a high molecular weight colonic cancer mucin, and this fragment with CSAp immunoreactivity is of approximately 120,000 molecular size (Shochat et al. 1981). Earlier tissue studies revealed that CSAp is present in colorectal tissues, including normal, benign diseased, and malignant, as well as in some mucinous cystadenocarcinomas of the ovary (Pant et al. 1977). After developing a solid-phase radioassay for CSAp (Pant et al., unpublished results), we have found, in our preliminary study, that it is elevated in 52% of patients with colorectal cancer, 20% of patients with pancreatic cancer, and 10% of patients with benign gastrointestinal diseases (Table 8). Other tumor types investigated to date have not shown elevations in more cases than was true for normal individuals. Thus, CSAp appears to be restricted to gastrointestinal lesions, particularly colorectal cancer. An important question is what the relationship is of CSAp to an antigen which has a higher level of sensitivity yet a lower specificity for colorectal cancer. The antigen for comparison was CEA, and Figure 1 shows such a comparison between CEA and CSAp positivity or negativity in 31

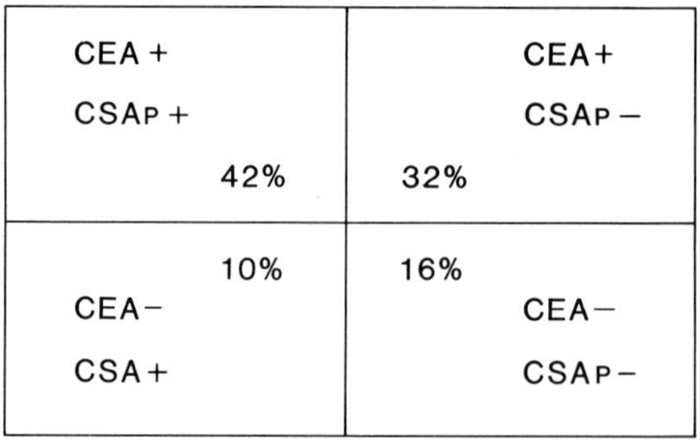

CEA + CSAp + 42%	CEA+ CSAp − 32%
10% CEA− CSA+	16% CEA− CSAp−

FIG. 1. Comparative analysis of plasma CEA and serum CSAp elevations in 31 colorectal cancer patients, using cutoffs of 5.0 ng/ml and 10.0 units for CEA and CSAp, respectively.

colorectal cancer patients. As was to be expected, CEA elevations (plasma values above 5 ng/ml) were present in a higher percentage of these patients than was true for CSAp. Both were positive or negative in a total of 58% of the cases, while a discordance between the two markers was noted in 42% of the patients. Since CEA is elevated in many more types of cancer than CSAp is, and since the elevations for CSAp are less frequent in benign gastrointestinal diseases and in the normal population than for CEA, it would seem that the added specificity of CSAp would improve upon the CEA assay results in the diagnosis of colorectal cancer. However, this point remains to be proven by clinical testing, and we are currently engaged in this evaluation.

Radioimmunodetection

Although none of these tumor markers has been found to be specific or distinct for cancer, the evidence indicates that they are in fact quantitatively increased with certain neoplastic conditions. In this circumstance, could these tumor antigens serve as targets for radioactive antibodies, which in turn could be detected by external scintigraphy? This approach is the method of cancer radioimmunodetection (Goldenberg 1978b, Goldenberg et al. 1978). We have undertaken clinical studies of cancer radioimmunodetection. To date we have studied approximately 300 patients with CEA radioactive antibodies, and another 50 patients with antibodies against AFP and against human chorionic gonadotropin. Our results with these three different tumor markers have appeared elsewhere (Goldenberg et al. 1978, Goldenberg et al. 1980a, b, c, Kim et al. 1980a, b). Our methods have been described in detail in these publications. Briefly summarized, purified CEA (or the appropriate marker to be localized) is used to immunize goats. The antiserum obtained several months later is purified through an automated affinity-chromatography system in which CEA cross-reactive antigens are removed and the antibody is adsorbed onto a CEA-affinity column. The result is that the antibody's CEA immunoreactivity is increased from approximately 30% to over 70% (Goldenberg et al. 1979). Thereafter the antibody IgG is isolated and labeled by the chloramine-T procedure with I-131. The radioactive antibody is now ready for injection into the patient. The patient is first evaluated by skin testing for hypersensitivity to goat IgG, and thereafter is put on a daily oral application of potassium iodide to reduce thyroid uptake of the radioactive iodine. The dose of radioactive antibody administered ranges from 2 to $3 \mu g$ of antibody IgG per kg of body weight, which amounts to 1–2 mCi of I-131 per patient. In order to compensate for circulating and interstitial nonspecific radioactivity, we have developed a subtraction method involving the administration of technetium components a short while before imaging the patients (Goldenberg et al. 1978, DeLand et al. 1980). In this way, the 140 keV of Tc is subtracted from the 364 keV image of I-131, resulting in the tumor-associated scan.

Our overall radioimmunodetection results in the first 142 patients studied with radioactive CEA antibodies are presented in Table 9. When analyzing

Table 9. *CEA Radioimmunodetection Results According to Tumor Sites*

Primary Diagnosis	No. of Pts.	Sensitivity (True-positive Rate)		Specificity (True-negative Rate)	
		No. +/Total	%	No. +/Total	%
Colorectal cancer	37	35/41	85	61/62	98
Ovarian cancer	19	21/24	88	19/21	90
Lung cancer	13	12/17	71	13/14	93
Mammary cancer	6	9/14	64	9/9	100
Pancreatic cancer	6	4/8	50	5/6	83
Cervical cancer	15	19/21	90	17/17	100
Other uterine cancers	5	9/10	90	4/4	100
Gastric cancer	4	5/6	83	6/6	100
Unknown origin	9	8/9	89	13/13	100
Miscellaneous cancers	26	17/30	57	41/41	100
Lymphoma	2	0/4	0	3/3	100

various body sites in which no evidence of tumor could be obtained by other clinical methods, a true-negative rate (specificity) of between 83% and 100% was found among the various tumor types. The sensitivity, or true-positive rate, varied from 50% in a small number of patients with pancreatic cancer to 90% in patients with cervical and other uterine cancers. Colorectal cancer has shown a sensitivity of 85%, whereas gastric cancer has a true-positive rate of 83%.

In Table 10 an analysis of the plasma CEA and radioimmunodetection results in 37 colorectal cancer patients is given. Radioimmunodetection scans were positive in nine of ten primary tumors evaluated prior to surgery, constituting a 90% sensitivity rate. Further, 26 of 31 confirmed metastatic sites were revealed by radioimmunodetection, indicating a sensitivity for metastatic disease of 84%. Four of the five metastatic sites not detected by radioimmunodetection were located in the lungs and measured less than 2 cm in diameter. Two patients showed tumor localization without confirmatory evidence of tumor being present or absent, and these were therefore excluded from our computation. Twenty-nine of 37 of the colorectal cancer patients had elevated plasma CEA levels at the onset of the study, but those with normal levels did not always have an absence of advanced disease, as revealed by radioimmunodetection. Indeed, five patients with normal plasma CEA titers had true-positive localization of tumors by radioimmunodetection. Interestingly, the level of circulating CEA did not seem to prevent successful tumor radioimmunodetection, even when values as high as 5,600 ng/ml were present. Positive tumor localization was achieved in various organs commonly involved with metastatic colorectal cancer, particularly the liver (Figure 2). Using the same technology, we have been able to locate hepatocellular and other tumors producing AFP after administering radioactive AFP antibodies to the patients (Goldenberg et al. 1980b, Kim et al. 1980b).

Our radioimmunodetection results indicate that truly cancer-specific mark-

Table 10. *Plasma CEA and Radioimmunodetection Results In 37 Colorectal Cancer Patients**

Patient	Plasma CEA (ng/ml)[a]	Radioimmunodetection Results Primary site	Radioimmunodetection Results Secondary sites
108	2210.0	O[b]	+, abdomen (1)[c]; + liver (1); ? +, mediastinum (1)
92	16.4	O	−, lung (1)
136	2.8	O	N
86	2.1	O	+, abdomen (1)
90	1190.0	O	+, liver (1)
152	3150.0	O	+, abdomen (1); +, liver (1)
5	10.7	+ (1)	N
73	2.5	+ (1)	N
81	80.0	O	N
84	48.0	O	N
40/84[d]	116.0	O	N
24	2.1	O	N
21	116.0	O	+, liver (1)
189	612.0	O	N
206	1.4	O	N
42	3.3	O	N
57	10.3	+ (1)	+, abdomen (1); +, liver (1)
64/78	0.8	+ (1)	N
195	12.2	O	+, liver (1); −, abdomen (1)
191	9.0	O	+, abdomen (1)
126	62.0	O	N
244	2.1	O	+, abdomen (1); −, lung (1)
250	0	O	−, lung (1)
203	188.0	O	+, abdomen (1); +, lung (1)
150	40.0	+ (1)	+, liver (1); +, lung (1)
128	16.1	+ (1)	+, lung (1)
87	154.0	O	+, liver (1)
46	152.0	O	+, abdomen (1)
26	0.9	+ (1)	N
38	68.0	+ (1)	N
60	5600.0	+ (1)	+, liver (1)
83	5.4	O	+, abdomen (1); +, submandible (1)
85	9.0	O	N
20	11.7	O	+, liver (1)
255	17.5	O	?+, abdomen (1)
6	0.3	O	+, abdomen (2)
262	212.0	− (1)[e]	+, liver (1)

[a]A value above 2.5 ng/ml is considered abnormal.

[b]+, tumor identified; −, tumor missed; O, tumor excised; N, no tumor identified or missed; ?+, positive scan without confirmatory clinical data available.

[c]Numbers in parentheses, number of tumor sites imaged.

[d]Patients with 2 numbers underwent a repeat radioimmunodetection study.

[e]Incomplete study, since lateral view not scanned.

*From Goldenberg et al. 1980a.

ers are not required for in vivo detection and localization of tumors. The identification and development of more tumor-specific antibodies, perhaps by means of hybridoma technology, should therefore afford even better opportunities for improved cancer radioimmunodetection. Since tumors are composed of heterogeneous populations of cells, some of which differ in their

Anti - CEA   Scan

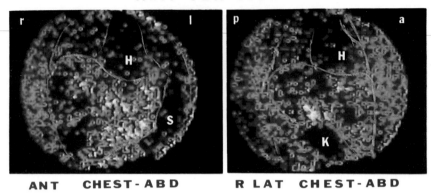

ANT   CHEST - ABD   R LAT   CHEST - ABD

FIG. 2. Immune scintiscan of a 54-year-old male with a history of Dukes' B adenocarcinoma of the ascending colon (1977) and now presenting with metastasis to the liver. Both views (anterior chest and abdomen; right lateral chest and abdomen) show multiple areas of abnormal radioactivity (white spots) in right and left lobes of the liver. Liver scintigraphy and ultrasound confirmed radioimmunodetection findings. This patient had a plasma CEA titer of 185 ng/ml and received 150 μg of anti-CEA IgG labeled with I-131 (1.94 mCi total dose); H, heart, S, stomach, K, kidney.

distribution of molecular markers, the use of combinations of different radioactive antibodies should result in better tumor detection and resolution. We have evaluated this proposition in our experimental animal system for human colorectal cancer, the GW-39 tumor model (Goldenberg et al. 1966), which consists of a human colonic carcinoma serially propagable in various sites of unconditioned, adult hamsters. This tumor system produces both CEA (Goldenberg and Hansen 1972) and CSAp (Pant et al. 1977). Interestingly, CSAp radioactive antibodies given alone in the GW-39 tumor system show localization ratios which far exceed those found previously with CEA antibodies in the same tumor model (Gaffar et al. 1981). In fact, as much as 9% of the injected antibody could be localized in the tumors four days after being administered. Moreover, when CSAp antibodies were combined with CEA antibodies, the CEA radioimmunodetection results improved considerably while the localization efficacy of CSAp antibodies remained essentially the same (Gaffar et al. 1981). Thus, it appears that the mixture of these two antibodies would be more effective in tumor radioimmunodetection than either alone, since more than one molecular target for radioactive antibodies are being exploited. Hence, future advances in cancer radioimmunodetection will include mixtures of antitumor antibodies directed against different tumor markers.

Prospects for Radioimmunotherapy

It has long been thought that the same markers used for immunodiagnosis, immunodetection, and immunolocalization could serve as targets for selected therapy mediated by appropriate antibodies. In biliary or liver cancers, Order and his co-workers have claimed success by multimodal treatment including high-dose radioactive antibodies to ferritin or CEA (Ettinger et al. 1979, Order et al. 1980). In order to evaluate whether the radioactive antibody by itself has therapeutic effects in colorectal cancer, we undertook experiments in the GW-39 tumor system. Many years ago, we showed that this tumor model is very refractive to most drugs used in the management of colorectal cancer, as well as to external X-irradiation therapy (Goldenberg and Ammersdörfer 1970). However, administering 1 mCi of I-131-labeled anti-CEA IgG as a single dose to animals bearing GW-39 tumors results in significant tumor growth inhibition (Goldenberg et al., unpublished results). Moreover, 84% of the animals were able to survive for an extended period of time if they received the radioactive specific antibody preparation, whereas poorer results could be obtained when cold antibody or when radioactive normal goat IgG was given. Since the GW-39 human colonic carcinoma system was predictive of our clinical findings in tumor radioimmunodetection (Goldenberg et al. 1974), it is not unreasonable to assume that these experimental therapeutic results might also have clinical applicability.

CONCLUDING REMARKS

Moertel recently wrote, "The oncologist should continue to regard all management of colorectal cancer today as experimental in nature so that we can build treatment of substantive benefit for the patient tomorrow" (Moertel 1978). From this viewpoint, it is understandable that the repertoire of tumor markers capable of monitoring colorectal and other gastrointestinal cancer patients may have only limited clinical value in the management of these patients. Nevertheless, these tumor markers do play a role as very sensitive indicators of tumor response to therapy, and in this capacity might serve to reduce patient exposure to ineffective therapeutic trials. Since some markers appear to have greater gastrointestinal specificity while others have more tumor sensitivity, combination marker tests attempting to complement both extremes may afford better opportunities for using these markers in gastrointestinal cancer diagnosis. Although a gastrointestinal, tumor-specific marker has not as yet been identified, it should be appreciated that all of the studies discussed herein involved the use of polyclonal antibodies directed against tumor-associated substances. With the advent of hybridoma-derived monoclonal antibodies recognizing tumor-specific markers, it is to be expected that further progress in the immunological approach to cancer detection, diagnosis, and therapy will be forthcoming.

ACKNOWLEDGMENTS

I am grateful to Drs. S. J. Bennett, S. A. Gaffar, K. D. Pant, and D. Shochat for their collaboration in research covered in this paper. Our studies have been supported by grants CA-15799 (through the National Large Bowel Cancer Project), CA-17742, and CA-25584, and contract NCI-NO1-CB-64011-35, awarded by the National Cancer Institute, Department of Health and Human Services.

REFERENCES

Abelev, G. I. 1971. Alpha-fetoprotein in ontogenesis and its association with malignant tumors. Adv. Cancer Res. 14:295–358.

Abelev, G. I., S. D. Perova, N. I. Khramkova, Z. A. Postnikova, and I. S. Irlin. 1963. Transplantation 1:174–180.

Bara, J., A. Paul-Bardais, F. Loisillier, and P. Burtin. 1978. Isolation of a sulfated glycopeptidic antigen from human gastric tumors: Its localization in normal and cancerous gastrointestinal tissues. Int. J. Cancer 21:133–139.

DeLand, F. H., E. E. Kim, G. Simmons, and D. M. Goldenberg. 1980. Imaging approach in radioimmunodetection. Cancer Res. 40:3046–3049.

Ettinger, D., L. Dragon, J. L. Klein, M. Sgagias, and S. E. Order. 1979. Isotopic immunglobulin in an integrated multimodal treatment program for a primary liver cancer. A case report. Cancer Treat. Rep. 63:131–134.

Gaffar, S. A., K. D. Pant, D. Shochat, S. J. Bennett, and D. M. Goldenberg. 1981. Experimental studies of tumor radioimmunodetection using antibody mixtures against carcinoembryonic antigen (CEA) and colon-specific antigen-p (CSAp). Int. J. Cancer 27:101–105.

Gelder, F. B., C. J. Reese, A. R. Moossa, T. Hall, and R. Hunter. 1978. Purification, partial characterization, and clinical evaluation of a pancreatic oncofetal antigen. Cancer Res. 38:313–324.

Gilbertsen, V. A., and O. H. Wangensteen. 1962. A summary of thirteen years' experience with the second look program. Surg. Gynecol. Obstet. 114:438–442.

Gold, D. V. 1979. Colonic mucoprotein antigen (CMA), in Compendium of Assays for Immunodiagnosis of Human Cancer, R. B. Herberman, ed. Elsevier North Holland, Inc., New York, pp. 231–236.

Gold, D. V., and D. M. Goldenberg. 1980. Antigens associated with human solid tumors, in Cancer Markers. Diagnostic and Developmental Significance, S. Sell, ed. Humana Press, Clifton, New Jersey, pp. 329–369.

Gold, D. V., and F. Miller. 1974. Characterization of human colonic mucoprotein antigen. Immunochem. 11:369–375.

Gold, P., and S. O. Freedman. 1965. Specific carcinoembryonic antigens of the human digestive system. J. Exp. Med. 122:467–481.

Goldenberg, D. M. 1976. Oncofetal and other tumor-associated antigens of the human digestive system. Current Top. Pathol. 63:289–342.

Goldenberg, D. M. 1978a. Carcinoembryonic antigen and other tumor-associated antigens in colon cancer diagnosis and management, in Colon Cancer, E. Grundmann, ed. Gustav Fischer Verlag, Stuttgart, pp. 163–178.

Goldenberg, D. M. 1978b. Immunodiagnosis and immunodetection of colorectal cancer. Cancer Bull. 30:213–218.

Goldenberg, D. M. 1979. Carcinoembryonic antigen in the management of colorectal cancer. Acta Hepato-Gastroenterol. 26:1–3.

Goldenberg, D. M., and E. Ammersdörfer. 1970. Synergistic effects of x-rays and drugs on a human tumor xenograft, GW-39. Eur. J. Cancer 6:73–80.

Goldenberg, D. M., F. DeLand, E. Kim, S. Bennett, F. J. Primus, J. R. van Nagell, Jr., N. Estes, P. DeSimone, and P. Rayburn. 1978. Use of radiolabeled antibodies to carcinoembryonic antigen for the detection and localization of diverse cancers by external photoscanning. N. Engl. J. Med. 298:1384–1388.

Goldenberg, D. M., and H. J. Hansen. 1972. Carcinoembryonic antigen present in human colonic neoplasms serially propagated in hamsters. Science 175:1117–1118.

Goldenberg, D. M., E. E. Kim, F. H. DeLand, S. Bennett, and F. J. Primus. 1980a. Radioimmunodetection of cancer with radioactive antibodies to carcinoembryonic antigen. Cancer Res. 40:2984–2992.

Goldenberg, D. M., E. E. Kim, F. DeLand, E. Spremulli, M. O. Nelson, J. P. Gockerman, F. J. Primus, R. L. Corgan, and E. Alpert. 1980b. Clinical studies on the radioimmunodetection of tumors containing alpha-fetoprotein. Cancer 45:2500-2505.

Goldenberg, D. M., E. E. Kim, F. H. DeLand, J. R. van Nagell, Jr., and N. Javadpour. 1980c. Radioimmunodetection of cancer using radioactive antibodies to human chorionic gonadotropin. Science 208:1284-1286.

Goldenberg, D. M., K. D. Pant, and H. L. Dahlman. 1976a. Antigens associated with normal and malignant gastrointestinal tissues. Cancer Res. 36:3455-3463.

Goldenberg, D. M., K. D. Pant, and H. L. Dahlman. 1976b. A new oncofetal antigen associated with gastrointestinal cancer. Proc. Am. Assoc. Cancer Res. 17:155.

Goldenberg, D. M., D. F. Preston, F. J. Primus, and H. J. Hansen. 1974. Photoscan localization of GW-39 tumors in hamsters using radiolabeled anticarcinoembryonic antigen immunoglobulin G. Cancer Res. 34:1-9.

Goldenberg, D. M., F. J. Primus, and F. DeLand. 1979. Tumor detection and localization with purified antibodies to carcinoembryonic antigen, *in* Immunodiagnosis of Cancer, Part 1, R. B. Herberman and K. R. McIntire, eds. Marcel Dekker, Inc., New York, pp. 265-304.

Goldenberg, D. M., S. Witte, and K. Elster. 1966. GW-39: A new human tumor serially transplantable in the golden hamster. Transplantation 4:760-763.

Häkkinen, I. 1979. FSA, *in* Compendium of Assays for Immunodiagnosis of Human Cancer, R. B. Herberman, ed. Elsevier North Holland, Inc., New York, pp. 241-246.

Häkkinen, I. P. T., O. Jarvi, and J. Gironroos. 1968. Sulphoglycoprotein antigens in the human alimentary canal and gastric cancer. An immunohistochemical study. Int. J. Cancer 3:572-581.

Hansen, H. J., J. J. Snyder, E. Miller, J. P. Vandevoorde, O. N. Miller, L. R. Hines, and J. J. Burns. 1974. Carcinoembryonic antigen (CEA) assay. A laboratory adjunct in the diagnosis and management of cancer. Hum. Pathol. 4:139-147.

Herlyn, M., Z. Steplewski, D. Herlyn, and H. Koprowski. 1979. Colorectal carcinoma-specific antigen: Detection by means of monoclonal antibodies. Proc. Natl. Acad. Sci. USA 76:1438-1442.

Herrera, M. A., T. M. Chu, and E. D. Holyoke. 1976. Carcinoembryonic antigen (CEA) as a prognostic and monitoring test in clinically complete resection of colorectal carcinoma. Ann. Surg. 183:5-9.

Hirai, H., S. Nishi, and H. Watabe. 1972. Radioimmunoassay of α-fetoprotein, *in* Protides of Biological Fluids, 20th Colloquium, H. Peeters, ed. Pergamon Press, New York, pp. 579-587.

Hirszfeld, L., W. Halber, and J. Laskowski. 1929. Untersuchungen über die serologischen Eigenschaften der Gewebe. II. Mitteilung. Ueber serologische Eigenschaften der Neubildungen. Z. Immunitätsforsch. 64:81-113.

Holyoke, E. D., T. M. Chu, and G. P. Murphy. 1975. CEA as a monitor of gastrointestinal malignancy. Cancer 25:830-836.

Hunter, R., F. Gelder, and A. R. Moossa. 1979. Pancreatic oncofetal antigen (POA), *in* Compendium of Assays for Immunodiagnosis of Human Cancer, R. B. Herberman, ed. Elsevier North Holland, Inc., New York, pp. 247-250.

Ishii, M. 1977. Study on a new basic fetoprotein associated with various types of malignant neoplasia. Igakuno Ayumi 100:344-346.

Ishii, M. 1979. Clinical usefulness of basic fetoprotein for immunodiagnosis of human cancer, *in* Compendium of Assays for Immunodiagnosis of Human Cancer, R. B. Herberman, ed. Elsevier North Holland, Inc., New York, pp. 45-50.

Ishii, M., and M. Hattori. 1976. Purification of basic fetoprotein and immunodiagnosis of human cancer by a radioimmunoassay of serum basic fetoprotein. Proc. Jpn. Cancer Assoc. 35:205.

Kawasaki, H., K. Imasato, and E. Kimoto. 1971. Immunohistological studies on gastric mucosal glycoprotein in gastric carcinoma. Gann 62:171-176.

Kim, E. E., F. H. DeLand, S. Casper, R. L. Corgan, F. J. Primus, and D. M. Goldenberg. 1980a. Radioimmunodetection of colorectal cancer. Cancer 45:1243-1247.

Kim, E. E., F. H. DeLand, M. O. Nelson, S. Bennett, G. Simmons, E. Alpert, and D. M. Goldenberg. 1980b. Radioimmunodetection of cancer with radiolabeled antibodies to α-fetoprotein. Cancer Res. 40:3008-3012.

Köhler, G., and C. Milstein. 1975. Continuous cultures of fused cells secreting antibodies of predefined specificity. Nature 256:495-497.

Mach, J.-P., H. Vienny, P. Jaeger, B. Haldemann, R. Egely, and J. Pettavel. 1978. Long-term follow-up of colorectal carcinoma patients by repeated CEA radioimmunoassay. Cancer 42:1439–1447.

Martin, E. W., Jr., M. Cooperman, and J. P. Minton. 1979. A retrospective and prospective study of serial CEA determinations in the early detection of recurrent colon cancer, in Compendium of Assays for Immunodiagnosis of Human Cancer, R. B. Herberman, ed. Elsevier North Holland, Inc., New York, p. 215.

Mayer, R. J., M. B. Garnick, G. D. Steele, Jr., and N. Zamcheck. 1978. Carcinoembryonic antigen (CEA) as a monitor of chemotherapy in disseminated colorectal cancer. Cancer 42:1428–1433.

McIntire, K. R., C. L. Vogel, A. Primack, T. A. Waldmann, and S. K. Kyalwazi. 1976. Effect of surgical and chemotherapeutic treatment on alpha-fetoprotein levels in patients with hepatocellular carcinoma. Cancer 37:677–683.

McIntire, K. R., T. A. Waldmann, C. G. Moertel, and V. L. W. Go. 1975. Serum α-fetoprotein in patients with neoplasms of the gastrointestinal tract. Cancer Res. 32:1941–1946.

Moertel, C. G. 1978. Chemotherapy of colorectal cancer, in Colon Cancer, E. Grundmann, ed. Gustav Fischer Verlag, Stuttgart, pp. 207–216.

Olweny, C. L. M., T. Toa, E. Katongole-Mbidde, J. Mugerwa, S. K. Kyalwazi, and H. Cohen. 1975. Treatment of hepatocellular carcinoma with adriamycin. Cancer 36:1250–1257.

Order, S. E., J. L. Klein, D. Ettinger, P. Alderson, S. Siegelman, and P. Leichner. 1980. Phase I-II study of radiolabeled antibody integrated in the treatment of primary hepatic malignancies. Int. J. Radiat. Oncol. Biol. Phys. 6:703–710.

Pant, K. D., H. L. Dahlman, and D. M. Goldenberg. 1977. A putatively new antigen (CSAp) associated with gastrointestinal and ovarian neoplasia. Immunol. Commun. 6:411–421.

Pant, K. D., H. L. Dahlman, and D. M. Goldenberg. 1978. Further characterization of CSAp, an antigen associated with gastrointestinal and ovarian tumors. Cancer 42:1626–1634.

Pant, K. D., and D. M. Goldenberg. 1979. Colon-specific antigen-p (CSAp), in Compendium of Assays for Immunodiagnosis of Human Cancer, R. B. Herberman, ed. Elsevier North Holland, Inc., New York, pp. 225–229.

Podolsky, D. K., M. M. Weiser, K. J. Isselbacher, and A. M. Cohen. 1978. A cancer-associated galactosyltransferase isoenzyme. N. Engl. J. Med. 299:703–705.

Potter, T. P., Jr., J. D. Jordan, and T. A. Jordan. 1979. TennaGen assay, in Compendium of Assays for Immunodiagnosis of Human Cancer, R. B. Herberman, ed. Elsevier North Holland, Inc., New York, pp. 217–224.

Potter, T. P., Jr., T. Jordan, J. D. Jordan, and H. Lasater. 1978. Tennessee antigen (TennaGen): Characterization and immunoassay of a tumor associated antigen, in Prevention and Detection of Cancer, Part II, Detection, High Risk Markers, Detection Methods and Management, H. E. Nieburgs, ed. Marcel Dekker, New York, pp. 467–490.

Purves, L. R., C. Manso, and F. O. Torres. 1973. Serum α-fetoprotein levels in people susceptible to primary liver cancer in southern Africa. Gann Monogr. Cancer Res. 14:51–66.

Pusztaszeri, G., C. A. Saravis, and N. Zamcheck. 1976. The zinc glycinate marker in human colon carcinoma. J. Natl. Cancer Inst. 56:275–277.

Rapp, W., M. Windisch, P. Peschke, and K. Wurster. 1979. Purification of human intestinal goblet cell antigen (GOA), its immunohistological demonstration in the intestine and in mucus producing gastrointestinal adenocarcinomas. Virchows Arch. [Pathol. Anat.] 382:163–177.

Saravis, C. A., S. K. Oh, G. Pusztaszeri, W. Doos, and N. Zamcheck. 1978. Present status of the zinc glycinate marker (ZGM). Cancer 42:1621–1625.

Shochat, D., R. L. Archey, K. D. Pant, H. L. Dahlman, D. V. Gold, and D. M. Goldenberg. 1981. Characterization of colon-specific antigen-p (CSAp) and isolation of immunologically active tryptic peptides. J. Immunol. 126:2284–2291.

Silver, H. K. B., J. Deneault, P. Gold, W. G. Thompson, J. Shuster, and S. O. Freedman. 1974. The detection of α_1-fetoprotein in patients with viral hepatitis. Cancer Res. 34:244–247.

Smith, J. B. 1971. Occurrence of alpha-fetoprotein in acute viral hepatitis. Int. J. Cancer 8:421–424.

Sugarbaker, P. H., W. D. Bloomer, E. D. Corbett, and J. T. Chaffey. 1976. Carcinoembryonic antigen (CEA) monitoring of radiation therapy for colorectal cancer. Am. J. Roentgenol. 127:641–644.

Waldmann, T. A., and K. R. McIntire. 1974. The use of a radioimmunoassay for alpha-fetoprotein in the diagnosis of malignancy. Cancer 34:1510–1515.

Wanebo, H. J., R. Bhaskar, C. M. Pinsky, R. G. Hoffman, M. Stearns, M. J. Schwartz, and H. F. Oettgen. 1978. Preoperative carcinoembryonic antigen level as a prognostic indicator in colorectal cancer. N. Engl. J. Med. 299:448-451.

Witebsky, E. 1930. Zur serologischen Spezifität des Carcinomgewebes. Klin. Wochenschr. 2:58-63.

Witebsky, E., N. L. Rose, and S. Shulman. 1956. Studies of normal and malignant tissue antigens. Cancer Res. 16:831-841.

Gastrointestinal Cancer, edited by
John R. Stroehlein and
Marvin M. Romsdahl.
Raven Press, New York © 1981.

Advances in Gastrointestinal Interventional Radiology

Jesus Zornoza, M.D.

Department of Diagnostic Radiology,
The University of Texas System Cancer Center
M. D. Anderson Hospital and Tumor Institute, Houston, Texas

Traditional diagnostic techniques in the evaluation of patients with gastrointestinal carcinoma have played a definite role in the detection and staging of disease. More recently, ultrasound and computed tomography (CT) have made possible the visualization of certain organs which previously required the use of contrast material or radionuclides. The applications of these diagnostic modalities have been augmented by the development of percutaneous biopsy techniques (Zornoza et al. 1977) and the therapeutic applications of various diagnostic procedures such as the percutaneous drainage of the biliary system in patients with obstructive jaundice.

PERCUTANEOUS ASPIRATION BIOPSY

Despite the development of a variety of diagnostic modalities such as percutaneous transhepatic cholangiography (PTC), endoscopic retrograde cholangiopancreaticography (ERPC), ultrasound, and computed tomography (CT), the diagnosis of pancreatic, hepatic, and other intra-abdominal masses is still difficult. Percutaneous aspiration biopsy of these mass lesions provides a cytologic diagnosis, sparing the higher risk of exploratory surgery and cost to patients with unresectable or recurrent malignant disease. The technique is safe, simple, and accurate provided certain precautions are observed.

Technique

Percutaneous aspiration biopsies are performed with commercially available 19 to 22 gauge, 10-15 cm spinal-type needles (Figure 1). The localization of the tumor target can be obtained by a wide variety of radiographic techniques. In general the simplest imaging method that adequately delineates the tumor area should be used. Localizing methods most often used for biopsy guidance include angiography (Goldstein and Zornoza 1978), ultrasound (Smith et al. 1974, Yamanaka and Kimura 1979, Cohen 1979), CT (Haaga 1979), and fluoros-

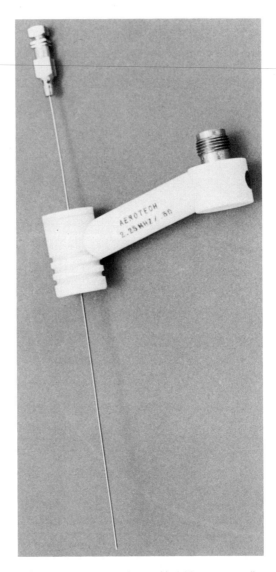

FIG. 1. Aspiration transducer with a 22 gauge needle.

copy (Pereiras et al. 1978, Goldstein and Zornoza 1978). The vast majority of our biopsies have been performed under fluoroscopic guidance. A few have been done under angiographic, ultrasonic, or CT control.

Once the lesion has been localized, the skin is prepared and draped in the usual manner. The easiest approach is usually the anterior abdominal wall, but a flank approach may be selected for lesions located in the posterior segment of the right hepatic lobe. The needle is introduced to the appropriate depth as determined from the preliminary studies; usually, a sensation of resistance is felt when the tumor mass is reached. The specimen is obtained by rotating and moving the needle up and down in order to loosen cells. Suction is applied with a 10 ml plastic syringe connected to the needle. Two to four needle passes are usually made to insure adequate cytologic material. The specimens are placed in a preservative solution (Mucolexx). All smears are stained by the Papanicolaou technique.

Relative contraindications include bowel dilatation and abnormal bleeding. Ascites and obstructive jaundice were not regarded as contraindications.

Indications

The most common indications for aspiration biopsy in the case of suspected pancreatic carcinoma are: (1) patients with lesions involving the pancreatic head who have undergone biliary decompression surgery, but from whom no biopsy specimen was obtained (Figure 2), and (2) patients with lesions of the body and tail of the pancreas, with clinical and radiological evidence of unresectability (Figure 3).

Aspiration biopsy of the liver is indicated in the following: (1) patients with ascites or jaundice, in whom a Menghini biopsy is contraindicated, and (2)

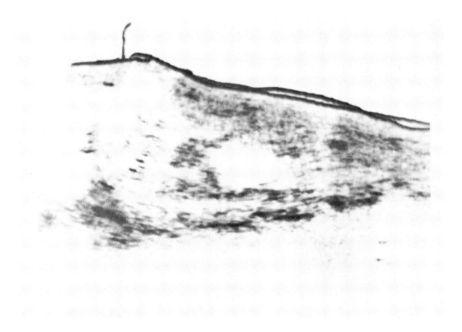

FIG. 2. A 53-year-old male had previous surgery to relieve jaundice but a biopsy was not obtained. Longitudinal ultrasonogram demonstrates a 5 cm mass in the area of the head of the pancreas. The sonographic examination aided biopsy localization, particularly in the assessment of depth.

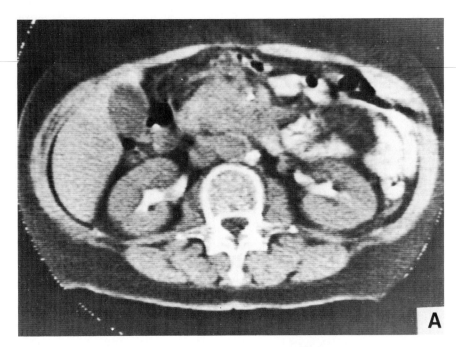

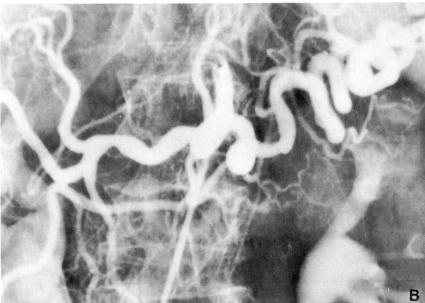

FIG. 3. A 71-year-old male with weight loss and a palpable abdominal mass. **A.** CT of the abdomen demonstrates mass in front of the aorta displacing the bowel loops; the mass is most likely pancreatic in origin. **B.** Celiac angiogram reveals encasement of the splenic artery and the common hepatic artery as well as neovascularity. Percutaneous needle aspiration biopsy revealed pancreatic adenocarcinoma.

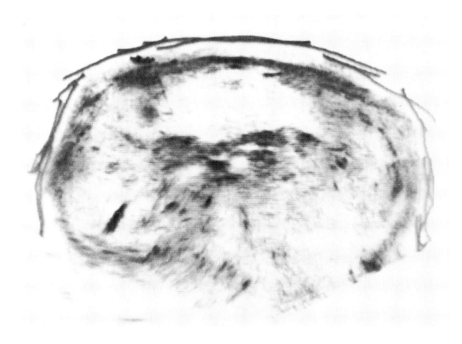

FIG. 4. A 74-year-old female with the diagnosis of cloacogenic carcinoma of the rectum and chronic myelogenous leukemia. Transverse sonogram shows a hypoechoic mass involving the left lobe of the liver. Percutaneous needle biopsy revealed metastatic adenocarcinoma.

patients with focal lesions of the liver, involving the left lobe (Figure 4) or the posterior segment of the right lobe (Figure 5). CT is the best guiding method for these types of lesions because of the excellent image resolution and the anatomic delineation of the target lesion and the needle.

Discussion

The technique of percutaneous aspiration biopsy of the pancreas and liver is relatively simple and easily learned. The most important variable to success with this technique is cytopathologic support.

The greatest experience with individual organ aspiration biopsy has been achieved with pancreatic carcinoma. The results in our series (Zornoza 1980) of 60% correct diagnosis are similar to data reported by others (Ferrucci et al. 1980b, Pereiras et al. 1978, Ihse et al. 1979). No false-positive diagnoses were obtained. Negative cytologic material in the presence of pancreatic carcinoma is usually related to necrotic and/or scirrhous areas in the tumor.

Although conventional liver biopsy techniques remain the procedure of choice in patients with diffuse parenchymal liver disease, aspiration guided

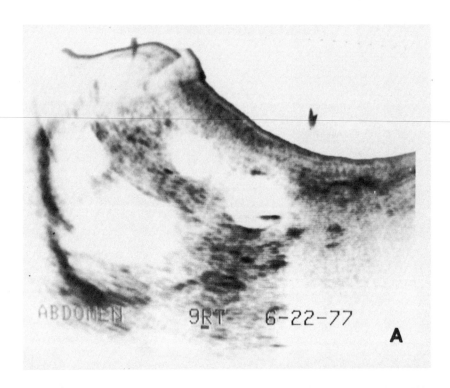

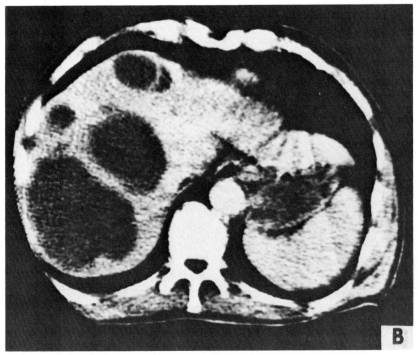

FIG. 5A and B. See legend on facing page.

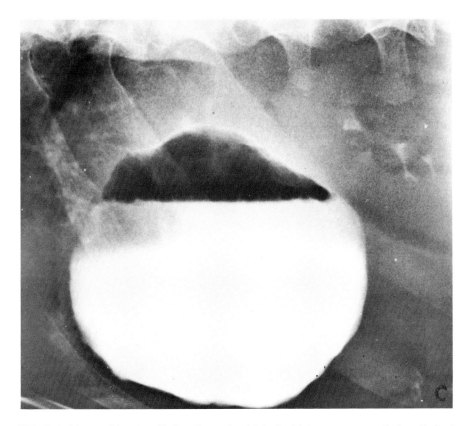

FIG. 5. A 64-year-old male with the diagnosis of intestinal leiomyosarcoma. **A.** Longitudinal sonogram of the liver shows multiple anechoic masses, one of them with a fluid level. **B.** CT of the liver demonstrates multiple low attenuation lesions. **C.** Lateral decubitus radiograph after injection of contrast material into cystic mass showing nodularity and irregularity of the wall. Aspirated fluid revealed metastatic leiomyosarcoma.

biopsies appear to be the method of choice for focal lesions of the liver and lesions located in the left lobe of the liver or the posterior segment of the right lobe. Our overall success rate of 83% compares favorably with several other series (Haaga 1979).

Depending upon the location of the mass to be biopsied, the needle usually traverses hollow viscera as well as major vascular structures. To date only minor complications related to this approach have been reported. There were also no sequelae resulting from the percutaneous puncture of three pancreatic pseudocysts in our series. Usually the biopsied site is not evident when the patients have surgery after the percutaneous procedure. A case of needle track seeding with malignant cells after aspiration biopsy has been documented and may be related to the unusual number of needle passes made to obtain a diagnosis (Ferrucci et al. 1980b).

In summary, percutaneous aspiration biopsy is a safe and accurate technique that can provide a histologic diagnosis of pancreatic, hepatic, and other intra-abdominal masses. With new improvements in localizing methods, such as ultrasound and CT, smaller lesions can be biopsied with larger needles, consequently obtaining more definite diagnoses.

BILIARY DRAINAGE

Percutaneous transhepatic biliary drainage (PTBD) is a new nonsurgical method for decompression of an obstructed biliary system. The risk of surgery on jaundiced patients with tumors of the extrahepatic bile duct or pancreas is high, but it may be reduced by presurgical bile drainage. In tumors close to the liver, surgery is usually not feasible, and adequate biliary decompression can be obtained by transhepatic catheterization of an intrahepatic bile duct.

Techniques developed for introducing catheters transhepatically into the portal system have been applied to the catheterization of the biliary tree (Ring et al. 1978, Ferrucci et al. 1980a, Mori et al. 1977, Nakayama et al. 1978, Molnar and Stockum 1974, Kaude et al. 1969, Tylen et al. 1977, Hoevels et al. 1978). Using this approach, catheters and guide wires can be manipulated within the bile ducts and advanced through obstructing lesions in order to achieve an external as well as an internal drainage. This procedure has proved to be as effective as a surgically performed biliary bypass operation. Complications related to surgery can be eliminated.

Technique

Preparation of the patient is practically the same as that for percutaneous transhepatic cholangiography (PTC) and, in most instances, a conventional diagnostic fine needle PTC is the required first step. Routine measures include a check of the bleeding parameters, sterile precautions, coverage with antibiotics, and consent form.

Fine needle PTC is performed from the right upper lateral abdomen by means of the Chiba needle technique (Okuda et al. 1974). The opacification of the biliary duct will determine the presence of an obstruction, and permits selection of an optimal segment for catheterization. If it is decided that PTBD is indicated, a 15 cm 18 gauge cannula with a Teflon sheath is then introduced into the liver. The large cannula is advanced into the intended biliary duct under fluoroscopic control while the patient holds his breath (Figure 6). Satisfactory puncture is indicated by free flow of bile as the sheath is slowly withdrawn. Once the sheath is confirmed to be intraductal, a 0.038 inch safety guide wire is inserted through the sheath and into the bile duct system. Special

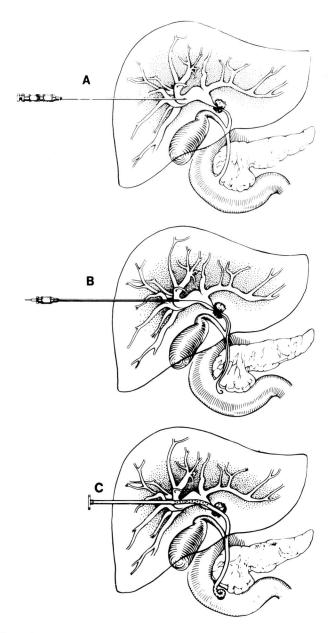

FIG. 6. Schematic representation of the technique for catheterization and drainage of obstructed bile ducts. **A.** The biliary ducts are punctured using an 18 gauge Teflon sheath needle. **B.** The needle is removed and a guide wire is manipulated into the duct toward the obstruction. **C.** Using Seldinger technique, a catheter is advanced over the guide wire. Side holes above and below the obstruction allow external as well as internal drainage.

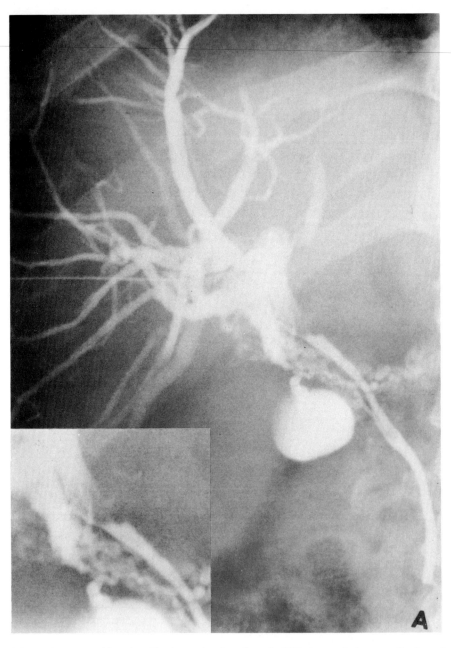

FIG. 7. A 65-year-old male with obstructive jaundice. **A.** PTC demonstrates opacification of intrahepatic and extrahepatic biliary ducts. Insert demonstrates detail of an intraluminal mass at the common hepatic duct. (*cont.*)

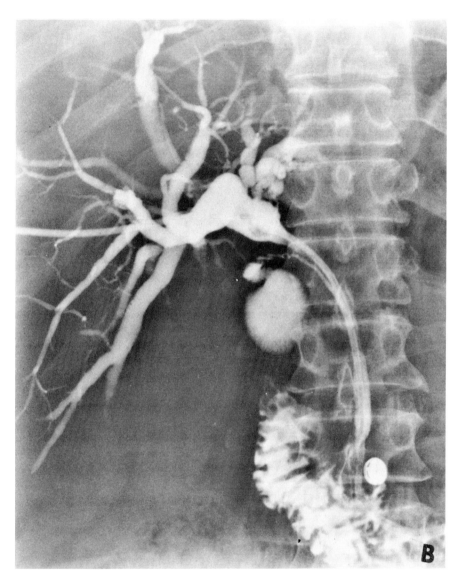

FIG. 7 (*cont.*). **B.** An 8.3 French catheter was introduced transhepatically through the obstruction. The pigtail configuration anchors the catheter in the duodenum.

guide wires can be used when sharp turns or severe strictures are encountered. After the guide wire has been advanced as intended, the Teflon sheath is removed and a tapered, pigtail 8.3 French catheter with multiple side holes is advanced over the guide wire. To facilitate the passage of the catheter, several Teflon vessel dilators may be used. During this maneuver, the patient may experience considerable pain; therefore, a dose of intravenous analgesic is usually administered beforehand.

If the guide wire cannot be advanced past the obstruction, a catheter should be left in place in the intrahepatic duct and external drainage established. For internal drainage, the guide wire should be advanced through the obstruction and the catheter usually positioned with its tip through the ampulla of Vater in the descending duodenum (Figure 7). If catheterization is successful, the guide wire is removed and the catheter is affixed on the skin. The catheter is allowed to drain externally for two to three days. If no complications occur, the catheter can be clamped so that the bile can flow into the duodenum. When only external drainage can be achieved, and to compensate for the loss of bile, desiccated bile tablets should be administered orally.

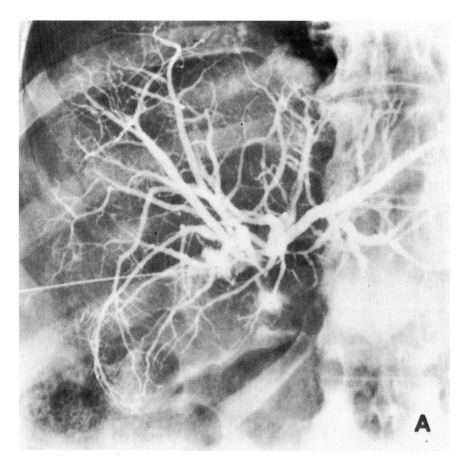

FIG. 8. A 65-year-old female with obstructive jaundice and breast carcinoma. **A.** Transhepatic cholangiogram demonstrates obstruction of the porta hepatis. (*cont.*)

Complications

Major complications occur in approximately 4% of the cases, and minor complications have been reported in as many as 24% (Ferrucci et al. 1980a). Cholangitis is the most frequent complication and occurs in approximately 15% of the cases. A frequent minor complication is malfunctioning of the catheter. The most common problem is catheter occlusion caused by detritus or blood clot. Catheter dislodgement occurs in approximately 5% of the cases. Sepsis, drainage of duodenal contents, and unrelieved jaundice are other common complications that can be avoided by good postprocedural catheter care.

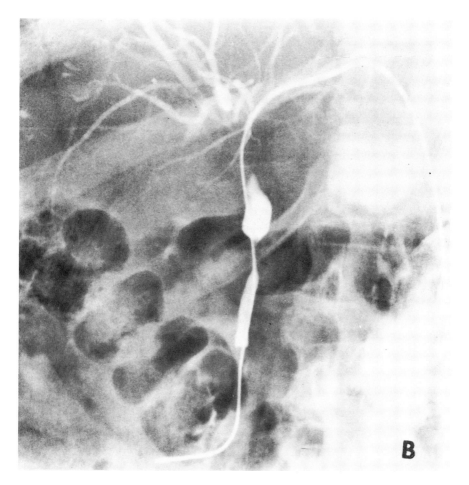

FIG. 8. (*cont.*). **B.** Using a left approach, a guide wire was passed below the obstruction and into the duodenum. (*cont.*)

Discussion

Malignant tumors of the extrahepatic bile duct and pancreatic region often are unsuspected until late in the course of the disease, with the main symptom being jaundice. Approximately 80% to 90% of such patients will be found to have surgically unresectable tumors. Radical surgery in such advanced stages is not possible; however, palliative biliary bypass is mandatory. Various surgical methods for biliary drainage are available, but the operative mortality approaches 30%. PTBD offers an alternative to the surgical bypass procedure for the relief of obstructive jaundice resulting from an inoperable malignant tumor (Figure 8). Also, preoperative decompression of jaundice in patients

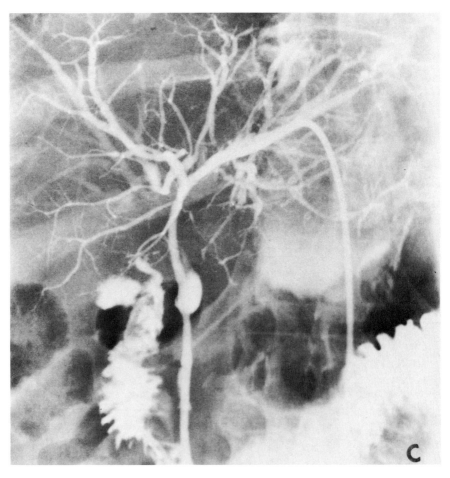

FIG. 8. (*cont.*). **C.** An 8.3 French catheter was advanced through the obstruction into the distal common bile duct, allowing for internal as well as an external drainage.

with operable carcinoma of the pancreatic or duodenal region can be achieved, thus reducing the mortality rate of radical pancreatic resection.

Histologic confirmation of the diagnosis of malignant disease can also be obtained without surgery in many cases. A thin needle aspiration biopsy of the obstructed area can be performed (Ferrucci et al. 1980b), and brush biopsies can also be obtained through the transhepatic catheter (Mendez et al. 1980). In certain situations, internal endoprosthesis can be introduced through the area of obstruction (Hoevels and Ihse 1979). This would eliminate the major problem in bile drainage through a percutaneous catheter; that is, the high frequency of infectious processes of the biliary tract. However, the optimal type of endoprosthesis is not yet available and further experience is needed to resolve this problem.

REFERENCES

Cohen, M. M. 1979. Early diagnosis of pancreatic cancer using ultrasound and fine needle aspiration cytology. Am. Surg. 45:715–717.

Ferrucci, J. T., P. R. Mueller, and W. P. Harbin. 1980a. Percutaneous transhepatic biliary drainage. Radiology 135:1–13.

Ferrucci, J. T., J. Wittenberg, P. R. Mueller, J. F. Simeone, W. P. Harbin, R. H. Kirkpatrick, and P. D. Taft. 1980b. Diagnosis of abdominal malignancy by radiologic fine-needle aspiration biopsy. A. J. R. 134:840–843.

Goldstein, H. M., and J. Zornoza. 1978. Percutaneous transperitoneal aspiration biopsy of pancreatic masses. Am. J. Digest. Dis. 23:840–843.

Haaga, J. R. 1979. New techniques for CT-guided biopsies. A. J. R. 133:633–641.

Hoevels, J., and I. Ihse. 1979. Percutaneous transhepatic insertion of a permanent endoprosthesis in obstructive lesions of the extrahepatic bile ducts. Gastrointest. Radiol. 4:367–377.

Hoevels, J., A. Lunderquist, and I. Ihse. 1978. Percutaneous transhepatic intubation of bile ducts for combined internal-external drainage in preoperative and palliative treatment of obstructive jaundice. Gastrointest. Radiol. 3:23–31.

Ihse, I., B. M. Toregard, and M. Akerman. 1979. Intraoperative fine needle aspiration cytology in pancreatic lesions. Ann. Surg. 190:732–734.

Kaude, J. V., C. H. Weidenmier, and O. F. Agee. 1969. Decompression of bile ducts with percutaneous transhepatic technic. Radiology 93:69–71.

Mendez, G., Jr., E. Russell, J. U. Levi, H. Koolpe, and M. Cohen. 1980. Percutaneous brush biopsy and internal drainage of biliary tree through endoprosthesis. A. J. R. 134:653–659.

Molnar, W., and A. E. Stockum. 1974. Relief of obstructive jaundice through percutaneous transhepatic catheter—A new therapeutic method. A. J. R. 122:356–367.

Mori, K., A. Misumi, M. Sugiyama, M. Okabe, T. Matsuoka, J. Ishii, and M. Akagi. 1977. Percutaneous transhepatic bile drainage. Ann. Surg. 185:111–115.

Nakayama, T., A. Ikeda, and K. Okuda. 1978. Percutaneous transhepatic drainage of the biliary tree. Technique and results in 104 cases. Gastroenterology 74:554–559.

Okuda, K., K. Tanikawa, T. Emura, S. Kuratomi, S. Jinnouchi, K. Urabe, T. Sumikoshi, Y. Kanda, Y. Fukuyama, H. Musha, H. Mori, Y. Shimokawa, F. Yakushiji, and Y. Matsuura. 1974. Nonsurgical percutaneous transhepatic cholangiography—Diagnostic significance in medical problems of the liver. Am. J. Digest. Dis. 19:21–36.

Pereiras, R. V., W. Meiers, B. Kunhardt, M. Troner, D. Hutson, J. S. Barkin, and M. Viamonte. 1978. Fluoroscopically guided thin needle aspiration biopsy of the abdomen and retroperitoneum. A. J. R. 131:197–202.

Ring, E. J., J. A. Oleaga, D. B. Frieman, J. W. Husted, and A. Lunderquist. 1978. Therapeutic applications of catheter cholangiography. Radiology 128:333–338.

Smith, E. H., R. J. Bartrum, Jr., and Y. C. Chang. 1974. Ultrasonically guided percutaneous aspiration biopsy of the pancreas. Radiology 112:737–738.

Tylen, U., J. Hoevels, and J. Vang. 1977. Percutaneous transhepatic cholangiography with external drainage of obstructive biliary lesions. Surg. Gynecol. Obstet. 144:13–18.

Yamanaka, T., and K. Kimura. 1979. Differential diagnosis of pancreatic mass lesion with percutaneous fine-needle aspiration biopsy under ultrasonic guidance. Digest. Dis. Sci. 24:694–699.

Zornoza, J. 1981. Abdomen, *in* Percutaneous Needle Biopsy, J. Zornoza, ed. Williams & Wilkins Co., Baltimore, pp. 102–144.

Zornoza, J., K. Jonsson, S. Wallace, and J. M. Lukeman. 1977. Fine needle aspiration biopsy of retroperitoneal lymph nodes and abdominal masses. An updated report. Radiology 125:87–88.

Gastrointestinal Cancer, edited by
John R. Stroehlein and
Marvin M. Romsdahl.
Raven Press, New York © 1981.

Pathology, Staging, and Prognostic Implications of Gastrointestinal Cancer

Basil Clifford Morson, D.M., F.R.C.Path.

St. Mark's Hospital, London, England

GASTRIC CANCER

Microscopic Appearances

The histological classification of gastric adenocarcinoma is made difficult because the complex structure of the gastric mucosa, both normal and intestinalized, is reflected in the wide variety of tumors which may arise from it. Not only are there marked differences between the appearance of separate carcinomas but also often considerable variety within individual tumors, either in structure, differentiation, or both. Traditional classifications have divided gastric adenocarcinoma into a bewildering number of groups based on such purely descriptive features as glandular differentiation, amount and type of stroma, and mucin production. It is often not clear from the literature whether different authors using a particular term are referring to the same group of tumors.

Because of these problems, Stout (1942) was of the opinion that detailed histological classifications were of little benefit and that a knowledge of the gross appearance of the tumors was more valuable in diagnosis and assessment of prognosis. Other pathologists have pursued a more optimistic policy, and two relatively recent classifications, those of Lauren (1965) and of Mulligan and Rember (1974), warrant consideration.

The Lauren classification which is based on a histological study of 1,344 gastrectomy specimens collected at the University of Turku, Finland, between 1945 and 1964 cuts across the classical descriptions and allocates gastric carcinoma into two main groups, intestinal type and diffuse type. The criteria for this division are based on the histology and cytology of the carcinomas, secretion of mucus, and mode of growth. These characteristics differ in degree from one to another and occasionally one or more are absent in a particular tumor.

In general terms, intestinal type carcinomas have a glandular pattern, usually accompanied by papillary formation or solid components. They are made up of rather large, pleomorphic cells with large, hyperchromatic nuclei often showing mitoses. The cells lining glandular lumina are well polarized columnar cells usually with a prominent brush border. When secretion is present it tends to occur focally in the cytoplasm of only scattered cells; if extracellular, it is located chiefy in the glandular lumina. By contrast, diffuse type carcinomas are made up of scattered solitary or small clusters of cells or, if of a more solid cellular appearance, the individual cells are only loosely attached to each other. Glandular lumina are uncommon and if present small and indefinite. Individual cells are small and fairly uniform with indistinct cytoplasm and regular, only faintly hyperchromatic, although often pyknotic, nuclei without many mitoses. In the occasional tumors with gland formation the lining cells are unpolarized, and surface differentiation of brush border type, if present, is sparse and uneven. The vast majority of tumors show mucin secretion over extensive areas in nearly all of the tumor cells and intracellular secretion is evenly distributed throughout the cytoplasm. If extracellular, secreted mucus is dispersed in the stroma.

The mode of growth in the two types of tumors differs. Intestinal carcinomas usually are well defined and show variation in structure of the tumor between the center and the periphery. Inflammatory cell infiltration is usually profuse. Diffuse carcinomas have a more uniform structure and are not so well defined, with a tendency to spread widely in the mucosa. Connective tissue proliferation is more marked and inflammatory cell infiltration less prominent than in intestinal cancers.

Solid and mucinous tumors occur in both groups but can be distinguished on structural grounds.

Of the 1,344 tumors described by Lauren, 53% were intestinal, 33% diffuse, and the remaining 14% unclassified, including tumors which were atypical or too poorly differentiated to categorize.

Analysis of the two main groups showed a 2:1 male-to-female preponderance in the intestinal group, with the mean age of the patients being 55.4 years. In the diffuse carcinoma group the sex ratio was approximately 1:1 and the mean age of the patients 47.7 years. The frequency and extent of intestinal metaplasia were more marked in the intestinal type carcinomas and were present in all age groups. Macroscopically, 60% of the intestinal type tumors were described as polypous or fungating, 25% excavating, and 15% infiltrating (linitis plastica type), whereas the corresponding figures for diffuse carcinoma were 31%, 26%, and 43%. Of the 153 patients to whom curative treatment was given, those with intestinal type carcinoma had a more favorable prognosis, with 43% surviving for more than three years compared to 35% of the patients with diffuse type. On the basis of these characteristics, Lauren suggested that intestinal type and diffuse type carcinomas might have a differing etiology and pathogenesis.

The classification of Mulligan and Rember (1974), recently updated by Mulligan (1975), is based on a histological analysis of 297 gastric carcinomas in 290 patients seen at the Colorado General Hospital between 1927 and 1973. It divides gastric carcinoma into three groups: mucous cell carcinoma, present in 131 patients (45.2% of the total); pylorocardiac gland cell carcinoma in 82 patients (28.3%); and intestinal cell carcinoma in 68 patients (23.4%). In the latter group, five patients had two primary tumors each and one had three separate primary tumors. In nine patients (3.1%) the tumor was unclassified.

The essential difference between the two classifications is the recognition by Mulligan and Rember of the pylorocardiac gland cell carcinoma as a distinct group. Grossly, these tumors are usually well demarcated and fungate into the lumen of the stomach, or are sometimes widely ulcerated and fibrosed. Satellite foci adjacent to the main carcinoma are infrequent compared with the other two types. The tumors tend to be located in the antrum or at the cardia, and as their name suggests are presumed to arise from pyloric and cardiac gland epithelial cells deep in the gastric mucosa. The male-to-female ratio of 4.13 for this type of tumor compared with 2.81 for the whole series leads Mulligan to suggest that hematogenous stimuli, for example steroid hormones, may be important in their genesis. Microscopically, small and large glands lined by variably stratified or singly oriented low to tall cylindrical cells are present. Papillary infolding is sometimes conspicuous or the lining cells may be flattened by inspissated secretion so that an endothelial or mesothelial appearance results. With single cell orientation there is often striking vacuolation giving rise to clear cells which stain brilliantly with the PAS reagent so that the glands resemble secretory endometrium. The prognosis of this type of tumor is intermediate between the other two types.

Mulligan and Rember describe two patterns of intestinal cell carcinoma based on glandular differentiation and often coexisting in the same tumor, but without prognostic significance.

Another feature of the classification is the smaller percentage of unclassified tumors. The description of mucous cell carcinoma coincides with the diffuse type in the Lauren classification, whereas the intestinal type of Lauren includes both the intestinal cell and pylorocardiac gland cell carcinoma of Mulligan and Rember. The incidence and severity of intestinal metaplasia in those specimens in which adequate sampling of grossly noncancerous mucosa was done were 80% in intestinal cell carcinoma, 43% in pylorocardiac gland cell carcinoma, and 37.5% in mucous cell carcinoma.

The value of both classifications is in their simplicity. As mentioned earlier, the Lauren classification has been widely used in epidemiological studies, and evidence that the intestinal type is more widespread in high-risk areas has been produced. Both classifications emphasize the importance of intestinal metaplasia as an associated lesion of gastric cancer (Morson 1955). In our experience there have been two main drawbacks to the use of the Lauren classification for routine purposes. The first is that in a considerable proportion of cases both types of pattern are seen in the same tumor, especially when extensive sampling of the tumor is carried out. Second, when applied to a series of cases, the five-year survival rate for both types was approximately the same (Hawley et al. 1970). While of considerable interest from the point of view of histogenesis, we have found difficulty in distinguishing histologically the pylorocardiac gland cell carcinomas from the intestinal type, unless obvious clear cells are present. Mulligan (1975), using a modification of the Dukes' classification (Dukes 1932) in staging 266 gastric carcinomas, found only 7.6% of mucous cell carcinomas confined to the stomach, compared to 22.2% of pylorocardiac gland cell carcinomas and 41.3% of intestinal cell carcinomas. In evaluating the prognosis of these different types of tumor, however, he did not take staging into account; therefore, it was not apparent whether the differing prognosis described was related to differences in biological behavior of the tumors or merely reflected differences in their degree of spread at the time of presentation.

In a study (Stemmermann and Brown 1974) of five-year survival in Hawaiian Japanese with gastric carcinoma, and using the Lauren classification, when Stages 2 and 3 in each group were combined, using the TNM system (Kennedy 1970), there was a 27.4% five-year survival in the intestinal group compared with a 9.9% five-year survival in the diffuse group.

One group of gastric tumors with a seemingly good prognosis is the so-called indolent mucoid carcinoma (Brander et al. 1974). In a series of 574 cases this type formed only 1% of resected carcinomas and 12% of mucoid carcinomas (defined on the basis of 50% or more of the tumor in sections being composed of epithelial mucus, either intracellular or extracellular). It was composed of lakes of extracellular mucus in which tumor cells floated either singly or in groups, often as tubules or ribbons of well-differentiated cells. The edge of the tumor had a rounded or "pushing" appearance (Monafo et al. 1962). This tumor corresponds to the intestinal type mucinous carcinoma (Inberg et al. 1973).

EARLY GASTRIC CANCER

Early gastric cancer is defined as a carcinoma which is confined to the mucosa or the mucosa and submucosa, regardless of the presence of lymph node metastasis. It must be emphasized that this is a classification of the gross or macroscopic appearances. Early gastric carcinoma can also be subdivided by microscopic criteria into two groups, intramucosal carcinoma and submucosal carcinoma, both with potential for lymph node metastasis. It is now doubtful whether, for the stomach, the expression carcinoma in situ can ever be used with confidence, because it is difficult and often impossible to be sure whether neoplastic cells have passed across the basement membrane of the crypts into the lamina propria of the mucous membrane. Invasion of the latter only, without extension into the submucosal layer, is commonly observed by Japanese pathologists who have had great experience with early gastric cancer.

Surface carcinoma and superficial carcinoma are terms which have been used synonymously with intramucosal carcinoma. The expression superficial spreading carcinoma was introduced (Stout 1942) to describe that type of carcinoma which spreads superficially in the mucosa and submucosa without penetrating the deep muscle layers until it has covered a considerable surface area. It could be regarded as an early manifestation of linitis plastica. It has little relevance to the classification of early gastric carcinoma. It is important to have international agreement on the nomenclature and classification of tumors, and the Japanese method should be adopted as a worldwide practice.

The classification of early gastric cancer was agreed upon at a meeting of the Japan Gastroenterological Endoscopic Society in 1962 (Murakami 1971). Early gastric cancer was divided into three main groups and three subgroups on the basis of the macroscopic appearances at endoscopy and in gastrectomy specimens (Figure 1) as follows:

Type I. *The protruded type.* The tumor projects clearly into the lumen and includes all polypoid, nodular, and villous tumors. Perhaps the best nomenclature for the English literature would be protuberant or polypoid rather than protruded.

Type II. *The superficial type.* This is further subdivided into three subgroups:
Type II(a). Elevated above the surrounding mucosa. In carefully prepared gastrectomy specimens this is seen as a flat, plaque-like lesion, well circumscribed, and raised up above the surrounding mucosa by only a few millimeters.
Type II(b). Flat. No abnormality is macroscopically visible, although some color change may be visible endoscopically and in very carefully prepared gastrectomy specimens.
Type II(c). Depressed. The surface is slightly depressed below adjacent mucosa for not more than the thickness of the submucosa. Surface erosion may be apparent from a thin covering of exudate.

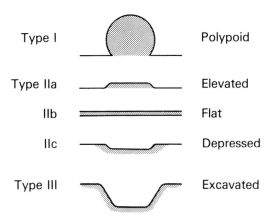

Type I	Polypoid
Type IIa	Elevated
IIb	Flat
IIc	Depressed
Type III	Excavated

FIG. 1. Macroscopic classification of early gastric carcinoma.

Type III. *Excavated type*, which is essentially ulceration of variable depth
into the gastric wall. This is rarely seen in pure form and is almost
always combined with any of the other types.

The Japanese invariably use the symbols of the classification and this
becomes complex when a lesion has features of more than one type. Some
combinations of types are more common than a single type, and all possible
combinations of the five types have been described. The dominant macroscopic feature is placed first. Thus, early gastric cancer can be described as
I + IIc, or IIc + III, or IIa + IIc, etc. Combinations of three types are also
seen.

For many pathologists this classification, using numerals and alphabetical
letters as symbols in various combinations, has seemed complex to the point
of being indigestible. Perhaps it is better that they should look at the classification in Figure 1 and use the descriptive terms rather than the symbols, but the
latter are essential for the description of combinations of types.

This Japanese classification, and its modifications introduced by European
authors, is now being widely adopted and it is essential that pathologists
should understand and become familiar with it. This is necessary not only for
reporting purposes but also because the classification has relevance for the
histogenesis of carcinoma of the stomach. The endoscopist and radiologist as
well as the surgeon and the gastroenterologist who is especially concerned
with the diagnosis and treatment of gastric cancer require this sophisticated
service from the pathologist.

It is important to remember that the type III early gastric carcinoma refers
to the ulceration or excavation and not to the state of the surrounding mucosa.
Thus, the designation of type III carcinoma should seldom be used alone but
in combination with another type such as III + IIc, for example.

The classification of early gastric cancer can be used for lesions of any size,
although most of them are about 2.0 cm in diameter or less. Larger areas of up
to 5 cm in diameter are not uncommon. Most early gastric cancer will be found
in the antrum and along the lesser curvature of the stomach. This is why it is so
important that pathologists be particularly alert for macroscopic abnormalities in these areas. About 10% of gastrectomy specimens for early gastric
cancer will show multifocal lesions.

The relative frequency of the different macroscopic types of early gastric
cancer varies with different authors and with different countries. The protuberant (type I) carcinomas account for between 10% and 15%, but the
incidence given by European authors (Elster et al. 1975, Johansen 1976) is
somewhat higher than that of the Japanese (Nagayo 1968). Superficial (type II)
carcinoma is more common than type I but these are mostly type IIc (superficial depressed); slightly elevated and flat varieties of type II are relatively
much less common. However, European authors report a much higher incidence of all superficial types of early gastric cancers than their Japanese

colleagues. It has already been pointed out that type III early gastric cancer in its pure form is rare, but all combinations with the other types are common. Thus, the combination forms, not unexpectedly, account for about 75% of all early gastric cancers reported in Japan and between 40% and 50% in the main European publications (Elster et al. 1975, Johansen 1976, Nagayo 1968). The excavating type of early gastric cancer is more commonly seen in Japan than in Europe, although usually in combination with other types. This should not be taken to mean that all excavating lesions are ulcer-cancers in the sense that the carcinomas arose from previously benign peptic ulcers. There is considerable disagreement among Japanese authors about the frequency of ulcer-cancer in Japan, but if strict criteria (Newcomb 1932) are observed the incidence is low (Nakamura et al. 1967). This low incidence would conform with the current opinion of North American and European pathologists.

The relative incidence of the various types and combinations of types of early gastric carcinoma in different geographical areas could have epidemiological importance. This is one reason why the Japanese classification should be adopted as a worldwide practice.

Histology of Early Gastric Cancer

Types I (protuberant) and IIa (superficial elevated) early gastric carcinoma are almost invariably well-differentiated adenocarcinomas. Among the type IIc (superficial, flat), well-differentiated, poorly differentiated, signet-ring cell, and undifferentiated carcinomas are all seen but the degree of differentiation in any one lesion is often variable (Elster et al. 1975). The relative frequency of poorly differentiated and undifferentiated carcinomas is much higher among the type III (excavated) early gastric cancers than any of the other types in the classification. In general, then, elevated carcinomas are usually well-differentiated, flat ones contain all histological types, and depressed and excavating cancers have the highest incidence of poorly differentiated and undifferentiated carcinomas.

It must be emphasized that the gastric mucosa has to be very carefully scrutinized for evidence of intramucosal carcinoma, especially in the case of type II early gastric cancers. Invasion of the lamina propria only by undifferentiated or signet-ring carcinoma cells in particular can be missed very easily. For this reason multiple sections of the mucosa around gastric ulcers should be examined for signs of intramucosal carcinoma. Similarly, very careful scrutiny of gastric biopsies is essential. Mucin stains can be helpful in the detection of isolated clumps of undifferentiated carcinoma cells in the lamina propria.

This is perhaps the right moment to return to the problems of differentiating between epithelial atypia in gastric mucosa, carcinoma in situ, intramucosal carcinoma, and what many pathologists would call an adenoma of the stomach.

Epithelial atypia (or dysplasia) is useful for the description of cellular changes which fall short of the full criteria for the diagnosis of carcinoma in situ. The latter must exist at some stage in the progression of epithelial dysplasia of gastric mucosa into invasive carcinoma but, as already stated, it is usually impossible to be certain that the neoplastic cells have not passed across the basement membrane of the crypts into the lamina propria without serial sectioning of the entire lesion, which is impracticable. Probably the phase of carcinoma in situ in the stomach is an extremely short one.

For the reasons given it is recommended that the expression carcinoma in situ be dropped in favor of intramucosal carcinoma, provided this is used only when invasion of the lamina propria has been demonstrated. For doubtful cases it is essential to examine multiple sections through the tissue. Even then, invasion may not be demonstrated and the pathologist is in a dilemma. The Japanese have recognized this problem and have introduced the expression "borderline lesion." For the purist this is an unsuitable expression for the description of a histological appearance, but it does illustrate the problem. Study of the Japanese literature suggests that what the Japanese are describing might be called an adenoma by many European and North American pathologists. Although polypoid adenomas of the stomach do occur they are rare compared with their counterparts in the colon. They are usually tubulo-villous or villo-glandular in their histological structure. The borderline lesion of the Japanese pathologists appears to us more like a slightly elevated or even flat adenoma and would correspond to a type IIa or IIb early gastric cancer. It could be called intramucosal adenoma in order to distinguish it from polypoid adenoma. The macroscopic or endoscopic classification thus has some relevance to the problems of classification of gastric polyps, especially the neoplastic group or 'adenomas'. The Japanese are currently observing the borderline lesion by regular gastric biopsy to see how it behaves. There is some evidence that it progresses to invasive carcinoma only slowly and in some cases possibly not at all, rather like the adenoma-carcinoma sequence in the large intestine (Murakami 1971, Muto et al. 1975).

Spread and Prognosis

Lymph node metastases are present in 90% of autopsies of patients with gastric carcinomas and in 70% of surgical resections (Stout 1943). The nodes most commonly involved are those along the lesser curve, followed by those on the greater curve. There is also early involvement of nodes in the porta hepatis and around the celiac axis. Supraclavicular node involvement, though well recognized clinically, is not common. It is important for the surgeon to remove, and the pathologist to examine, all nodes, however small, since even the smallest apparently uninvolved node may contain secondary growth, and there is evidence that prognosis depends on the number of nodes involved.

The diagnosis of carcinoma of the stomach is still regarded by many as a

Table 1. *Lymph Node Involvement and Survival Rate in 139 Patients with Resectable Gastric Carcinoma*

Node involvement	Total cases	Five-year survivors	Percentage
Nodes not involved	37	15	40.5
Nodes involved	102	12	11.8
Total	139	27	19.4

death warrant. This is quite unjustified. A report from the Mayo Clinic (Cutler 1969) gives a 10-year survival rate in surgically treated cases of 20%, which is similar to the crude five-year survival figure for our own small series of cases (Table 1). However, these are figures for advanced gastric cancer, which is the stage most commonly seen in Western Europe and North America. In Japan about 30% of all gastrectomies for carcinoma of the stomach are for early gastric cancer, as defined by Japanese researchers. This appears to be the result of greatly improved methods of diagnosis by radiology, endoscopy, biopsy, and exfoliative cytology.

Prognosis bears no clear relationship to macroscopic type of growth, location of tumor, or duration of symptoms prior to surgical treatment (Brooks et al. 1965, Urban and McNeer 1959, Brown et al. 1961). It depends mostly on the presence or absence of involved lymph nodes. The prognosis is significantly better when no lymph nodes are involved, and better than average when only one or two nodes are affected (Harvey et al. 1951) (Tables 1 and 2). A careful search for, and histological examination of, all lymph nodes must be made, as absence of enlargement in size is no criterion for freedom from metastasis.

The incidence of lymph node metastasis in early carcinoma varies with the depth of penetration into the wall of the stomach. In cases of intramucosal carcinoma, lymph node involvement is exceptional but can occur. Only one example is reported in 32 cases. In contrast, the same author (Kidokoro 1971) found a 12% incidence of metastasis to regional nodes in a large series of submucosal cancers collected from 22 hospitals. Advanced gastric cancer has a very high frequency of lymph node involvement of the order of 60%-70%.

Table 2. *Numbers of Involved Nodes and Survival Rate in 102 Patients with Gastric Carcinoma*

Survival	Total cases	Average nodes involved
Under five years	90	8.1
Over five years	12	4.2

The five-year survival rate after surgical treatment for early gastric carcinoma is about 95% (Kidokoro 1971). Recurrence after treatment for intramucosal carcinoma is very rare, and most of the deaths are found in patients who have had invasion into the submucosa. Even so, the survival rate of this group averages about 93%.

These figures should be considered in the light of the fact that in Japan about 30% of gastrectomies for cancer are carried out for early carcinoma. This means that the prognosis of gastric cancer can be very greatly improved if the disease is detected at an early stage of development. If this Japanese achievement is to be matched by European and North American researchers, it is essential that we improve our methods of detection of early gastric cancer and make these facilities available to a much larger number of patients than hitherto.

COLORECTAL CANCER

Modern operations for cancer of the colon and rectum are based on meticulous studies of the spread of cancer in surgical specimens and the relationship between pathology and prognosis after surgical treatment (Grinnell 1953, Galante et al. 1967, Dukes 1940).

The Dukes' classification was introduced at St. Mark's Hospital in 1928 and is now accepted all over the world as a valuable guide to prognosis. The Dukes' A case (15% of all patients undergoing surgery) is one in which the intestinal cancer has spread into the tissues of the bowel wall but not beyond the muscularis propria, and where there are no lymph node metastases. It is known today, after many years of follow-up, that a patient with cancer of the colon or rectum at the Dukes' A stage can be almost invariably cured of his disease by appropriate surgical treatment. A Dukes' B case (35% of all patients undergoing surgery) is one in which the growth has spread beyond the muscularis propria into the pericolic or perirectal tissues in continuity, but where there are no regional lymph node metastases. Such patients can be told that they have, on the average, about a 70% chance of being cured of their disease. Once the lymph nodes are involved (Dukes' C cases), the prognosis becomes poor irrespective of the extent of direct spread; only about one in three patients survives five years. At surgery, about 50% of all cancers are in this stage. The importance of early diagnosis of cancer of the colon and rectum is obvious from a study of the Dukes' classification.

Local Spread

Direct spread of the primary tumor in continuity occurs along those tissue planes which provide the least resistance. The submucosa is composed of loose connective tissue which is readily involved, but the muscularis propria offers considerable resistance to infiltration by malignant cells because of its dense structure. As a result, adenocarcinoma tends to spread through those gaps in the muscle through which the blood supply to the mucous membrane travels. It is also quite common to see infiltration along the myenteric plexus between the circular and longitudinal layers. Beyond the muscularis propria the soft adipose and connective tissues of the serosa or mesenteric border offer little resistance; however, the peritoneal membrane is a tough structure which often remains intact despite being stretched over the carcinomatous mass. It is unusual to find much direct upward or downward spread in continuity in the submucosal layer beyond the visible borders of the tumor, in contrast to what is usually seen in gastric or esophageal carcinoma. However, extensive downward intramural spread of rectal cancer can occur with tumors of a high grade of malignancy, which is the main reason why low anterior resection for high grade rectal cancer should be avoided (Quer et al. 1953). The relationship between local spread in continuity and prognosis after surgical treatment has been described. In cases without lymph node metastases the corrected five-year survival rate was 90% with slight spread, 80% with moderate spread in continuity, and 57% with deeply invasive tumors. It is clearly important to describe the extent of local spread of the carcinoma in surgical specimens of intestinal cancer because this is a remarkably accurate guide to prognosis. The relationship of local spread to prognosis is also affected by the grade of malignancy of the primary tumor; there is a much higher incidence of high grade tumors in surgical specimens showing extensive local spread than in those showing slight or moderate extension.

Lymphatic Spread

Carcinoma can be seen permeating lymphatic channels, particularly in the submucosal and extramural tissues. The distinction between lymphatics and capillaries is often difficult. This problem is discussed later, in the section on venous spread.

Lymph node metastasis appears to be a progressive process in which carcinoma spreads from node to node. It is rare to find involved nodes at a distance from the primary tumor and unaffected nodes intervening. In the great majority of cases of carcinoma of the colon and rectum, lymphatic spread follows the most direct route to the regional lymph nodes. If these become involved, lymph flow can be blocked and so-called retrograde lymphatic metastasis may then arise (Grinnell 1966). This is only apparent in advanced cancer and is associated with a very poor prognosis.

The presence of lymph node metastases in a surgical specimen of colonic or rectal cancer (Dukes' C cases) greatly worsens prognosis. The five-year survival rate is reduced to about 30% compared with an 80% survival for cases without involved nodes (Dukes' A and B cases combined). The prognosis also varies with the number of involved lymph nodes. Thus, the five-year survival rate is about 60% with only one node affected, 35% with two to five nodes involved, and only 20% when six or more nodes are affected. The influence of lymph node involvement on prognosis is also closely related to the grade of malignancy of the primary tumor and the extent of local spread. There is a progressive increase in the percentage of cases with lymphatic metastases when passing from low to average and on to high grade of malignancy.

Spread to the inguinal lymph nodes occurs in rectal cancer. In the St. Mark's Hospital series of surgical specimens only 2% of all rectal cancers showed involvement of inguinal nodes, but if cancers of the lower third of the rectum are taken alone the figure rises to 7%. Inguinal node involvement mostly occurs when the hemorrhoidal glands are already affected.

Sinus cell hyperplasia of regional lymph nodes occurs in about one third of surgical specimens for cancer of the colorectum. It has been suggested that this could be an indication of host resistance (Wartman 1959). Using the WHO protocol (Cottier et al. 1972, 1973) the morphology of lymph nodes in colorectal cancer among five-year survivors compared with non-survivors showed no differences (Price, unpublished data). Conversely, another study of lymph node histology in carcinoma of the sigmoid colon did show a relationship between lymph node histology and survival after surgical treatment (Patt et al. 1975). Further studies are clearly indicated.

Venous Spread

Surgical specimens should always be very carefully examined for evidence of permeation of veins by carcinoma. This can take the form of so-called visible venous spread or may be detected only in microscopic preparations (Dukes and Bussey 1958, Dukes 1940).

Dissection of the mesenteric vessels may reveal evidence of massive permeation of the regional veins by tumor cells. It appears as if the malignant tumor, having found a path of least resistance, has pushed a root-like process along the lumen. Inspection of veins close to the primary growth can also reveal lesser degrees of visible venous permeation. Particularly close observation should be made of the submucosal venous plexus at the margins of the primary growth.

Examination of a surgical specimen of intestinal cancer should include sections of the growing edge of the tumor where it is spreading through the bowel wall, as well as blocks of tissue taken from the margin of the growth on its mucosal aspect. In a personally studied series of more than 700 surgical specimens of rectal cancer, 50% showed spread of cancer into regional veins. The incidence of submucosal venous spread only was 15%, and in 35% there was evidence of permeation of extramural vessels. The incidence of venous spread was greatest in specimens where there was also involvement of regional lymph nodes and when the primary tumor was of a high grade of malignancy (Talbot et al. 1980).

In our experience the presence of submucous venous spread only has little or no effect on prognosis. Permeation of extramural veins appears to have a serious effect, however, reducing the five-year survival rate from 55% to about 30% (Carroll 1963). This is particularly true for growth found within thick-walled extramural veins, which are defined as veins with a muscular wall. It has also been shown that extramural venous spread is associated with a high incidence of metastatic spread to the liver and other sites both at the time of operation and in the follow-up period. Again, this is particularly so if growth was found within thick-walled extramural veins. It is clear, however, that the presence of growth within veins, and even massive permeation of such vessels, does not mean that malignant embolism has occurred or that distant metastases will inevitably develop. Some explanation for this can be found from microscopic examination of veins permeated by carcinoma.

The distinction between vein, capillary, and lymphatic can be difficult. The presence of smooth muscle within the wall of a vessel, red blood cells in the lumen, and a companion artery or arteriole are usually sufficient to identify the vessel as a vein; however, it is sometimes impossible to distinguish between a capillary and a lymphatic. It is particularly interesting to observe the histology at the growing point of venous permeation by carcinoma. The growth is often covered by a platelet thrombus, beneath which there is organizing granulation tissue covering the tumor. This appearance is particularly characteristic of well-differentiated adenocarcinoma, while undifferentiated cells usually lie free within the lumen of the vein. It is obvious that free malignant cells will readily pass into the portal circulation, whereas a tongue of differentiated adenocarcinoma can become strangulated by thrombosis within the lumen of the vein or break off to form an embolus. The latter by this time may have its own blood supply, which would make its survival as a metastasis more likely.

Prognosis

About one half of all patients with carcinoma of the colon and rectum can be cured by appropriate surgical treatment (Grinnell 1953, Galante et al. 1967, Muir 1956, Hughes 1963, Shepherd and Jones 1971). However, there are reports of lower cure rates from some centers (Dukes et al. 1948). Differences in survival rates can often be explained by variations in the selection of cases and methods of statistical analysis. It is important, for example, to make a distinction between the results of treatment in centers specializing in rectal and colonic surgery and those from general hospitals. The crude five-year survival rate is a far less accurate way of measuring the cure rate than is survival "corrected" for differences in age and sex as well as deaths from intercurrent disease. Allowance must also be made for the resectability rate, whether the operation was palliative because of the presence of locally inoperable growth or distant metastases, or radical in the sense that the surgeon believed that he had completely removed the primary tumor and all known metastases. Obviously the postoperative mortality rate also has to be taken into account. However, apart from these surgical considerations the results of treatment of cancer of the colon and rectum depend on the grade of malignancy and the extent of spread of the carcinoma in the surgical specimen. In the foregoing pages it has been shown how, for example, the Dukes' A case has a virtually 100% chance of cure, but that once lymph node metastasis has taken place the cure rate drops to about 30%. It is clearly important that pathologists should examine surgical specimens of intestinal cancer in considerable detail with special emphasis on the grade of malignancy, the extent of local spread in continuity, the presence of venous spread, and the number of involved lymph nodes (Slaney et al. 1968). The Dukes' classification is used throughout the world as a valuable guide to prognosis and should be reported as part of the examination of every surgical specimen of intestinal cancer.

EARLY COLORECTAL CANCER

Adenocarcinoma of the colon and rectum has no potential for lymph node metastasis until it has invaded across the line of the muscularis mucosae into the submucosal layer. This is in contrast to gastric cancer in which it has been shown that intramucosal carcinoma has potential for such metastasis. The difference in behavior is because the gastric mucosa has a rich supply of lymphatics whereas the colorectal mucous membrane has few, if any, until the level of the muscularis mucosae is reached (Fenoglio et al. 1973). As long as neoplastic cells are confined within the mucosa, the term "adenoma" is used. Early colorectal cancer must then be defined as invasion into the submucosal layer. It has been shown that if spread in continuity is confined to the submucosal plane of the bowel wall which, of course, includes the stalk of a polyp, then the risk of lymph node metastasis having already taken place is of the order of only a few percent with all but very poorly differentiated carcinomas, which are uncommon anyway. However, once growth has spread into the muscularis propria it is of the order of about 10% (Morson 1966). With spread in continuity beyond the muscularis propria into the pericolic or perirectal tissues, the figure is greatly increased to about 60%. These facts have been used to show that local excision has an important part to play in the treatment of early cancer of the colorectum (Morson et al. 1977).

Many early colorectal cancers present as malignant polyps, which means a spherical tumor on a stalk that can usually be removed easily at sigmoidoscopy or colonoscopy. Others may be quite large tumors, mostly consisting of adenoma but in which there is a focus of early cancer. Some are all adenocarcinoma but independent of surface size and shape have not spread deeper than the submucosal layer. Of course, such histological information is only obtained when the tumor has been removed for histological examination.

A recent report has confirmed that a policy of local excision for early colorectal carcinoma can be very successful, with a 100% cure rate in carefully selected cases (Morson et al. 1977). The policy is based on complete local excision or total biopsy of the tumor in the first place, whether by an intrarectal approach or via the colonoscope. If it is a tumor on a stalk, it can be placed directly in fixative. Flat or sessile tumors, including large specimens, should be pinned out on cork, taking care to demonstrate the surgical margins of excision. Careful preparation of the specimen is an essential prerequisite to histologic examination. This involves multiple step sections through the whole tumor to detect the presence of invasive carcinoma across the line of the muscularis mucosae, the depth of invasion, and the completeness of local excision. The grade of the carcinoma should also be assessed.

The policy practiced at St. Mark's Hospital has been to advise local excision only for those tumors in which excision appeared to be complete and the carcinoma was not poorly differentiated. Any decision as to whether to perform a further radical operation is the responsibility of the surgeon or endoscopist, but this should be made in close collaboration with the pathologist. In recent years, and particularly since the advent of therapeutic colonoscopy, there has been an increasing place for local excision in the treatment of early colorectal cancer. It is also interesting that in the St. Mark's Hospital series of 143 cases, no less than 78.3% of these early carcinomas showed histological evidence of origin from benign adenoma.

Thus, the concept of early colorectal cancer is different from that of early gastric cancer and this has important implications for treatment. It must be emphasized that the expression early colorectal cancer is not meant to imply a stage in histogenesis, but rather cancer which is essentially curable, in an analogous way to the use of early gastric cancer in Japan (Murakami 1971).

REFERENCES

Brander, W. L., P. R. G. Needham, and A. D. Morgan. 1974. Indolent mucoid carcinoma of stomach. J. Clin. Pathol. 27:536.

Brooks, V. S., J. A. H. Waterhouse, and D. J. Powell. 1965. Carcinoma of the stomach: A 10 year survey of results and factors affecting prognosis. Br. Med. J. i:1577.

Brown, C. H., M. Merlo, and J. B. Hazard. 1961. Clinical study of 5-year survivors after surgery for gastric carcinoma: Report of 58 patients including 12 fifteen-year survivors. Gastroenterology 40:188.

Carroll, S. E. 1963. The prognostic significance of gross venous invasion in carcinoma of the rectum. Can. J. Surg. 6:281.

Cottier, H., J. Turk, and L. Sobin. 1972. A proposal for a standardised system of reporting human lymph node morphology in relation to immunological function. Bull. WHO 47:375 and J. Clin. Pathol. (1973), 26:317.

Cutler, S. J. 1969. Trends in cancer of the digestive tract. Surgery 65:740.

Dukes, C. E. 1932. The classification of cancer of the rectum. J. Pathol. Bact. 35:323.

Dukes, C. E. 1940. Cancer of the rectum: An analysis of 1000 cases. J. Pathol. Bact. 50:527.

Dukes, C. E., H. J. R. Bussey, and G. W. Lamb. 1948. The examination and classification of operation specimens of intestinal cancer. Bull. Inte. Ass. Med. Mus. 28:55.

Dukes, C. E., and H. J. R. Bussey. 1958. The spread of rectal cancer and its effect on prognosis. Br. J. Cancer 12:309.

Elster, K., F. Kolaczek, K. Shimamoto, and H. Freitag. 1975. Early gastric cancer experience in Germany. Endoscopy 7(3):5.

Fenoglio, C. M., G. I. Kaye, and N. Lane. 1973. Distribution of human colonic lymphatics in normal hyperplastic and adenomatous tissue. Its relationship to metastasis from small carcinomas in pedunculated adenomas. Gastroenterology 64:51.

Galante, M., J. Englebert, and W. S. Fletcher. 1967. Cancer of the colon. Ann. Surg. 165:732.

Grinnell, R. S. 1953. Results in treatment of carcinoma of the rectum. Surg., Gynecol. Obstet. 96:31.

Grinnell, R. S. 1966. Lymphatic block with atypical retrograde lymphatic metastases and spread in carcinoma of the colon and rectum. Ann. Surg. 163:272.

Harvey, H. D., J. B. Titherington, A. P. Stout, and F. B. St. John. 1951. Gastric carcinoma. Cancer 4:717.

Hawley, P. R., P. Westerholm, and B. C. Morson. 1970. Pathology and prognosis of carcinoma of the stomach. Br. J. Surg. 57:877.

Hughes, E. S. R. 1963. Results of treatment of carcinoma of the colon and rectum. Br. Med. J. ii:9.

Inberg, M. V., P. Lauren, J. Vuori, and S. J. Viikari. 1973. Prognosis in intestinal-type and diffuse gastric carcinoma with special reference to the effect of the stromal reaction. Acta Chir. Scand. 139:273.

Johansen, A. A. 1976. Early gastric cancer. Current topics in pathology, *in* Monograph on Pathology of the Gastrointestinal Tract, B. C. Morson, ed. Springer-Verlag, Berlin, pp. 1–47.

Kennedy, B. J. 1970. TNM classification for stomach cancer. Cancer 26:971.

Kidokoro, T. 1971. Frequency of resection, metastasis and five-year survival rate of early gastric carcinoma in a surgical clinic, *in* Gann Monograph on Cancer Research: Early Gastric Cancer, Vol. II, T. Murakami, ed. University Park Press, Baltimore, pp. 45–49.

Lauren, P. 1965. The two histological main types of gastric carcinoma: Diffuse and so-called intestinal-type carcinoma. Acta Pathol. Microbiol. Scand. 64:31.

Monafo, W. W., G. L. Karuse, and J. G. Medina. 1962. Carcinoma of the stomach. Morphological characteristics affecting survival. Arch. Surg. 85:754.

Morson, B. C. 1955. Carcinoma arising from areas of intestinal metaplasia in the gastric mucosa. Br. J. Cancer 9:377.

Morson, B. C. 1966. Factors influencing the prognosis of early cancer of the rectum. Proc. R. Soc. Med. 59:607.

Morson, B. C., H. J. R. Bussey, and S. Samoorian. 1977. Policy of local excision for early cancer of the colorectum. Gut 18:1045.

Muir, E. G. 1956. Results of treatment in carcinoma of the colon and rectum. Br. Med. J. ii:742.

Mulligan, R. M. 1975. Histogenesis and biologic behaviour of gastric carcinoma, *in* Gastrointestinal and Hepatic Pathology Decennial, 1966–1975, S. C. Sommers, ed. Appleton-Century-Crofts, New York, pp. 31–101.

Mulligan, R. M., and R. R. Rember. 1974. Histogenesis and biologic behaviour of gastric carcinoma. Arch. Pathol. 58:1.

Murakami, T. 1971. Pathomorphological diagnosis: Definition and gross classification of early gastric cancer, *in* Early Gastric Cancer, Gann Monograph on Cancer Research II, T. Murakami, ed. University of Tokyo Press, Tokyo, pp. 53–55.

Muto, T., H. J. R. Bussey, and B. C. Morson. 1975. The evolution of cancer of the colon and rectum. Cancer 36:2251.

Nagayo, T. 1968. Mode of origin of gastric mucosal cancer with special reference to that of "superficial spreading type," *in* Gann Monograph on Cancer Research: Epidemiological, Experimental and Clinical Studies on Gastric Cancer, R. Kinosita, T. Nagayo, and T. Tanaka, eds. Maruzen Co., Tokyo, pp. 113–122.

Nakamura, K., H. Sugano, K. Takagi, and A. Fuchigami. 1967. Histopathological study on early carcinoma of the stomach: Some considerations on the ulcer-cancer by analysis of 144 foci of the superficial spreading carcinoma. Gann 58:377.

Newcomb, W. D. 1932. The relationship between peptic ulceration and gastric carcinoma. Br. J. Surg. 20:279.

Patt, D. J., R. K. Brynes, J. W. Vardiman, and L. W. Coppleson. 1975. Mesocolic lymph node histllogy is an important prognostic indicator for patients with carcinoma of the sigmoid colon: An immunomorphologic study. Cancer 35:1388.

Quer, E. A., D. C. Dahlin, and C. W. Mayo. 1953. Retrograde intramural spread of carcinoma of the rectum and rectosigmoid. Surg., Gynecol. Obstet. 96:24.

Shepherd, J. M., and J. S. P. Jones. 1971. Adenocarcinoma of the large bowel. Br. J. Cancer 25:680.

Slaney, G., J. A. Waterhouse, and J. Powell. 1968. Cancer of the colon and rectum and its response to treatment. Gut 9:730.

Stemmermann, G. N., and C. Brown. 1974. A survival study of intestinal and diffuse types of gastric carcinoma. Cancer 33:1190.

Stout, A. P. 1942. Superficial spreading type of carcinoma of the stomach. Arch. Surg. 44:651.

Stout, A. P. 1943. Pathology of carcinoma of the stomach. Arch. Surg. 46:807.

Talbot, I. C., S. Ritchie, M. H. Leighton, A. O. Hughes, H. J. R. Bussey, and B. C. Morson. 1980. The clinical significance of invasion of veins by rectal cancer. Br. J. Surg. 67:439.

Urban, C. H., and G. McNeer. 1959. The relation of the morphology of gastric carcinoma to long and short term survival. Cancer 12:1158.

Wartman, W. B. 1959. Sinus cell hyperplasia of lymph nodes regional to adenocarcinoma of the breast and colon. Br. J. Cancer 13:389.

Gastroesophageal and Pancreatic Cancer

Gastrointestinal Cancer, edited by
John R. Stroehlein and
Marvin M. Romsdahl.
Raven Press, New York © 1981.

Gastroesophageal Cancers: An Overview

John R. Stroehlein, M.D.

Department of Medicine, The University of Texas System Cancer Center
M. D. Anderson Hospital and Tumor Institute, Houston, Texas

Since the last Clinical Conference devoted to gastrointestinal cancers, held in 1966, many improvements have occurred in identification of premalignant conditions, accuracy of diagnosis, and selective forms of therapy for esophageal and gastric cancer. Advances have in some ways been more substantive in these conditions than for many forms of gastrointestinal cancer. It is therefore paradoxical that cancers of the esophagus and stomach are not overly emphasized in the United States, with much of the literature in these areas coming from abroad. This is due partly to the relatively small incidence of esophageal and gastric cancer, the limitations of therapy—some perceived and many real—and a decreasing incidence of gastric cancer. The above notwithstanding, these diseases are very important to the health of the nation since esophageal cancer is expected to affect approximately 8,800 individuals and claim 8,100 lives during the coming year. Gastric cancer, despite a decreasing incidence, is still expected to affect roughly 23,900 persons and take 13,000 lives (American Cancer Society 1980). In view of improvements in identification of premalignant disorders, diagnosis, and therapy, these diseases are no less important for the individual physicians who care for patients with esophageal and gastric disorders. We have therefore tried to identify some of the important aspects of diagnosis and treatment, and these will be discussed in more detail during following presentations.

We have already heard of the geographical variations in incidence of these cancers and some potential etiological considerations. Additional pathological or anatomic conditions related to development of esophageal and gastric cancer have now been recognized and are attracting increased attention. For esophageal cancer these include a remarkably increased incidence of squamous cell carcinoma in association with head and neck squamous cell cancer (Goldstein and Zornosa 1978, Weaver et al. 1979) and the development of adenocarcinoma from Barrett's esophagus wherein a sequence of metaplasia—dysplasia—carcinoma is now accepted (Dees et al. 1978, Haggitt 1978). Both situations have considerable implications in diagnosis, surveillance, and therapy and will be discussed in more detail during the next two reports.

Meanwhile our attention in gastric cancer has focused on an accepted classification of early gastric carcinoma which was first proposed by the Japanese Gastroenterological Endoscopy Society and modified temporarily by the Japanese Research Society for Gastric Cancer. Early gastric cancer is, by definition, confined to the mucosa and submucosa and morphologically classified as being polypoid (type I), superficial (type II-a-c), or excavated (type III). Recognition of the morphological characteristics has also been described in the Western literature and has contributed to roentgenographic and endoscopic diagnosis of these lesions (Morson 1977). When diagnosed early, gastric cancer has a 90% five-year survival rate which makes accurate recognition very important (Arima and Shimura 1978, Miller et al. 1979, Serck-Hanssen 1979, Sugiura et al. 1979).

In addition to characterization of early gastric cancer, the past two decades have brought about an appreciation of an increased risk for developing differentiated gastric cancer in the presence of intestinal metaplasia (Kawai and Ida 1977, Salas 1977, Nakahara 1978) and an increased risk for gastric cancer occurring in the gastric stump 15 years following partial gastrectomy for benign peptic ulcer disease (Serck-Hanssen et al. 1977, DeBoer et al. 1978, Hellers et al. 1979). Diagnostic aspects of these and other gastric lesions, including problems associated with differentiating benign from malignant ulcers, will be described in more detail during a subsequent presentation. It is important to recognize that the diagnostic capabilities which will be described have greatly enhanced diagnostic accuracy. These techniques, including air contrast roentgenographic examination and refinements in fiberoptic endoscopy with directed biopsy and cytology, have contributed markedly to our appreciation of early gastric cancer and our understanding of the natural history of upper gastrointestinal cancers and their premalignant counterparts. They have also helped in evaluating response to therapy and identifying early local recurrence. The highly developed accuracy of these diagnostic tests (Laufer et al. 1975, Graham et al. 1979, Kasugai et al. 1978, Maruyama 1979, Treichel 1979) has made effective early screening of high risk groups possible (Hiraoka et al. 1978, Sugiura 1979, Serck-Hanssen 1979). These modalities also offer the opportunity for future research studies related to precancerous conditions and precancerous lesions (Morson et al. 1980).

Despite the recognition of risk factors and the potential for early diagnosis, few groups in the United States are at sufficient risk to justify widespread use of screening techniques. Thus most diseases are not well localized when clinically identified. Those that are offer the possibility for surgical cure, as will be discussed. Unfortunately therapeutic limitations do exist for most patients with esophageal cancer, and these contribute to the debate regarding surgical versus nonsurgical management (Moertel 1978a, Parker 1978). Selection of patients and results of surgery for esophageal squamous cell carcinoma in the M. D. Anderson experience will be discussed in more detail, and combined modalities such as surgery plus radiation therapy will be described.

In a large, nonrandomized survey of 239 patients with esophageal cancer, combination of these modalities improved the outlook for patients treated with preoperative radiotherapy for esophageal squamous cell carcinoma (Nakayama 1979); however, definitive work has yet to be accomplished. Despite the favorable outlook for selected patients with esophageal cancer treated surgically, many are not suitable candidates for surgical treatment, and palliative forms of therapy have to be considered. These will not be specifically covered during the course of this session except as they pertain to radiation therapy or resection used for palliation with beneficial results (Piccone et al. 1979). Palliative management has been summarized recently by others (Payne 1979). Rather than debating which modality of therapy is preferable, reports will focus on patient selection for therapy and factors which contribute to complications of therapy.

In the case of gastric cancer there is no debate as to the primary therapy, which currently is surgical; however, the indications for surgery and the type of surgical approach that will provide the best results for the most patients has become well established only within the past few years. Appropriate surgical management for gastric cancer will be discussed in detail. More aggressive surgical approaches should be reserved for selected clinical situations, including fundal lesions or those with direct involvement of adjacent organs. Palliative care should be directed to the symptomatic patient and provided by resection as opposed to bypass where feasible (Buchholtz et al. 1978, Giuli 1979, Ekbom and Gleysteen 1980). For both esophageal and gastric surgery, nutritional support has proven to be of considerable value in reducing postoperative complications. In previous years surgical therapy would have been prohibited for many patients. Nutritional assessment, principles of application, and illustrations of effectiveness of nutritional support have already been discussed.

In the field of chemotherapy some improvements have been made in the management of gastric cancer. Results of adjuvant treatment programs for gastric adenocarcinoma in the United States are anxiously awaited. The chemotherapy of esophageal and gastric lesions, which will be presented in more detail, shows some promise in the improvement of chemotherapeutic management of upper gastrointestinal cancer. Diagnostic accuracy, nutritional support, and selection of surgical or radiation therapy alternatives have already been reasonably well established and for the time being fully developed. Unless a greater percentage of individuals at increased risk can be more accurately identified and placed under surveillance through the application of screening tests, with resultant diagnosis of esophageal and gastric cancer at a very early stage, further improvements in survival are going to depend largely on improvements in our chemotherapeutic management of these disorders. At present a number of agents with activity against esophageal and gastric neoplasms have been developed, and the use of combination therapy for gastric cancer has been shown to increase the response rates. However, many forms of combination therapy have not significantly improved survival (Moertel 1978b). A recent report, which will be updated during the discussion on chemotherapy for gastric cancer, has demonstrated the potential for improved survival using a combination of 5-fluorouracil, Adriamycin, and mitomycin (MacDonald et al. 1980). The efficacy of this regimen is now being tested for less advanced conditions, and also including adjuvant therapy. Further controlled studies are needed to assess the long-term effects of adjuvant chemotherapy; however, there is some indication that adjuvant chemotherapy may improve survival for gastric cancer patients (Koyama 1978).

Better characterization of prognostic factors should aid in selection of patients for therapy at all stages of disease, although in some studies prognostic variables have not been effective indicators of response to therapy. Radiation in combination with chemotherapy has been used to treat esophageal cancer and gastric cancer. This combination is primarily limited by toxicity; however, in patients who tolerate therapy it may produce some improvement in long-term results. These and other combination modalities including immunotherapy are likely to receive attention in further studies because of early reports in these areas of investigation.

It is hoped that the technical improvements and our increased understanding of esophageal and gastric cancer which enhance diagnosis, as well as the development of supportive measures which enhance the therapeutic options (particularly as they pertain to surgical management) will serve as a sound foundation for future improvements in the care of patients with these disorders. The following discussions represent our attempt to present current knowledge in many of these areas, recognizing full well our deficiencies but seeking to establish achievements and build upon the existing foundations to develop more effective therapy through quality care, insightful observations, and sound basic and clinical investigations.

REFERENCES

American Cancer Society. Cancer Facts and Figures. 1980. American Cancer Society. New York 1980.

Arima, S., and H. Shimura. 1978. Clinicopathological study on 100 early gastric cancer cases. Gastroenterol. 13:244–254.

Buchholtz, T. W., C. E. Welch, and R. A. Malt. 1978. Clinical correlates of resectability in gastric carcinoma. Ann. Surg. 188:711–715.

DeBoer, J., K. Huibregtse, and G. N. Tytgat. 1978. Gastric carcinoma after partial gastrectomy. Tijdschr Gastroenterol. 21:157–166.

Dees, J., M. Van Blankenstein, and M. Frankel. 1978. Adenocarcinoma in Barrett's esophagus: A report of thirteen cases. Gastroenterol. 74:1119.

Ekbom, G. A., and J. J. Gleysteen. 1980. Gastric malignancy: Resection for palliation. Surgery 88:476–481.

Giuli, R. 1979. Surgical treatment of stomach cancers. Review of 759 operations. Sem. Hop. Paris 55:801–805.

Goldstein, H. M., and J. Zornoza. 1978. Association of squamous cell carcinoma of the head and neck with cancer of the esophagus. Am. J. Roentgenol. 131:791–794.

Graham, D. Y., J. T. Schwartz, G. D. Cain, and F. Gyorkey. 1979. How many biopsies are enough? Gastrointest. Endosc. 25:39–40.

Haggitt, R. 1978. Adenocarcinoma complicating columnar epithelial lined (Barrett's) esophagus. Am. J. Clin. Pathol. 70:1–5.

Hellers, G., O. Bergstrand, S. Ewerth, and K. Nilsell. 1979. The incidence of cancer in the resected stomach. A preliminary report of a population study. Acta Chir. Scand. (Suppl.) 493:11.

Hiraoka, T., S. Endo, K. Umeda, A. Oshima, R. Suzuki, Y. Morikawa, K. Ban, and H. Imazu. 1978. Effect of stomach examination screening on decrease in gastric cancer deaths in Nose town. Kosei no. Shihyo 25:3–14.

Kasugai, T., S. Kobayashi, and N. Kuno. 1978. Endoscopic cytology of the esophagus, stomach and pancreas. Acta Cytol. (Baltimore) 22:327–330.

Kawai, K., and K. Ida. 1977. Endoscopical diagnosis of intestinal metaplasia and evaluation as precancerous lesion. Digestion 16:251.

Koyama, Y. 1978. The current status of chemotherapy for gastric cancer in Japan with special emphasis on mytomycin C. Recent Results Cancer Res. 63:135–147.

Laufer, I., J. E. Mullens, and J. Hamilton. 1975. The diagnostic accuracy of barium studies of the stomach and duodenum-correlation with endoscopy. Radiology 115:569.

MacDonald, J. S., P. S. Schein, P. V. Woolley, B. S. Tarilyn Smythe, W. Ueno, D. Hoth, F. Smith, M. Boiron, C. Gisselbrecht, R. Brunet, and C. Lagarde. 1980. 5-Fluorouracil, doxorubicin and mitomycin (FAM) combination chemotherapy for advanced gastric cancer. Ann. Intern. Med. 93:533–536.

Maruyama, M. 1979. Early gastric cancer, *in* Double Contrast Gastrointestinal Radiology with Endoscopic Correlation, I. Laufer, ed. W. B. Saunders Co., Philadelphia, pp. 241–287.

Miller, G., P. Froelicher, M. Kaufmann, and W. Maurer. 1979. Ten years endoscopic diagnosis of early gastric cancer in Europe. Z. Krebsforsch 93:99–107.

Moertel, C. G. 1978a. The case against surgery. Am. J. Digest. Dis. 23:735–736.

Moertel, C. G. 1978b. Chemotherapy of gastrointestinal cancer. N. Engl. J. Med. 299:1049–1052.

Morson, B. C. 1977. The Japanese classification of early gastric cancer, *in* The Gastrointestinal Tract, J. H. Yardley, B. C. Morson, and M. R. Abell, eds. The Williams and Wilkins Co. Baltimore, pp. 176–183.

Morson, B. C., M. Sobin, E. Grundmann, M. Johansen, T. Nagayo, and A. Serck-Hanssen. 1980. Precancerous conditions and epithelial dysplasia in the stomach. J. Clin. Pathol. 33:711–721.

Nakahara, K. 1978. Special features of intestinal metaplasia and its relation to early gastric carcinoma in man: Observation by a method in which leucine aminopeptidase is used. J. Natl. Cancer Inst. 6:693–702.

Nakayama, K. 1979. Cancer of the thoracic esophagus. Gan. 22:31–40.

Parker, E. F. 1978. Carcinoma of the esophagus: Is there a role for surgery? The case for surgery. Am. J. Digest. Dis. 23:730–734.

Payne, W. S. 1979. Palliation of esophageal carcinoma. Ann. Thorac. Surg. 28:208–209.

Piccone, V. A., N. Ahmed, S. Grosberg, and H. H. LeVeen. 1979. Esophagogastrectomy for carcinoma of the middle third of the esophagus. Ann. Thorac. Surg. 28:369–377.

Salas, J. 1977. Precancerous lesions of the stomach in Costa Rica. Patologia (Mex) 15:63–79.

Serck-Hanssen, A. 1979. The detection of early gastric carcinoma. Scand. J. Gastroenterol. (Suppl.) 14:106–110.

Serck-Hanssen, A., E. Schrumpf, J. Stadaas, S. Aune, J. Myren, and M. Osnes. 1977. Mucosal changes in the gastric stump 20–25 years after resection for ulcer: A follow-up study. Digestion 16:273.

Sugiura, H., S. Kobayashi, and T. Kasugai. 1979. Present status of the diagnosis of minute carcinoma of the stomach. Gastroenterol. Endosc. 21:717–721.

Treichel, J. 1979. Double contrast radiography of the stomach. Technique and results in early gastric cancer. J. Radiol. 60:299–305.

Weaver, A., S. M. Fleming, T. C. Knechtges, and D. Smith. 1979. Triple endoscopy: A neglected essential in head and neck cancer. Surgery 86:493–497.

Gastrointestinal Cancer, edited by
John R. Stroehlein and
Marvin M. Romsdahl.
Raven Press, New York © 1981.

Pathology of Adenocarcinoma of the Esophagus and Gastroesophageal Region, and "Barrett's Esophagus" as a Predisposing Condition

J. Leslie Smith, Jr., M.D.

*Department of Pathology, The University of Texas System Cancer Center
M. D. Anderson Hospital and Tumor Institute, Houston, Texas*

While this session of the conference is on "Recent Advances in Gastroesophageal Cancer," this presentation deals more specifically with advances in pathology. As a basis for discussion, consideration will be given briefly to the classification of malignant epithelial neoplasms of the esophagus and stomach. Following this, attention will be focused on questions related to adenocarcinoma of the esophagus and gastroesophageal region, with emphasis given to the "Barrett's" or "columnar epithelium-lined" esophagus and its predisposition to the development of cancer.

CLASSIFICATION OF MALIGNANT ESOPHAGEAL AND GASTRIC EPITHELIAL TUMORS

The classification of malignant esophageal and gastric epithelial tumors has not changed significantly over many years. The vast majority of malignant esophageal tumors encountered continue to be squamous carcinomas, and as such do not present significant diagnostic problems histologically unless they are poorly differentiated. More uncommon primary carcinoma types include carcinosarcoma or pseudosarcoma (Osamura et al. 1978). Tumors of this type present cytologic and histologic features similar to tumors arising from squamous mucosal surfaces of other sites, as well as skin, and which have been considered by some to be variants of squamous carcinoma. There have been several reports in recent years of an "oat cell" carcinoma variant (Reid et al. 1980, Rosen et al. 1975). Some of these tumors have exhibited squamous differentiation as well as the "oat-cell" pattern and have been considered to be squamous carcinoma variants also, although further confirmation is indicated. There is no question that the tumors mentioned are true esophageal tumors. Primary adenocarcinomas of the esophagus are rare, as will be discussed, and are much less common than would be indicated by the frequency with which the diagnosis is made from biopsy specimens or even some surgical specimens. Concepts regarding adenocarcinoma of, or involving, the esophagus have been clarified in recent years, and the data and information presented will provide additional documentation in this regard.

The vast majority of malignant epithelial tumors of the stomach are adenocarcinomas of gastric glandular origin. Much less frequent are those of endocrine cell origin, i.e., carcinoid or similar tumors. It is not the purpose, nor within the scope, of this presentation to discuss in detail the gross and morphologic types of gastric carcinomas and their histologic variants. Attention will be devoted to gastric adenocarcinomas arising in the region of the gastroesophageal junction. Their mode of spread will be considered, as will problems that can arise in the histopathologic evaluation of these tumors and their distinction from primary esophageal tumors.

MATERIAL

As of this writing, 1,008 patients with the diagnosis of carcinoma of the esophagus have been seen at M. D. Anderson Hospital and Tumor Institute. Of these patients, 873 have been diagnosed and coded as having squamous carcinoma or squamous carcinoma variants, and 135 have been coded as having adenocarcinoma. Based on these data, adenocarcinoma would constitute 13.4% of all esophageal carcinomas, a figure higher than will be shown to be real. The majority of the diagnoses coded as "adenocarcinoma of the esophagus" were based, however, on biopsy specimens. These were from patients whose tumors were found to be unresectable and who were treated by other modalities. Thus the true histogenesis was not proven. Our institution, being a referral institution, is one in which a high proportion of advanced disease is encountered.

In our files, however, 46 surgical specimens were located which had been diagnosed as adenocarcinoma of the esophagus or esophagogastric junction. The findings in these cases will form the basis for this presentation.

ADENOCARCINOMA OF THE ESOPHAGUS
AND ESOPHAGOGASTRIC JUNCTION

A diagnosis of adenocarcinoma of the esophagus is an incomplete diagnosis if it does not document the histogenesis of the tumor. Theoretically, adenocarcinoma of the esophagus would most likely be expected to arise from (1) the mucous-secreting glands of the esophagus, or (2) from "heterotopic gastric tissue." In reality, the majority of the "adenocarcinomas of the esophagus" diagnosed from esophageal biopsy specimens are (3) adenocarcinomas of gastric mucosal origin, in the region of the gastroesophageal junction, with secondary involvement of the esophagus. It now appears that the most frequent "true" primary adenocarcinoma of the esophagus is (4) adenocarcinoma which arises from the "columnar epithelium-lined esophagus" or Barrett's esophagus. Each of the above will be considered separately.

Tumors of Mucous-Secreting Gland Origin

Of the 46 surgical specimens studied only one was identified as an adenocarcinoma of mucous-secreting gland origin, indicating, as other reports have shown, that these are rare tumors. The tumor was present in the lower third of the esophagus of a 65-year-old black male. It was nodular, fairly well defined, and measured 4.5 cm in greatest dimension. The nodule extended into the lumen of the esophagus and was covered by superficially eroded or ulcerated mucosa. A 3.5 cm zone of normal esophageal mucosa was present between the tumor and the esophagogastric junction. Histologically, the patterns of the tumor ranged from a well-differentiated adenocarcinoma pattern, closely resembling that of normal mucous-secreting glands (Figure 1), to a virtually undifferentiated pattern. In areas the pattern suggested some degree of squamous differentiation. The range of patterns reported for tumors arising in mucous-secreting glands has been similar to that of tumors arising in salivary glands, including mucoepidermoid and adenoid cystic carcinoma types.

Adenocarcinoma of "Heterotopic Gastric Tissue" Origin

The concept that heterotopic gastric tissue occurs in the esophagus has been accepted for decades, and origin of adenocarcinoma from such tissues has been reported (Morson and Belcher 1952). Undoubtedly, many of the

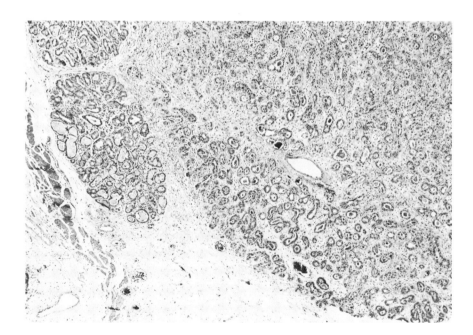

FIG. 1. Primary adenocarcinoma of the esophagus of mucous-secreting gland origin, well-differentiated. Mucous-secreting glands with cellular atypia are present on the left.

tumors which have been considered to have arisen in heterotopic gastric tissue have arisen from mucosa which now would be considered to be of the specialized columnar epithelium-lined mucosa of Barrett's type. The question of adenocarcinoma arising in true heterotopic gastric tissue has thus become somewhat clouded. In the present study there were no tumors which presented convincing evidence of origin from true heterotopic gastric tissue.

Adenocarcinoma of Gastric Mucosal Origin with Secondary Involvement of the Esophagus

Thirty-two of the 46 "esophageal" adenocarcinomas were proven to be of gastric mucosal origin. The tumors in question involved the distal esophagus and esophagogastric junction; in most instances they suggested, grossly, an esophageal rather than a gastric tumor. The explanation for this phenomenon lies in the distribution of lymphatics and the lymphatic spread of tumors in the lower esophagus. There is direct continuity of the lymphatics of the stomach and esophagus. One set of lymphatics is in the submucosa and the other in the smooth muscle layers. Adenocarcinoma cells of tumors arising in the esophagogastric region spread proximally in these lymphatics, with the establishment of metastatic tumor in these levels. Submucosal metastatic tumor may initially be focal or multifocal in distribution. A continuous layer or band-like distribution of submucosal tumor may develop. The esophageal squa-

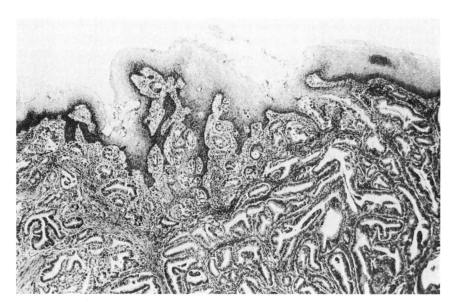

FIG. 2. Esophageal tissue exhibiting submucosal extension of tumor from an adenocarcinoma arising in the gastric cardia at gastroesophageal junction.

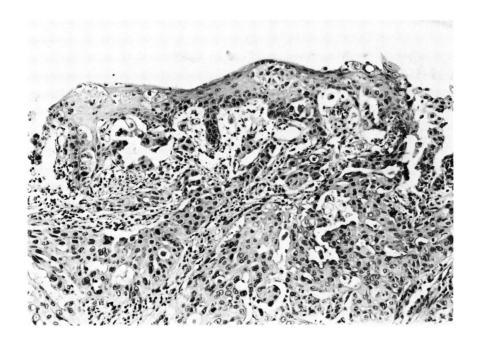

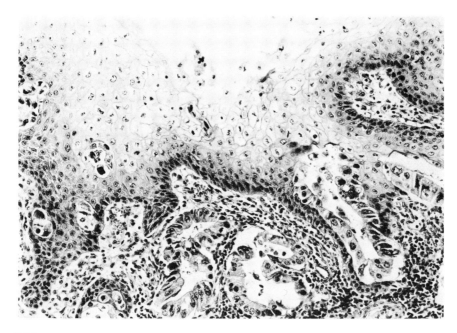

FIGS. 3 and 4. Penetration of the squamous mucosa of the esophagus by adenocarcinoma in the submucosa of gastric origin. Such patterns may simulate or suggest origin in the esophagus.

mous mucosa, as a result, appears to be undermined by tumor, a feature observed in some area of all tumors of this type in this study (Figure 2). With continued proliferation of the submucosal tumor, the squamous mucosa is encroached upon and frequently penetrated by tumor. At the points of early penetration the tumor may appear to be related to, or even arise from, the mucosa, a feature which could be interpreted in a biopsy specimen as support for an interpretation of primary esophageal tumor (Figures 3 and 4). Continued proliferation, penetration, and attenuation of the mucosa results in mucosal ulceration. The ulceration is at first focal or multifocal with intervening zones of normal mucosa (Figure 5). The zones of mucosa become smaller, eventually disappearing with the formation of larger tumor ulcerations. The esophageal wall may be circumferentially involved or a portion of the wall may be involved. With the mode of spread, as described, it is possible for tumor ulceration to develop in the esophagus with normal squamous mucosa being present between the ulceration and the site of origin in the gastric mucosa at the esophagogastric junction.

Adenocarcioma Arising in the Columnar Mucosa of Barrett's Esophagus

It has now become generally accepted that chronic or prolonged gastroesophageal reflux can result in the replacement of squamous mucosa of the esophagus, generally the lower esophagus, by columnar epithelium. Barrett

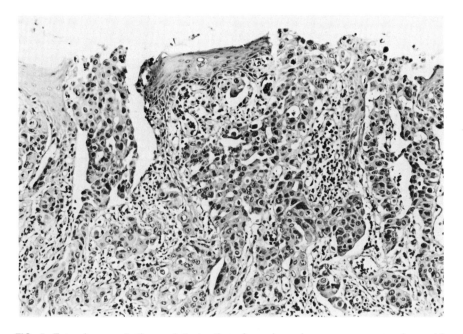

FIG. 5. Extensive penetration and destruction of esophageal squamous mucosa by gastric adenocarcinoma which has undermined the esophageal mucosa.

described this type of mucosa in 1950, and today it bears his name (Barrett 1950). It was initially believed that a congenitally short esophagus was the explanation for the presence of this mucosa, but experimental data have supported the concept that it represents mucosal metaplasia secondary to injury or damage by chronic reflux. A high frequency of hiatal hernia has been reported in patients with this change (Haggitt et al. 1978), and there is a report of its occurrence in a patient with scleroderma of the esophagus (Cameron and Payne 1978), observations which would support the reflux etiology concept. In recent years there have been numbers of reports documenting origin of adenocarcinoma from this mucosa, and it is presently felt that its presence predisposes an individual to the development of carcinoma (Shafer 1971, Hawe et al. 1973, Naef et al. 1975, Berenson et al. 1978).

Of the 46 patients in this study, nine have been interpreted as having had adenocarcinoma arise in columnar mucosa of Barrett's type. There was a tenth patient whose lower esophagus was lined by Barrett's type mucosa, but whose tumor arose from mucosa of the gastric cardia. The Barrett's mucosa of seven patients lined the lower third of the esophagus. The lesion of one patient was in the mid-esophagus and of another in the upper third. Eight of the nine patients were male, and all were Caucasian. The ages ranged from 37 to 84 years, with a mean age of 61 years. Hiatal hernias were recorded in four patients. Five of the patients have died from their disese, with survival times ranging from three to 15 months. Five were still living at 5 to 17 months following surgery. These were more recent patients on whom follow-up will be needed. The prognosis overall for patients with these tumors is extremely poor.

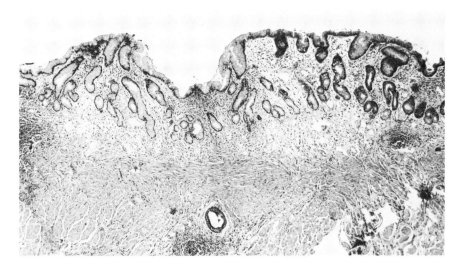

FIG. 6. Columnar mucosa of Barrett's type lining the esophagus. Normal esophageal anatomic landmarks such as the mucous-secreting gland duct and the type of muscularis as seen here document the tissue as being esophageal rather than gastric.

For a tumor to be interpreted as arising from esophageal columnar mucosa of Barrett's type, it must be shown that benign columnar mucosa is present and that it is, in fact, lining the esophagus (Figure 6). This identification is necessary because columnar mucosa of Barrett's type closely simulates gastric fundic mucosa. A good gross description of the specimen is essential, including documentation of the specific sites from which tissue sections are obtained. It is also possible to establish that columnar-lined mucosa is from the esophagus by identifying normal anatomic structures of the esophagus such as the mucous-secreting glands or ducts.

The histologic pattern of the columnar epithelium is variable. Paull et al. (1976) have described three types. These are (1) the specialized columnar epithelium which resembles intestinal mucosa with a villiform surface, goblet cells, and mucous glands, but no Paneth cells (Figure 7); (2) a junctional epithelium resembling gastric cardiac mucosa with mucous-secreting glands and no parietal cells, and (3) a gastric fundic-type epithelium containing parietal cells, chief cells, and mucous cells. They described the specialized columnar epithelium as being present generally in the proximal portion of the involved area and the gastric fundic-type epithelium being present distally, with the junctional type interposed between the two. In the present study there were instances where there was more than one type in one section, and

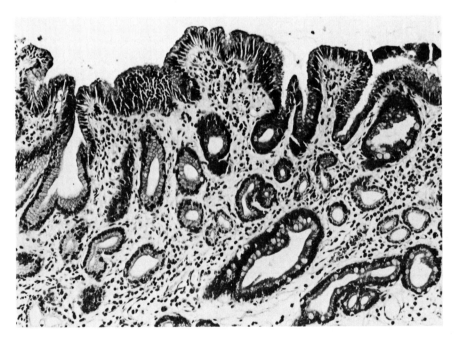

FIG. 7. Specialized columnar epithelium of Barrett's type which resembles intestinal mucosa with a villiform surface, goblet cells, and mucous glands, but no Paneth cells.

the dividing line between the types was not always sharp. In all cases the columnar epithelium was associated with inflammation ranging from slight to marked. The degree of inflammation was variable even within the same lesion. It is of interest that the specialized columnar epithelium, resembling intestinal mucous, together with the gastric type epithelium and chronic inflammation produce a pattern similar to that of chronic atrophic gastritis with intestinal metaplasia, although they lack the Paneth cells usually found in intestinalized gastric mucosa (Figure 8). It is recognized that chronic atrophic gastritis with intestinal metaplasia is predisposed to the development of carcinoma and it appears that a similar predisposition is indicated by the presence of the specialized columnar epithelial pattern. Dysplasia, ranging from slight to carcinoma-in-situ, was present in the mucosa of all specimens. It was present not only in the immediate vicinity of the invasive tumor, but in remote mucosa as well. In some specimens multiple foci of severe dysplasia, carcinoma-in-situ, and invasive carcinoma were identified (Figure 9). The histologic patterns of the adenocarcinoma ranged from well-differentiated to undifferentiated and presented no unique or specific features.

SUMMARY

In summary, the most frequent explanation for a diagnosis of adenocarcinoma from an esophageal biopsy specimen is that of extension of the tumor from a primary carcinoma of the gastric cardia. Adenocarcinoma may arise

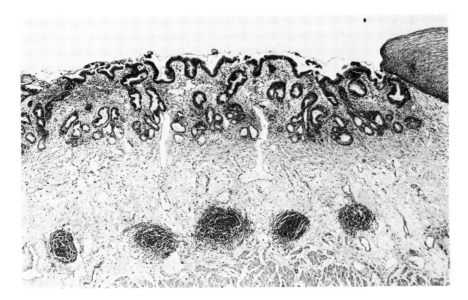

FIG. 8. Barrett's mucosa and chronic inflammation simulating chronic atrophic gastritis with intestinal metaplasia, although the Paneth cells are lacking.

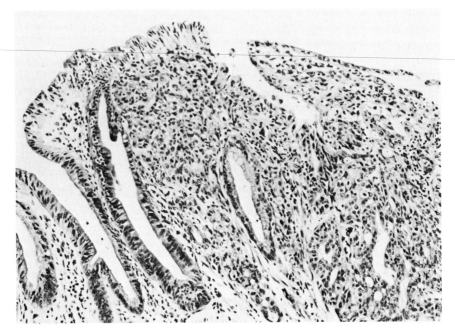

FIG. 9. Focus of carcinoma-in-situ and early invasive carcinoma within Barrett's mucosa of esophagus.

from the mucous-secreting glands of the esophagus, but this occurrence is rare. True primary adenocarcinomas of the esophagus, in our experience, although still rare, are most often explained by adenocarcinoma arising in the columnar epithelium-lined esophagus, the Barrett's esophagus. The columnar mucosa appears to represent a metaplastic change due to chronic reflux, and the evidence in this study supports the observations of others that the columnar mucosa is predisposed to malignant change.

REFERENCES

Barrett, N. R. 1950. Chronic peptic ulcer of the oesophagus and "oesophagitis." Br. J. Surg. 38:175–182.

Berenson, M. M., R. H. Riddell, D. B. Skinner, and J. W. Freston. 1978. Malignant transformation of esophageal columnar epithelium. Cancer 41:554–561.

Cameron, A. J., and W. S. Payne. 1978. Barrett's esophagus occurring as a complication of scleroderma. Mayo Clin. Proc. 53:612–615.

Haggitt, R. C., J. Tryzelaar, F. H. Ellis, and H. Colcher. 1978. Adenocarcinoma complicating columnar epithelium-lined (Barrett's) esophagus. Am. J. Clin. Pathol. 70:1–5.

Hawe, A., S. Payne, L. H. Weiland, and R. Fontana. 1973. Adenocarcinoma in the columnar epithelial lined lower (Barrett) oesophagus. Thorax 28:511–514.

Morson, B. C., and J. R. Belcher. 1952. Adenocarcinoma of the oesophagus and ectopic gastric mucosa. Br. J. Cancer 6:127.

Naef, A. P., M. Savary, L. Ozzello and F. G. Pearson. 1975. Columnar-lined lower esophagus: An acquired lesion with malignant predisposition. J. Thorac. Cardiovasc. Surg. 70:826–834.

Osamura, R. Y., K. Shimamura, J. Hata, N. Tamaoki, K. Watanabe, M. Kubota, S. Yamazaki, and T. Mitomi. 1978. Polypoid carcinoma of the esophagus. Am. J. Surg. Pathol. 2:201–208.

Paull, A., J. S. Trier, M. D. Dalton, R. C. Camp, P. Loeb, and R. K. Goyal. 1976. The histologic spectrum of Barrett's esophagus. N. Engl. J. Med. 295:476–480.

Reid, H. A. S., W. W. Richardson, and B. Corrin. 1980. Oat cell carcinoma of the esophagus. Cancer 45:2342–2347.

Rosen, Y., S. Moon, and B. Kim. 1975. Small cell epidermoid carcinoma of the esophagus. An oat-cell-like carcinoma. Cancer 36:1042–1049.

Shafer, R. B. 1971. Adenocarcinoma in Barrett's columnar-lined esophagus. Arch. Surg. 103:411–413.

Gastrointestinal Cancer, edited by
John R. Stroehlein and
Marvin M. Romsdahl.
Raven Press, New York © 1981.

Esophageal Cancer in the United States: Diagnostic Modalities and Surveillance of High-Risk Groups

Roland W. Bennetts, M.D.

Department of Medicine, The University of Texas System Cancer Center
M. D. Anderson Hospital and Tumor Institute, Houston, Texas

INTRODUCTION

The majority of epidemiological research in squamous cell carcinoma of the esophagus has consisted of descriptive studies, often with inadequate data bases, and has stressed sex and geographic inequalities. In the United States this means a doubling of prevalence rates for urban communities over rural communities, seemingly without relationship to industrialization. Also evident, as in many parts of the world, is a three- to fourfold increased prevalence in males over females and a twofold increased prevalance in non-whites compared to whites (Fraumeni and Blot 1977). Primarily because of its relative rarity and the dismal prospect of long-term survival, esophageal cancer has failed to capture the attention of clinical researchers. In 1980, 8,800 new cases of squamous cell carcinoma of the esophagus are expected; of these individuals, fewer than 5% will survive five years (American Cancer Society 1980).

GROUPS AT HIGH RISK

Cross-sectional and case-control prevalence studies have been of great use in isolating populations at probable higher risk for esophageal cancer. The best examples of this include research showing a thousandfold or more increased risk for esophageal carcinoma in individuals experiencing long-term survival after diagnosis of lye stricture (Appelqvist and Salmo 1980) or achalasia (Carter and Brewer 1975, Hankins and McLaughlin 1975). Retrospective cohort studies to more firmly establish the incidence of disease in specific presumed normal subpopulations have often weakened presumed associations and generally have not surveyed an adequate number of variables. Examples of this latter phenomenon are manifold, but include the three major presumed associations which are: condensed catechin tannins (Morton 1978), tobacco (Bradshaw and Schonland 1974, Jussawalla and Deshpande

1971, Kolonel 1979, Weir and Dunn 1970), and alcohol (Audigier et al. 1975, Bradshaw and Schonland 1974, Chilvers et al. 1979, Kolonel 1979). Entirely lacking in all of these latter studies is the screening to remove at entry all participants with subclinical disease. Therefore, the cohort studies not only have failed to yield weighting factors for the various risks, but have often merely exposed prevalence data.

There is, then, little data available for review that illuminates the usefulness of esophageal cancer screening. At a minimum, a long-term prospective incidence study of a screened, high-risk population adequately subgrouped for selected risk factors is required in order to establish true risk values. Subsequently, the value of the screening could be determined by grouping an initially screened population to receive either long-term screening at regular intervals or standard care. From Table 1, it can be seen that relatively few groups at high risk for esophageal carcinoma are of adequate size and risk to justify any type of screening maneuver. For example, if the entire population at risk for esophageal cancer associated with more than a decade of asbestos exposure were maximally screened annually, the following might be found: (1) one person annually would die as a result of the screening procedure; (2) 50 new carcinomas would be found in the first year and 20 to 30 annually thereafter; (3) five-year survival after therapy for esophageal cancer in this group might be trebled to 15%. Over any five-year period this would mean a gain of 12.5 lives at a loss of five other lives and a cost in excess of $100,000,000.

SCREENING TECHNIQUES

Effective screening of high-risk populations for esophageal cancer also assumes an acceptable method in an interested, compliant group. Certainly the ideal method should be easily tolerated, inexpensive, brief, and capable of

Table 1. *Squamous Cancer of the Esophagus: United States of America 1980**

Risk Factors	Risk Value	Group Size	Expected Cases	% of New Cases
Plummer-Vinson[†]	"Very High"	<100	<5	<0.05
Ionizing Radiation[‡]	25	>10,000	<5	<0.05
Tylosis[§]	10^5	600	<10	<0.1
Lye Stricture*[//]	10^3	5000	30	0.33
Asbestos[#]	25	100,000	30	0.33
Achalasia*	50	50,000	30	0.33
Head and Neck Cancer[¶]	10^3	36,200	400	5
Tannins, Tobacco* Alcohol	5	<10^6	8300	94

*See text for references
†(Wynder et al. 1957)
‡(Chudecki 1972)
§(Harper et al. 1970)
//(Leape et al. 1971)
#(Selikoff et al. 1973)
¶(Cahan et al. 1976, Goldstein and Zornoza 1978)

Table 2. *Screening for Esophageal Cancer**

Technique	Time	Cost ($)	Morbidity	Mortality	Sensitivity Early	Sensitivity Late	Specificity Early	Specificity Late
History	<5 minutes	10	0	0	0	0.9	0	0.5
Physical	<5 minutes	25	0	0	0	0.4	0	0
Serology†	<5 minutes	10	0	0	0	0.6	0	0
Scans†	60 minutes	>75	<0.05	0	0	0.8	0	0.8
Barium study	30 minutes	>50	0	0	0.4	1	0.6	0.8
Blind cytology†	5 minutes	25	<0.005	<0.0001	>0.6	0.95	0.90	0.90
Endoscopy	30 minutes	>100	<0.05	<0.0001	>0.5	0.95	0.90	0.90

*See text for references
†Experimental

diagnosing early lesions with high sensitivity and specificity. Table 2 illustrates an attempt to list the characteristics of currently available methods as can best be determined by literature review and the experience at M. D. Anderson Hospital and Tumor Institute.

Since a history and physical examination classically only reveal disease that is not only present but has already extended, they are necessarily inadequate in identifying patients with early lesions. The earliest symptom of esophageal cancer is an often misplaced sense of difficulty in the initiation or completion of deglutition. In time, this motor phenomenon is replaced by neoplastic obstruction with a better localized dysphagia and attendant regurgitation, aspiration, sialorrhea, and weight loss. Currently more than 90% of esophageal cancer patients will be diagnosed after the onset of such symptoms. The delay to diagnosis usually exceeds three months. Physical examination for staging includes testing for cranial nerve involvement, lymphadenopathy, and abdominal mass, as well as a rectal examination to check for blood loss and rectal shelf (Nelson 1974).

Barium contrast studies, especially double contrast studies, are extremely useful and provide a very sensitive evaluation of the mucosal surface of the esophagus (Yamada et al. 1972). There are at least three methods of generating double contrast esophagrams. Water, mineral oil, and air have been used to create a double contrast in standard barium esophagrams, but only air provides a safe, high quality result. Tube insufflation or eructation of air into the barium column is cumbersome and provides a nonuniform result, especially given a debilitated or obstructed patient. The method preferred and followed at the radiology clinic of M. D. Anderson Hospital is aeration of the swallowed barium by its ingestion through a vented straw. The choice of a thick barium mixture with excellent coating properties will enhance the air contrast. Preferred mixtures are of uniform particulates in very high density for initial air contrast, followed by standard mixtures for solid column examination. Lacking in the current experience is a large-scale prospective use of this test in a screening manner (Basu 1975). Besides some obvious limitations, repeated fluoroscopic examination, even with current image intensification, provides potential and unpredictable long-term morbidity.

Endoscopy, which is highly reliable and otherwise very attractive as a screening modality, is both expensive and time-consuming. However, it provides an excellent view of the mucosal surface as well as the possibility of directed cytological and biopsy sampling of the mucosa. Sensitivity and specificity data for flexible endoscopy of established disease are uniformly high in all series (Crespi et al. 1979, Nelson 1974), but its power as a test for early disease in screening high-risk groups remains untested. For many years there has been interest in applying topical agents, such as Lugol's solution (Mandard et al. 1980) or toluidine blue (Yoshida et al. 1976), to the mucosa to highlight the areas of subtle mucosal change. These studies, like the use of radioactive phosphorus and Geiger counter with endoscopy discussed later, remain experimental.

Relatively little has been done with regard to serological studies for esophageal cancer; certainly, patients with advanced disease have been screened for alpha fetoprotein, carcinoembryonic antigen titer (Wahren et al. 1979), and even chemiluminescence (Baraboy et al. 1980). As can be seen in Table 2, none of these latter methods has proved of great use. In the area of scans, work to date has been done with gallium (Kondo et al. 1979), cobalt labeled bleomycin (Suzuki et al. 1974), and CAT scanning (Daffner et al. 1979), which proves scanning to be useful as a staging device but not as a real screening tool. Radioactive phosphorus scanning of the esophagus has been done, much of it initially here at M. D. Anderson Hospital by Dr. Robert Nelson (Nelson and Lanza 1969). The chief limitations of this method seem to be its adaptation to use with the flexible instruments. The primary disadvantage is maintaining an open esophageal lumen and having a small enough Geiger counter which can thereby be exposed to the surface without contact. Research in this method remains interesting but at a standstill; therefore, this method is not available as a screening technique.

Blind cytology examinations which were common in the preendoscopy period in the United States are being used more extensively in other countries where esophageal carcinoma is a much greater health problem (Coordinating Group for Research on Esophageal Cancer 1976, Dowlatshahi et al. 1978). Of all the currently available and experimental methods for diagnosis of esophageal lesions, only blind cytology by minimally abrasive catheter comes close to meeting the stipulations for the ideal method (Galaktionov 1976). Double contrast barium studies are highly reliable as diagnostic studies but an expensive alternative to screening. Further experimentation with barium studies may prove them to be more sensitive and specific for early lesions (Yamada et al. 1972).

CONCLUSIONS

Although there are many groups at a high risk of developing esophageal carcinoma, there is little information with regard to the true annual incidence in any single group which would establish the frequency of examinations or cost effectiveness of major screening projects (Table 1). Certainly, for the 90% of new esophageal cancer patients who come from the less-than-high-risk (less than 1:1000) groups, screening is not currently applicable.

As botanists, chemists, and epidemiologists sift through the ever-accumulating prevalence data, preventive medicine measures will be brought to bear in the hope of altering the long-term trends in esophageal cancer incidence worldwide. This is the ultimate answer for the overwhelming majority of cases.

In the interim, we must isolate and screen available high-risk subgroups by experimental protocol to establish true incidence rates, screening schedules, and perhaps actual risk factors. Such experimental screening projects would involve highly informed patients who would be more willing to accept maximum intervention. In the Head and Neck Surgery Clinic at M. D. Anderson Hospital and Tumor Institute up to 600 new patients at high risk for esophageal cancer are seen annually. Given this ready access to a high-risk group, a long-term joint study between head and neck surgery and gastroenterology is being planned to investigate some of the above questions.

Lacking data, reasonable current recommendations are that all patients with lye stricture, achalasia, prior head and neck cancer, or tylosis be evaluated annually with endoscopy and brush cytology (Norton et al. 1980). An acceptable alternative would be to alternate endoscopy with double contrast X-ray studies at an annual review of history and physical examination.

Such ad hoc conservative, though aggressive, screening maneuvers are justified until prospective studies clarify their usefulness. For groups at lower known or presumed risk for squamous cell carcinoma of the esophagus, initial screening followed by counseling aimed at reducing risk is advised. It is our hope that within this decade, data from M. D. Anderson Hospital and Tumor Institute and other institutions interested in esophageal cancer will validate the screening methods for early disease, demonstrate the usefulness beyond the cost-benefit analysis of early diagnosis, and establish the true risk factors for esophageal cancer in high-risk populations.

REFERENCES

American Cancer Society. 1980. Cancer facts and figures 1980. New York, p. 9.

Appelqvist, P., and M. Salmo. 1980. Lye corrosion carcinoma of the esophagus. Cancer 45:2655–2658.

Audigier, J. C., A. J. Tuyns, and R. Lambert. 1975. Epidemiology of oesophageal cancer in France. Digestion 13:209–219.

Baraboy, V. A., V. L. Ganul, A. V. Evtushenko, L. V. Okulov, V. E. Orel, Y. A. Tatsy, and G. V. Chebotarev. 1980. Spontaneous chemiluminescence of serum in patients with cancer of esophagus and proximal stomach. Vopr. Onkol. 26(1):51–54.

Basu, S. 1975. Mass screening of gastrointestinal tract to detect carcinoma of stomach. J. Indian Med. Assoc. 64:327–329.

Bradshaw, E., and M. Schonland. 1974. Smoking, drinking and oesophageal cancer in African males of Johannesburg, South Africa. Br. J. Cancer 30:157–163.

Cahan, W. G., E. B. Castro, P. B. Rosen, and E. W. Strong. 1976. Separate primary carcinomas of the esophagus and head and neck region in the same patient. Cancer 37:85–89.

Carter, R., and L. A. Brewer. 1975. Achalasia and esophageal carcinoma. Am. J. Surg. 130:114–120.

Chilvers, C., P. Fraser, and V. Beral. 1979. Alcohol and oesophageal cancer. J. Epidemiol. Community Health 33:127–133.

Chudecki, B. 1972. Radiation cancer of the thoracic oesophagus. Br. J. Radiol. 45:303–304.

Coordinating Group for Research on Esophageal Cancer. 1976. Early diagnosis and surgical treatment of esophageal cancer under rural conditions. Chin. Med. J. 2:113–116.

Cook-Mozaffari, P. J., F. Azordegan, N. E. Day, A. Ressicaud, C. Sabai, and B. Aramesh. 1979. Oesophageal cancer studies in the Caspian littoral of Iran. Br. J. Cancer 39:293–309.

Crespi, M., A. Grassi, G. Amiri, N. Munoz, B. Aramesh, A. Mojtabai, and V. Casale. 1979. Oesophageal lesions in Northern Iran. Lancet 2:217–220.

Daffner, R. H., M. D. Halber, R. W. Postlethwait, M. Korobkin, and W. M. Thompson. 1979. CT of the esophagus. Am. J. Roengenol. 133:1051–1055.

Dowlatshahi, K., A. Daneshbod, and S. Mobarhan. 1978. Early detection of cancer of the oesophagus along Caspian littoral. Lancet 1:125–126.

Fraumeni, J. F., Jr., and W. J. Blot. 1977. Geographic variation in esophageal cancer mortality in the United States. J. Chronic Dis. 30:759–767.

Galaktionov, B. B. 1976. Abrasive sound for cytological investigation of esophageal disorders. Vopr. Onkol. 22(9):76–78.

Goldstein, H. M., and J. Zornoza. 1978. Association of squamous cell carcinoma of the head and neck with cancer of the esophagus. Am. J. Roentgenol. 131:791–794.

Hankins, J. R., and J. S. McLaughlin. 1975. The association of carcinoma of the esophagus with achalasia. J. Thorac. Cardiovasc. Surg. 69:355–360.

Harper, P. S., R. M. J. Harper, and A. W. Howel-Evans. 1970. Carcinoma of the oesophagus with tylosis. Q. J. Med. 39:317–333.

Jussawalla, D. J., and V. A. Deshpande. 1971. Evaluation of cancer risk in tobacco chewers and smokers. Cancer 28:244–252.

Kolonel, L. 1979. Smoking and drinking patterns among different ethnic groups in Hawaii. Natl. Cancer Inst. Monogr. 53:81–87.

Kondo, M., S. Hashimoto, A. Kubo, T. Kakegawa, and N. Ando. 1979. [67]Ga scanning in the evaluation of esophageal carcinoma. Radiology 131:723–726.

Leape, L. L., K. W. Ashcraft, D. E. Scarpelli, and T. M. Holder. 1971. Hazard to health—liquid lye. N. Engl. J. Med. 284:578–581.

Mandard, A. M., J. Tourneux, M. Gignoux, L. Blanc, P. Segol, and J. C. Mandard. 1980. In situ carcinoma of the esophagus. Endoscopy 12:51–57.

Morton, J. F. 1978. Economic botany in epidemiology. Econ. Bot. 32:111–116.

Nelson, R. S. 1974. Carcinoma of the esophagus, *in* Gastroenterology, H. L. Bockus, ed., Vol I. W. B. Saunders Co., Philadelphia, pp. 295–304.

Nelson, R. S., and F. L. Lanza. 1969. The clinical value of radioactive phosphorus in the diagnosis of esophageal cancer. Am. J. Digest. Dis. 14:538–544.

Norton, G. A., R. W. Postlethwait, and W. M. Thompson. 1980. Esophageal carcinoma: a survey of populations at risk. South. Med. J. 73:25–27.

Selikoff, I. J., E. C. Hammond, and H. Seidman. 1973. Cancer risk of insulation workers in the United States, *in* Biological Effects of Asbestos, P. Bogovski et al., eds. International Agency for Research on Cancer, Lyon, pp. 209–216.

Suzuki, Y., K. Hisada, T. Hiraki, and A. Ando. 1974. Clinical evaluation of tumor scanning with [57]Co-bleomycin. Radiology 113:139–143.

Wahren, B., J. Harmenberg, F. Edsmyr, P. Jakobsson, and S. Ingimarsson. 1979. Possible tumour markers in patients with oesophagus cancer. Scand. J. Gastroenterol. 14:361–365.

Weir, J. M., and J. F. Dunn. 1970. Smoking and mortality. Cancer 25:105–112.

Wynder, E. L., S. Hultberg, F. Jacobsson, and I. J. Bross. 1957. Environmental factors in cancer of the upper alimentary tract. Cancer 10:470–487.

Yamada, A., S. Kobayashi, B. Kawai, A. Fujimoto, and K. Nakayama. 1972. Study on x-ray findings of early oesophageal cancer. Australas. Radiol. 16:238–246.

Yoshida, M., T. Hayaski, and S. Suzuki. 1976. Endoscopic toluidine blue iodine method of the esophagus. Stomach Intest. 11:359 (abstract).

Gastrointestinal Cancer, edited by
John R. Stroehlein and
Marvin M. Romsdahl.
Raven Press, New York © 1981.

Screening and Diagnosis of Gastric Cancer

Robert S. Nelson, M.D.

Department of Medicine, The University of Texas System Cancer Center
M. D. Anderson Hospital and Tumor Institute, Houston, Texas

The incidence of adenocarcinoma of the stomach is decreasing in the United States, but remains high in various other parts of the world. Information from these geographical areas should give epidemiological clues which would assist in screening populations for improved early diagnosis. Histological changes in the gastric mucosa which seem to precede or accompany gastric cancer also might be of assistance in predicting occurrence.

The preoperative histological diagnosis of gastric cancer may now be made in almost all cases if proper procedures are carried out. The difficulty in early diagnosis remains that of determining which patients should be completely evaluated. The lack of early symptoms in many cases compounds the problem, as does physician and patient delay in the case of a symptomatic individual.

SCREENING PROCEDURES

Epidemiological Observations

Epidemiologists have long pointed out that there are differences in diet and environmental factors associated with a high rate of gastric cancer. They cite the low incidence among the maize-eating Bantu in Africa and the corn-eating Nigerians, with an increase when these races are transplanted into urban surroundings with changed diet (Oettle 1968). Cancer of the stomach decreases among Japanese transplanted to the United States, presumably because of differences in diet and undetermined environmental influences (Elsborg and Mosbech 1979).

Direct carcinogens are suspected of playing a part. Phenols present in smoke, soot, tar, and smoked foods may be factors in the increased incidence of gastric cancer in Finns and Icelanders, as well as in the drinking water of other populations (Dungal 1966). Some coal miners have a definitely increased tendency to develop gastric cancer compared to other miner groups (Matolo et al. 1972). Talc-treated rice has been conditionally incriminated as carcinogenic among the Japanese, and nitrosamines in areas, such as Chile, where sodium nitrate is used extensively as fertilizer are suspected of being at least a factor (Merliss 1972, Zaldivar 1970).

Theoretically, such observations should help point to populations most at risk, and these, in turn, could then undergo more routine and specific screening tests. It is hoped that changes in environment and diet might help to eliminate gastric cancer. Unfortunately, neither of these goals is at present close to attainment. With the diversity of ethnic groups and their mixing within the United States, a clear-cut picture becomes almost impossible. Only future studies will determine the practical value of these observations.

Practical Screening Mechanisms and Factors

Japanese Mass Screening Efforts

The Japanese have a very high incidence of gastric cancer in a rather homogeneous population, and mass screening attempts have been successful in evaluating large portions of the population. In 1965, for example, 333,531 individuals were examined in 104 hospitals and 51 public clinics. Gastric cancer was discovered in 46 of these individuals. Further experience has resulted in a small but steady increase in the number of early, potentially resectable cancers diagnosed. Between 1953 and 1971, a total of 734 cases of early gastric cancer were found. Of these, 61 were preliminarily diagnosed as advanced cancer and 182 as benign lesions, demonstrating the value of histological studies and surgery (Nagayo and Yokoyama 1974). No other country has undertaken a survey of this type.

Achlorhydria

Achlorhydria is frequently found in patients whose stomachs demonstrate gastric atrophy, atrophic gastritis (probably the precursor of atrophy), and intestinal metaplasia. The association is not absolute; however, various limited surveys have been done using "tubeless gastric analysis" in which a marker is swallowed and tests are run to determine the presence of acid. Those with anacidity can then be examined more fully or on a routine basis. Unfortunately, this type of analysis is grossly inaccurate, especially in the older age group. Many patients who develop gastric cancer still secrete acid. Nevertheless, patients over 45 years of age with authentic gastric atrophy showed a 1% incidence of gastric cancer on annual roentgenographic survey, according to one study (Flood and Lattes 1967). However, mass screening of entire populations is believed to be costly and essentially unrewarding. It appears that there are too many variables in determining achlorhydria to make this test the basis for mass screens.

Pernicious Anemia

The incidence of gastric cancer in different groups of patients with pernicious anemia has been variously recorded as 4%-21%. Whether this is due to nonspecific gastritic mucosal changes or to some other factor such as antibodies is unknown. All such patients should be thoroughly investigated if they become symptomatic. The question of routine investigation after the age of 45 or 50 years is an open one, and probably would result in few diagnoses (Elsborg and Mosbech 1979).

Previous Subtotal Resection or Gastroenterostomy

It has become increasingly evident that routine resections or gastroenterostomy in the treatment of peptic ulcerations disposes the patient to an increased risk of development of cancer in the remaining stomach. The incidence increases with the length of interval following surgery, and is thought to be caused by regurgitation of small bowel contents into the stump. Tumors typically occur in the vicinity of the anastomosis, and become much more frequent after the age of 50 years. Gastric and duodenal ulcer patients are equally at risk, and gastric cancer was found to be at least 6.3 times more common in patients who had had surgery (Papachristou et al. 1980).

Gastric Ulcer

There is no evidence that benign gastric ulcer, per se, predisposes to gastric cancer. Differentiation of benign ulcer from ulcerating cancer is imperative.

Polyposis

Occasional patients with congenital polyposis of the colon will be found to have polyps of the stomach. Among those with adenomatous polyps, a small number will develop carcinoma. Patients with one or more adenomatous polyps who do not have congenital polyposis also have an increased incidence of gastric cancer. This is more likely to arise from the mucosa itself than from polyps. In any case, histological proof of adenomatous polyposis is necessary for surveillance or regular follow-up.

Hiatus Hernia

There is no evidence that hiatus hernia predisposes to carcinoma of the stomach or esophagus. In either case, however, it may complicate the diagnosis of cancer.

DIAGNOSIS

Directed endoscopic biopsy for gastric lesions became possible approximately 14 years ago. Directed brush cytology was developed at the same time. The use of these two diagnostic modalities has revolutionized the preoperative diagnosis of gastric cancer. Their value varies only with the experience of the operator and the willingness of the physician to refer his patient for endoscopic biopsy. Properly applied, these techniques will allow a firm diagnosis of cancer, or a correct diagnosis of a benign condition in 98% of all patients suspected of having gastric cancer (Nelson 1970).

Gastric disease is still, however, first suspected because of an abnormal radiological study in the majority of patients, and diagnostic radiology is an excellent screening device. Properly performed with air contrast, it has a high degree of accuracy, even for small mucosal lesions. All gross roentgenographic findings must be confirmed by endoscopy and biopsy. In addition, if the cause for persistent symptoms is not suggested on the roentgenogram, endoscopy must still be employed to confirm a negative diagnosis.

Specific Clinical Situations

The relatively small occurrence rate of gastric cancer in the United States, as well as in some other countries, makes general survey methods impractical. The problem of diagnosis remains, however, and all efforts should be made to diagnose early or slow-growing tumors, as well as those of the more progressive type in a resectable state. This may not result in an appreciable lowering of mortality, since early cases will be rare, but it will certainly have a beneficial effect on morbidity and management as a whole.

Undiagnosed Upper Gastrointestinal Symptoms

All patients, especially those over the age of 50 years, who have persistent upper gastrointestinal complaints unexplained by X-ray examination, should have endoscopy. The smaller the gastric cancer, the more easily it may be missed or misinterpreted. Such lesions often require persistent and multiple biopsy attempts for clarification.

Gastric Atrophy, Achlorhydria, and Pernicious Anemia

The basic pathology in each of these conditions is metaplasia leading to intestinalization. Achlorhydria can be established only on maximum stimulation tests, which rules out "tubeless gastric analysis," and in most cases, the diagnosis of these conditions results only from previous examination. Symptomatic individuals in these categories should have a careful evaluation, including endoscopy.

Gastric Ulcer

Most gastric ulcers are discovered on X-ray examination, but this method misses approximately 15% of lesions. Patients with lesions seen or suspected on roentgenograms should have mandatory endoscopy. All ulcers found, whether in symptomatic individuals with negative roentgenograms or those with positive X-rays, should be routinely and thoroughly biopsied.

Previous Gastric Resection or Gastroenterostomy

This group of patients has not been properly considered as gastric cancer-prone in the past, but it represents a definite segment of this tumor in any large clinic. It is important that the primary physicians be aware of the risk, especially in those over the age of 50. Once again, negative X-rays are insufficient proof when the patient has persistent symptoms, and endoscopy should be routine.

Polyposis

Polyposis of any degree requires endoscopy with resection of available polyps for complete histological examination. If the polyps are multiple and prove on resection to be of the adenomatous variety, consideration must be given to gastric resection. If this is impossible because of poor risk features, routine endoscopy with removal of further polyps, biopsy of suspicious areas in the gastric mucosa, and brush cytology must be employed at intervals.

SUMMARY

There are numerous epidemiological clues as to the cause of gastric cancer in certain population groups in various parts of the world. Unfortunately, these trends are not consistent or definite enough to provide the basis of mechanisms for control of the disease, even in those countries with a high incidence. Gastric cancer must still be listed as potentially controllable, but not presently.

The diagnosis of gastric cancer has been markedly improved with the development of fiberoptic endoscopy with directed biopsy and brush cytology. The use of this method in all suspected cases will give a correct histological diagnosis in 98%. Those groups most at risk include patients with gastric ulcer, achlorhydria, pernicious anemia, polyposis, and previous subtotal gastric resection or gastroenterostomy. Also at high risk are patients over 50 years of age with undiagnosed upper gastrointestinal symptoms and those with a strong family history for cancer. No means should be spared in the investigation of such individuals when there are chronic symptoms. A high index of suspicion, plus careful patient orientation and investigation at the earliest level, may well have a definite effect on the treatment results in gastric cancer.

REFERENCES

Dungal, N. 1966. Stomach cancer in Iceland. Can. Cancer Conf. 6:441–450.

Elsborg, L., and J. Mosbech. 1979. Pernicious anemia as a risk factor in gastric cancer. Acta Med. Scand. 206:315–318.

Flood, C. A., and R. Lattes. 1967. Premalignant lesions of the stomach, in Cancer of the Gastrointestinal Tract. Year Book Medical Publishers Inc., Chicago, pp. 113–125.

Macdonald, E. J. 1974. Gastric cancer diagnosis. Epidemiological aspects. JAMA 228:884–886.

Matolo, N. M., M. R. Klauber, W. M. Gorishek, and J. A. Dixon. 1972. High incidence of gastric carcinoma in a coal mining region. Cancer 29:733–737.

Merliss, R. R. 1972. Talc-treated rice and Japanese stomach cancer. Science 173:1141–1142.

Nagayo, T., and H. Yokoyama. 1974. c. Gastric cancer diagnosis. Early phases and diagnostic features. JAMA 228:888–889.

Nelson, R. S. 1970. Endoscopy in gastric cancer, in Recent Results in Cancer Research, Rentchnick, P., ed. Springer-Verlag, New York, pp. 42–44.

Oettle, A. G. 1968. Discussion, in Epidemiological, Experimental, and Clinical Studies on Gastric Cancer, R. Kinosita, T. Nagayo, T. Tanaka, eds. Maruzen Co. Ltd., Tokyo, p. 33.

Papachristou, D. N., N. Agnanti, and J. G. Fortner. 1980. Gastric carcinoma after treatment of ulcer. Am. J. Surg. 139:193–196.

Zaldivar, R. 1970. Geographic pathology of oral, esophageal, gastric, and intestinal cancer in Chile. Z. Krebsforsch 75:1–13.

Gastrointestinal Cancer, edited by
John R. Stroehlein and
Marvin M. Romsdahl.
Raven Press, New York © 1981.

Operative Management of Carcinoma of the Esophagus

Clifton F. Mountain, M.D., Kamal G. Khalil, M.D.,* Marion J. McMurtrey, M.D., and O. Howard Frazier, M.D.

*Department of Surgery, The University of Texas System Cancer Center
M. D. Anderson Hospital and Tumor Institute, Houston, Texas*

An integrated and selective approach to the operative management of carcinoma of the esophagus is derived from understandings of the nature of this disease. Full weight is given to the fact that the overwhelming majority of patients present for treatment late in the course of their disease. The role of surgery is first to define the patient who has some potential for cure, and second to define the patient whose quality of life may be enhanced or whose longevity may be increased in the continuing presence of disease. The following dependent factors must be considered in the design of any treatment strategy:

1. the patient's physiologic condition;
2. the presence of serious complications such as tracheoesophageal fistula or acute aspiration pneumonitis;
3. primary tumor characteristics such as the level of origin and its uppermost extent, the esophageal length involved, and the degree of circumferential involvement;
4. the absence or presence and the location of lymph node involvement; and
5. prior gastric or colon resection for an unrelated condition, and the status of the colon regarding diverticulosis, polyps, etc.

Observations on the devastating nature of esophageal carcinoma with respect to the quality of life, the fact that many patients die without evidence of lymphatic or hematogenous metastasis, and the fact that improvement in both quality of life and median survival have been achieved with palliative bypass serve to justify an aggressive therapeutic approach, within reason. Restoration of good nutrition and a normal act of swallowing are the primary objectives in all possible cases. In selected instances, these objectives are combined with attempts to "cure" through the use of radical treatment.

---

*Current Address: 1213 Hermann Drive, Houston, Texas.

SEQUENCE OF TREATMENT

Nutritional Support

The first priorities in all patients under consideration for surgical management are to avoid bronchial aspiration and to effect a positive nitrogen balance. These goals are effectively achieved by intravenous hyperalimentation and an educational program which trains the patient to effectively expectorate oral secretions. This regimen is used where there is first-degree or total obstruction, and in patients with tracheoesophageal fistula or in whom pernicious vomiting is a critical problem. Patients with two out of three of the following findings are placed on hyperalimentation:

1. weight loss greater than 10% of usual weight,
2. serum albumin level equal to or less than 3.5 grams, and
3. nonreactivity to delayed recall skin antigens.

An anabolic state with weight gain is achieved with 45 calories per kilogram per day. In addition, it can be shown that there is a return to a more immunocompetent status as measured both by skin testing and in vitro studies (Frazier et al. 1977).

Nasogastric tube feeding is used as a less expensive alternative to hyperalimentation in patients with second-degree obstruction, but only if it fulfills the priority requirements. In less obstructed patients, nutritional requirements can usually be met with protein-supplemented oral feedings; a schedule of six equal feedings is usually well tolerated. By using elemental diet formulas, the colonic residue is markedly reduced and so is the bacterial flora. Both these effects benefit the surgical procedure if the colon is chosen for bypass.

Sequential Approach to Treatment

As soon as possible following the initiation of nutritional support, usually from one to three weeks, a series of sequential steps in definitive management are effected. A diagrammatic representation of the overall treatment strategy is shown in Table 1. The plan is structured so that any succeeding step can be eliminated if this is indicated by the dynamic course of the disease, and no potential therapeutic option is excluded by any preceding treatment. Patients are initially categorized for treatment planning into two groups, one able to undergo major surgery and another in which nonsurgical treatment is the primary option. Surgical candidates then undergo selective mesenteric arteriography, preoperative irradiation, and subsequent laparotomy.

The findings at exploration determine whether palliative esophageal bypass and further nonsurgical treatment are advisable or whether to proceed with thoracotomy and possible definitive resection. In those patients with lesions arising in the upper two thirds of the esophagus and who are amenable to definitive resection, colon interposition is followed by right thoracotomy and esophagectomy. Partial esophagogastrectomy with esophagogastrostomy,

Table 1. *Carcinoma of the Esophagus—Treatment Sequence*

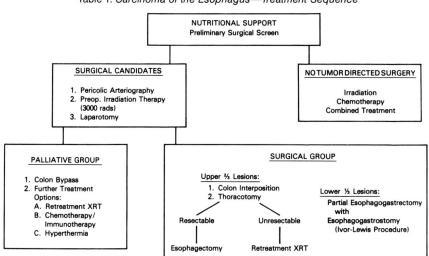

using the Ivor-Lewis approach, is the procedure of choice for lesions in the lower third of the esophagus (Lewis 1946, 1952).

Preliminary Surgical Screening

The essence of the surgical evaluative process is to assess therapy limitations according to primary tumor characteristics and regional extension or spread of the disease. A detailed description of diagnostic procedures appropriate for carcinoma of the esophagus will be found in the chapter by R. W. Bennetts (1981, see pages 137 to 142, this volume). From a surgical standpoint, the surgeon places primary emphasis on the studies that determine the option for surgical treatment. In sequence, the barium swallow and upper gastrointestinal series usually reveal the involved segment, although infrequently a tumor is diagnosed so early that no decrease in the size of the lumen is observed. Esophagoscopy provides a tissue diagnosis and further characterization of the lesion, particularly with regard to the uppermost level of disease extent. Distant metastatic scans are performed if these are indicated by other clinical and laboratory findings. Surgical candidates undergo the necessary physiologic studies related to operative risk and have routine mechanical lung function evaluation. A barium enema is necessary to identify any co-morbid disorders of the colon and to demonstrate any previous intra-abdominal surgery for other causes. Bronchoscopy is indicated for all lesions with the proximal extent at or above the tracheal bifurcation. Direct laryngoscopy is indicated in the presence of hoarseness or evidence of vocal cord paralysis.

The description of primary tumor classification as recommended by the American Joint Committee is shown in Table 2 (American Joint Committee

Table 2. *Esophagus—Primary Tumor Classification**

TO	No demonstrable tumor in the esophagus.
TIS	Carcinoma in situ.
T1	A tumor that involves 5 cm or less of esophageal length, that produces no obstruction, and that has no circumferential involvement and no extraesophageal spread.
T2	A tumor that involves more than 5 cm of esophageal length without extraesophageal spread, or a tumor of any size which produces obstruction or involves the entire circumference, but without extraesophageal spread.
T3	Any tumor with evidence of extraesophageal spread.

*American Joint Committee for Cancer Staging and End Results Reporting: *Manual for Staging of Cancer,* 1978, p. 65.

for Cancer Staging and End Results Reporting 1978). TO is used for retreatment classification and TIS represents carcinoma in situ. Increasing degrees of size or extensiveness are designated by T1, T2, and T3. Hoarseness, fixation of the larynx, coughing characteristic of respiratory distress following ingestion of liquids, deep boring chest pain at the level of the tumor site, and fever, which may indicate mediastinal involvement, are all clinical manifestations of extraesophageal spread indicative of a T3 disease situation, which is defined as follows:

1. recurrent laryngeal, phrenic, or sympathetic nerve involvement,
2. fistula formation,
3. involvement of the tracheal or bronchial tree,
4. vena cava or azygous vein obstruction, and
5. malignant effusion.

Mediastinal widening of itself is not considered evidence of mediastinal spread.

Clinically, the presence of a T3 lesion generally precludes planning for definitive resection; however, in those patients physiologically able to undergo major surgery, the option remains for palliative colon bypass to be followed by additional appropriate nonsurgical treatment.

Limited information as to lymph node spread is obtained clinically, with the exception of cervical or axillary involvement. Any nonsurgical evaluation is likely to underestimate the extent of disease with regard to lymph node status in the abdomen or mediastinum. The relationship of cervical, mediastinal, and abdominal lymph nodes to esophageal segments is illustrated in Figure 1 (Mountain and Hermes 1980), and the definitions for metastasis classification are shown in Table 3 (Adapted from American Joint Committee 1978).

The adjacent cervical lymph nodes are the regional nodal stations for the cervical esophagus; any lymph node involvement other than cervical or supraclavicular is regarded as distant metastasis, as is any metastasis to a distant site. For tumors arising in the thoracic esophagus, any cervical, supraclavicular, scalene, or abdominal lymph node involvement or metastasis to a distant site represents distant metastasis.

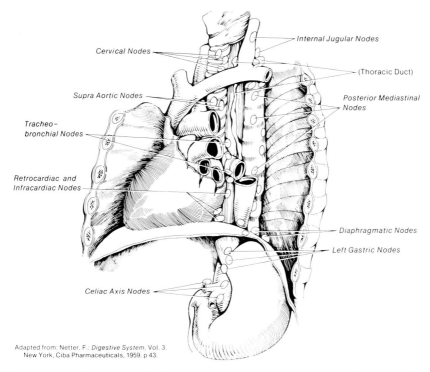

Cervical Nodes

Internal Jugular Nodes

(Thoracic Duct)

Supra Aortic Nodes

Posterior Mediastinal Nodes

Tracheo-bronchial Nodes

Retrocardiac and Infracardiac Nodes

Diaphragmatic Nodes

Left Gastric Nodes

Celiac Axis Nodes

Adapted from: Netter, F.: *Digestive System*, Vol. 3. New York, Ciba Pharmaceuticals, 1959. p 43.

FIG. 1. Relationship of mediastinal lymph nodes to esophageal segments. (Reproduced from Mountain and Hermes, 1980, with permission of G. K. Hall.)

No Tumor-Directed Surgery

Tumor-directed surgery is obviously eliminated from treatment planning in the presence of cardiopulmonary inadequacy or other debilitating physiologic conditions, including an uncorrectable nutritional imbalance or a short life

Table 3. *Esophagus Metastasis Classification**

SITE	REGIONAL NODAL STATIONS
Cervical Esophagus	Cervical or supraclavicular nodes, or both.
Thoracic Esophagus	Adjacent mediastinal lymph nodes.
	DISTANT METASTASIS
Cervical Esophagus	Lymph node involvement other than cervical or supraclavicular, or metastasis to a distant site.
Thoracic Esophagus	Any cervical, supraclavicular, scalene, or abdominal lymph nodes, or metastasis to a distant site.

*American Joint Committee for Cancer Staging and End Results Reporting: *Manual for Staging of Cancer,* 1978, p. 65.

Table 4. *Carcinoma of the Esophagus—Treatment Sequence*

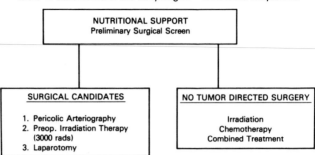

expectancy. Morbid disease such as cachexia, senility, severe pulmonary infection, cardiac abnormalities, hepatic damage, and impaired renal function carries increased morbidity and mortality risks, even in the presence of a clinically favorable tumor. For those patients whose disease remains regional, irradiation therapy is the treatment of choice. Further discussion of this modality for esophageal carcinoma will be found in the chapter by H. T. Barkley (1981, see pages 171 to 187, this volume). Chemotherapy and combined treatment may also be options for these patients (Table 4).

Those patients physiologically able to undergo major surgery are considered surgical candidates, not in the context of definitive resection, but rather for the second step in a treatment sequence that will now provide a means for normal alimentary function, whether or not further radical treatment can be considered.

Surgical Candidates

Selective Mesenteric Arteriography

For those patients considered appropriate surgical candidates, evaluation of the vascular supply to the colon by mesenteric arteriography is the next step (Table 4).

The most important factor in a successful colon interposition is an adequate blood supply. A long segment of normal bowel with an intact marginal artery or a completely anastomosing vascular arcade is required. In past years, we were plagued with dehiscence of the esophageal anastomosis in a considerable number of cases. Therefore, we undertook an evaluation of preoperative superior and inferior mesenteric arteriograms to determine if this information could enlighten the surgeon regarding the vascular supply and enable selection of a technically optimum segment of colon for reconstruction (Ventemeglia et al. 1977).

Selective routine preoperative mesenteric arteriograms were performed on 20 consecutive patients with carcinoma of the esophagus who were candidates for radical surgical treatment. An intact left marginal artery was present in all of the studies; however, in the right colon an adequate vascular arcade was present in only six cases. In Figure 2, the angiographic pattern as it relates to the planning of the operative procedure is shown. In this superior mesenteric arteriogram, the arrows show the interruption of the marginal artery at the level of the ascending colon. Right colon interposition is contraindicated in this instance. In prior experience, the incidence of significant breakdown of anastomosis in the neck when the right colon was used was 30% to 35%. This failure was undoubtedly due to an inadequate blood supply at the esophagocolonic anastomosis. An intact left marginal artery, as demonstrated by mesenteric arteriography, is shown in Figure 3. The entire segment of colon between the two sets of arrows would remain viable with colon interposition. The postoperative appearance of the colonic vasculature following successful colon interposition is shown in Figure 4. During the course of this study, only one patient of 19 undergoing left colon interposition developed anastomotic dehiscence in the neck, and the failure in this case was thought to be due to mesenteric venous obstruction.

Following review of mesenteric angiograms, all surgical candidates undergo preoperative [60]Cobalt radiotherapy, 3000 rads in two weeks. Upon completion of this treatment, laparotomy and colon interposition are performed if indicated.

The angiographic studies can save up to 45 minutes of operative time, because it is possible for the surgeon to know prior to laparotomy exactly

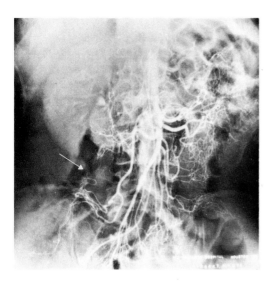
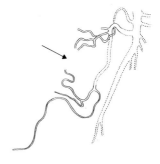

FIG. 2. Preoperative superior mesenteric arteriogram. Interruption of the marginal artery at the level of the ascending colon marked by arrows. Right colon interposition contraindicated. (Reproduced with permission of Ventemeglia, R., et al.: J. Thorac. Cardiovasc. Surg. 74:101, 1977.)

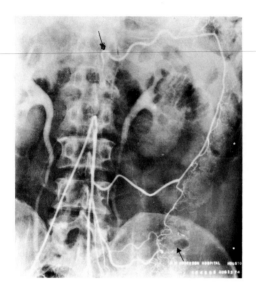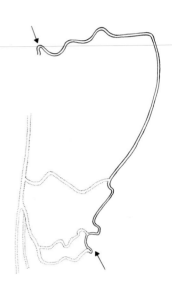

FIG. 3. Preoperative inferior mesenteric arteriogram. Extent of intact marginal artery marked by arrows. Good candidate for left colon interposition. (Reproduced with permission of Ventemeglia, R., et al.: J. Thorac. Cardiovasc. Surg. 74:102, 1977.)

where the vessels are and where they should be transected. This is one of the major factors contributing to success with colon interposition, which is illustrated diagrammatically in Figure 5.

The left colon has been mobilized and the right colon anastomosed to the sigmoid with colocolostomy. The left colon is swung on the middle colic artery in an antiperistaltic fashion so that the distal part of the left colon is now in the neck and the proximal part has been anastomosed to the stomach. Notice that the interposed colon is vertical; the cologastrostomy is not made at the fundus of the stomach, but rather in the prepyloric region. An esophagocolostomy is performed in the neck and a tube gastrostomy is placed for decompression of the stomach as a temporary relief valve. Pyloroplasty completes the operation. The interposed colon is substernal and extrapleural.

Another important point is that two surgical teams operate simultaneously, one in the cervical region and one in the abdomen. If the abdomen is free of disease at exploration, the patient is a candidate for subsequent esophagectomy. If there is evidence of extensive nodal involvement, minimal involvement which cannot be cleared with conviction, or liver involvement, the patient is placed in the palliative group.

Palliative Group

In the palliative group, the colon bypass achieves one of four major goals; namely, that swallowing function is restored as expediently as possible such that the patient enjoys the benefits of restored swallowing for as long as

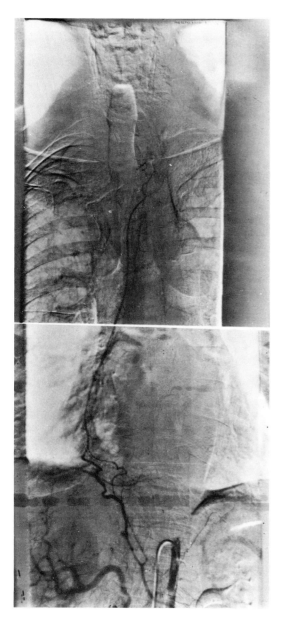

FIG. 4. Composite postoperative superior mesenteric arteriogram with a noninterrupted marginal artery extending from the middle colic artery to the neck. (Reproduced with permission of Ventemeglia, R., et al.: J. Thorac. Cadiovasc. Surg. 74:103, 1977.)

possible. Further, by the sequencing of the treatment used, other options remain for further therapy.

Retreatment irradiation is the option of choice where the disease remains regional to the field of treatment. This, because of the timing, represents a split course of therapy and has presented no problems with irradiation damage to the interposed colon.

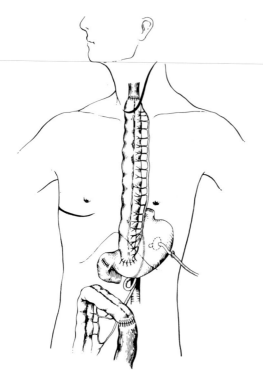

FIG. 5. Diagrammatic representation of retrosternal left colon interposition, pyloroplasty, gastrostomy, colocolostomy, and esophagocolic anastomosis. The marginal artery, noninterrupted, reaches the neck, fed by the middle colic artery. (Reproduced with permission of Ventemeglia, R., et al.: J. Thorac. Cardiovasc. Surg. 74:99, 1977.)

Surgical Group

Lesions in the Upper Two Thirds of the Esophagus

Table 5 describes the plan for those patients in the definitive surgical group. For lesions in the upper two thirds of the intrathoracic esophagus in the definitive group, colon interposition is followed by exploratory thoracotomy. Over 95% of all patients undergoing this sequence have had resectable tumors and have undergone total esophagectomy. In the event that the lesion is unresectable, retreatment irradiation remains an option.

Lesions in the Lower Third of the Esophagus

Patients with lesions of the lower third of the intrathoracic esophagus (Table 5) undergo esophagogastrectomy with esophagogastrostomy using the Ivor-Lewis procedure (Figure 6). The advantages of this procedure were noted by Lewis as follows:

1. accessibility to the upper two thirds of the esophagus is gained,
2. only the azygos vein has to be divided to lay bare the whole course of the esophagus, and
3. the aortic arch and, to a large extent, the descending aorta, instead of being an obstacle, becomes a safety barrier for the contralateral pleural cavity.

Table 5. *Carcinoma of the Esophagus—Treatment Sequence*

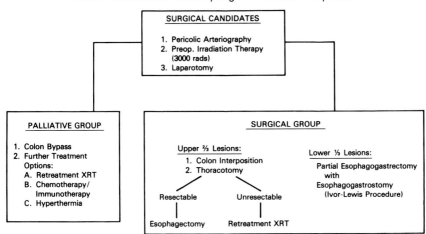

Others have noted that this approach permits more extensive resection, if necessary, and that upon completion of the surgery, the reconstructed stomach is in a more satisfactory position (Postlethwait 1979).

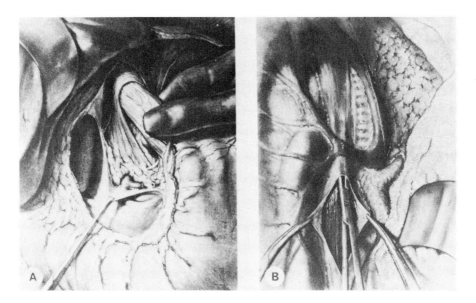

FIG. 6. Lewis technique has several advantages. **A.** Laparotomy permits identification of metastasis below the diaphragm prior to mobilization of the stomach. **B.** Right thoracotomy shows that only the azygos vein must be divided to expose the esophagus. (Reproduced from Postlethwait 1979, with permission of Appleton-Century-Crofts.)

RESULTS

If the application of a treatment sequence involving such a major procedure as colon interposition is to be rational, it must first of all be reasonably safe. In a review of 45 patients undergoing colon interposition and esophagectomy or colon interposition alone as a palliative procedure, there were two operative deaths for an operative death rate of 4.4%. One of the deaths was due to a stroke subsequent to esophagectomy following a palliative procedure; the other, in an elderly patient, was due to complications following treatment of a small-bowel obstruction secondary to intra-abdominal adhesions (Table 6).

The second consideration is relief of dysphagia, since this is the primary symptom for which the procedure is done. Restoration of swallowing ability was evaluated as good or very good in 95% of the cases.

The third consideration in this approach to management is morbidity. In 15 patients, there were no complications except reflux, which is universal but is not of itself regarded as a morbid condition. Each patient is individually instructed in regard to dealing with this problem.

A significant number of complications were encountered in the 80 major procedures performed (Table 7). However, the implications for the patient were not as formidable as the numbers imply. Only five of the problems required surgical intervention; one of the cervical leaks failed to heal spontaneously and one of the episodes of chylothorax required surgical intervention. Laparotomy and lysis of adhesions were performed in three cases. There were no deaths from infection.

The final outcome of this approach remains to be definitively assessed. However, for those patients having preoperative mesenteric arteriography

Table 6. *Carcinoma of the Esophagus*
Colon Interposition—Esophagectomy. Operative Mortality

	Number	Operative Deaths	%
Definitive Surgery			
Colon Interposition and Esophagectomy	27	1	3.7
Colon Interposition and Laryngopharyngectomy	5	—	—
Colon Interposition and Esophagogastrectomy	1	—	—
Subtotal	33	1	3.0
Palliative Surgery			
Palliative Colon Interposition	10	1	10.0
Palliative Colon Interposition and Thoracic Esophagectomy	2	—	—
Subtotal	12	1	8.3
Total	45	2	4.4

Table 7. *Carcinoma of the Esophagus*
Colon Interposition—Esophagectomy. Morbidity (N = 45)*

Complication	Number	Percentage
None	*15/43*	*34.9%*
Cervical 'Leak'	7/43	16.2%
Vocal Cord Palsy	4/43	9.3%
Infection	5/43	11.6%
Minor Pulmonary Embolism	3/43	6.9%
Chylothorax	4/43	9.3%
Small Bowel Obstruction	3/43	6.9%
Pneumonia	2/43	4.7%
Miscellaneous	6/43	13.9%

*Two postoperative deaths due primarily to stroke, ischemia.

and radiotherapy followed by colon interposition and esophagectomy, we anticipate achieving a survival rate at two years in excess of 50% and at five years of 35% to 40%.

In summary, a significant number of patients with esophageal carcinoma are amenable to disease control by current surgical and adjuvant modalities. The sequencing of treatment strategy to accommodate the dynamics of the disease affords individualized use of available therapeutic measures to achieve the most effective relief from devastating symptoms and to provide some potential for cure.

ACKNOWLEDGMENTS

The authors wish to acknowledge Kay E. Hermes, Senior Research Assistant, Section of Thoracic Surgery, for her contributions to the preparation of this manuscript; Ms. Ann Murphy, Assistant Epidemiologist, for statistical assistance and record review; Ms. P. J. Blotz for secretarial assistance; and the Department of Epidemiology, M. D. Anderson Hospital, for case listings.

REFERENCES

American Joint Committee for Cancer Staging and End Results Reporting. 1978. Staging of Cancer of the Esophagus, *in* Manual for Staging of Cancer, Cancer 1978, Chicago (Revised and Reprinted).

Barkley, H. T. 1981. Radiotherapy in the treatment of carcinoma of the esophagus, *in* Gastrointestinal Cancer, J. R. Stroehlein and M. M. Romsdahl, eds. Raven Press, New York, New York, pp. 171–187.

Bennetts, R. W. 1981. Esophageal cancer in the United States: Diagnostic modalities and surveillence of high-risk groups, *in* Gastrointestinal Cancer, J. R. Stroehlein and M. M. Romsdahl, eds. Raven Press, New York, New York, pp. 137–142.

Frazier, T. G., E. M. Copeland, K. G. Khalil, S. J. Dudrick, and C. F. Mountain. 1977. Intravenous hyperalimentation as an adjunct to colon interposition for carcinoma of the esophagus. Cancer 39:410–412.

Lewis, I. 1946. The surgical treatment of carcinoma of the esophagus. With special reference to a new operation for growths of the middle third. Br. J. Surg. 54:18.

Lewis, I. 1952. Carcinoma of the esophagus, *in* Gastroenterology, F. A. Jones, ed. Paul B. Hoeber, New York, p. 199.

Mountain, C. F., and K. E. Hermes. 1980. Cancer of the Esophagus: The Meaning of Lymph Nodes and Their Treatment—Esophagus, *in* Lymphatic System Metastasis, L. Weiss, H. A. Gilbert, I. Ballon, eds. K. G. Hall, Boston, pp. 250–261.

Postlethwait, R. W. 1979. Surgery of the Esophagus, Appleton-Century-Crofts, New York, p. 441.

Ventemeglia, R., K. G. Khalil, O. H. Frazier, and C. F. Mountain. 1977. The role of preoperative mesenteric arteriography in colon interposition. J. Thorac. Cardiovasc. Surg. 74:97–104.

Gastrointestinal Cancer, edited by
John R. Stroehlein and
Marvin M. Romsdahl.
Raven Press, New York © 1981.

The Surgical Management of Carcinoma of the Stomach

Richard G. Martin, M.D.

*Department of General Surgery, The University of Texas System Cancer Center
M. D. Anderson Hospital and Tumor Institute, Houston, Texas*

Although Avicenna first recognized and described the symptoms of carcinoma of the stomach in the eleventh century, it was not until January 29, 1881, that Dr. Theodore Billroth first performed successfully, on a human, a subtotal gastrectomy for carcinoma of the stomach. The patient died four months later of recurrent carcinoma. The same year Woelfler performed the first gastroenterostomy for cancer. By 1890, 41 gastric resections had been performed in the Billroth Clinic, with 19 successes. In 1896, two years after Billroth's death, Hans Haberkaut of Danzig reported that a total of 257 resections had been performed for cancer, with a mortality rate of 54.4%. Carl Schlatter, a Swiss surgeon, in 1897 performed the first total gastrectomy with end-esophagus-to-side jejunal anastomosis. One year later Dr. C. B. Brigham did the first successful total gastrectomy in America. It seems fitting that this symposium should take place on the eve of the hundredth anniversary of Dr. Billroth's surgical contribution to the treatment of gastric cancer.

ANATOMIC CONSIDERATIONS AND STAGING

The success of gastrectomy for carcinoma of the stomach depends mainly upon two factors: the first is the extent of penetration of the lesion into the gastric wall and the second is the degree of lymphatic spread. Extent of invasion and lymphatic metastasis are also determining factors in colon and rectal carcinoma. Because of the lymphatic drainage, the location of the lesion in the stomach becomes very important. Lesions in the prepyloric and antral area drain mainly along the lesser curvature of the stomach and around the duodenum, above and behind the head of the pancreas along the epiploic vessels and the short gastric vessels to the nodes in the area of the celiac artery. For lesions located in the fundus of the stomach, the lymphatics drain mainly to the paracardial nodes, the nodes along the lesser curvature, and those going along the short gastric vessels to the splenic hilum and the tail of the pancreas, then to the celiac group. Therefore, for lesions arising in the mid-portion of the stomach and the fundus, a total gastrectomy is the procedure of choice. These lymphatic pathways follow the major blood vessels supplying the stomach. Knowing that the prognosis depends upon the extent of invasion and the lymphatic involvement, a staging system has evolved using the TNM method of classification. The following is a postsurgical treatment TNM classification.

STAGE I: pT1 NO MO
             Tumor confined to the mucosa and submucosa (pT1). No metastasis in regional lymph nodes (NO). No distant metastasis (MO).

STAGE II: pT2 NO MO
             Tumor involving the mucosa and the submucosa, including the muscularis propria, and extending to or into the serosa, but not penetrating through the serosa (pT2). No metastasis in regional lymph nodes (NO). No distant metastasis (MO).
             pT3 NO MO
             Tumor penetrating through the serosa without invasion of contiguous structures (pT3). No metastasis in regional lymph nodes (NO). No distant metastasis (MO).

STAGE III: pT4 NO MO
             Tumor penetrates through the serosa with invasion of contiguous structures (pT4). No lymph nodes involved (NO). No distant metastasis (MO).
             pT1-3 N1 MO
             pT1-3 N2 MO
             pT1-3 N3 MO
             pT4 NO-3 MO
             Any involvement of the stomach wall as defined by pT1 to pT4 and including involvement of the intra-abdominal nodes resected for cure. No distant metastasis.

STAGE IV: pT4 NO3 MO
             pT1-3 N3 MO
             Tumor involving the stomach wall with invasion of contiguous structures (pT4) and any regional nodal involvement not resectable for cure, or M1 with any T and any N. Any carcinoma of the stomach with distant metastasis (M1), including those with TX or NX.

(Manual for Staging of Cancer, 1978.)

TECHNIQUE OF RESECTION

Gastrectomy is usually performed through a vertical midline incision; however, bilateral subcostal incisions or a right slash type incision extended into the chest may be used. If a total gastrectomy is contemplated, good exposure of the esophagus below the diaphragm is important. In general, the midline incision gives the best all-around exposure. After examining the abdomen thoroughly for distant metastasis and determining that gastrectomy is feasible, the procedure is carried out in the following manner. The omentum is freed from the transverse colon from the duodenal area to the spleen. It is then lifted upward and the lesser sac entered. The posterior aspect of the stomach is examined to determine the extent of tumor spread, if any, that would necessitate the tail of the pancreas being resected. The hepatoduodenal ligament is then dissected to remove all lymph nodes around the common duct and portal vein, exposing the hepatic artery and its right and left branches as well as the gastroduodenal and right gastric arteries. The right gastric artery is clamped and ligated. The dissection is carried down behind the duodenum, to include lymph nodes around this area and the head of the pancreas. The duodenum is divided 1 to 3 cm below the pylorus. After the duodenum is divided, the stomach can be lifted up and retracted to the right along with the spleen. The peritoneal attachments posterior to the spleen are cut allowing the spleen and the tail of the pancreas to be retracted upward into the wound. The tail of the pancreas is not resected unless there is obvious nodal metastasis in the hilum of the spleen. The portion of the pancreas taken is from the superior mesenteric vessels to the left. The nodes are dissected off of the hepatic artery to its origin at the celiac trunk. The splenic artery is ligated at an appropriate distance, depending on whether the tail of the pancreas is removed. If the pancreas is not removed, lymph nodes along the splenic artery are removed. The nodes about the celiac trunk are resected. The left gastric artery is clamped and ligated at its origin from the celiac trunk. The gastrohepatic ligament is dissected off from the base of the liver. All the tissue is retracted downwards and up out of the wound so that the paracardial lymph nodes may be dissected from around the lower end of the esophagus. The esophagus is freed up to the diaphragm, a right angle noncrushing clamp is applied to the lower esophagus, and the specimen is removed en bloc. The en bloc specimen consists of the regional lymph node drainage areas as well as those along the aorta in the area of the celiac trunk. This is a clean anatomical resection. In performing a subtotal gastric resection, the line of resection is from the esophagus at the lesser curvature junction, across the fundus of the stomach above the short gastric vessels, thus leaving a small cuff of stomach. In certain rare instances where a very small lesion is located in the prepyloric area, a less radical resection may be performed.

The type of reconstruction for gastrointestinal continuity depends upon the build of the individual and the preference of the surgeon. Several methods may be employed. They are an end-to-end esophagojejunostomy with a Rouxen Y anastomosis for duodenal drainage, a loop jejunal pouch end-to-side esophagojejuno anastomosis, a Hunt-Lawrence type pouch using the end-to-side jejunal loop, or a figure nine end-to-side jejunoesophageal anastomosis with a Rouxen Y. All of these procedures are acceptable.

Success depends upon good surgical technique, taking care to ensure no tension at the suture line and no leaks. A drain may be placed in the subphrenic space, especially if the tail of the pancreas has been resected. If a drain is placed in the subphrenic area, a sump type drain which is removed within 24 to 48 hours is the best. It should be emphasized at this time that the specimen removed be sent to the pathology laboratory for frozen section histological confirmation of tumor-free margins at the esophageal and duodenal lines of resection. If tumor should be present, a higher esophageal resection must be made. At times, it may be necessary to enter the chest and approach it through a thoracoabdominal incision.

INDICATIONS FOR GASTRIC RESECTION

Gastric resection, either radical subtotal or total gastrectomy, is indicated whenever possible for carcinoma of the stomach. The question is whether a radical procedure should be done for palliation. It is often difficult to define what will end up being palliation and what is going to be cure. The prognosis is poor for carcinoma of the stomach once lymph node metastasis has occurred. This is especially true if there are second station nodes involved, such as those around the celiac axis or the aorta. However, we have had patients with total gastrectomies, with 14 out of 14 positive lymph nodes, living well over six months following surgery. Certainly the cure rate would be very low in such cases, but palliation has been well worthwhile. Whenever possible, a gastric lesion should be resected rather than only a diverting gastroenterostomy done. It has been our experience that diverting gastroenterostomies of necessity have to be placed too high for good drainage, thus resulting in poor palliation. Difficulties arising from radical subtotal gastrectomy and total gastrectomy have been (1) the lack of a reservoir for ingested food, (2) reflux esophagitis, and (3) lack of caloric intake. Attempts are made to correct these with a suitable reservoir by performing a Rouxen Y or enterostomy low enough and far enough away from the gastroenterostomy or esophagoenterostomy to prevent reflux into the lower esophagus, although this is not always possible. Vitamin B_{12}, iron, and pancreatic enzymes are administered to all patients undergoing radical gastrectomy. Patients developing recurrent carcinoma of the gastric stump or those with carcinoma developing in the gastric stump following resection for ulcer disease, require laparatomy and total gastric resection whenever possible.

COMPLICATIONS FOLLOWING RADICAL SUBTOTAL OR TOTAL GASTRIC RESECTIONS

Anastomotic leak is the most important complication. This is true following either a Billroth I or Billroth II procedure, and it becomes even more significant following a total gastrectomy. One of the most difficult anastomoses to make is an esophagojejunostomy, either end-to-end or end-to-side. Great care must be taken when making this anastomosis. A two-layer closure is most often performed using an outer layer of silk and an inner layer of an absorbable suture. Stapling devices are available for those who are skilled in using this method. Good technical care is what is important. However, following stapling, the anastomotic site tends to remain open at all times thus causing more esophageal reflux.

The use of hyperalimentation pre- and postoperatively helps prevent leaks by improving nutrition; if a leak does occur, it can sustain the patient while the anastomosis heals. Preoperative hyperalimentation is especially indicated in an individual who has lost large quantities of weight and has a negative protein balance. Postoperatively, before a patient is fed solid food, it is routine to obtain a barium swallow to assure that no leak is present. If a leak should be present and it is small, hyperalimentation and nothing by mouth will frequently correct the situation. However, if a significant leak is present and a subdiaphragmatic collection of fluid is shown by x-ray examination, the subphrenic space must be surgically drained and the patient put on hyperalimentation (Figure 1). Usually the fistulous track will heal within ten days to two weeks. Care must be taken in placing the nasogastric tube at the time of total gastrectomy. It should be placed entirely through the anastomotic site and fastened in place. If for some reason, after surgery, the tube comes out, one should not try to insert it because the incidence of anastomotic leak is greatly increased by blindly reinserting the tube through the anastomotic site. In subtotal gastrectomies, the tube, if it is a large pouch, usually is placed in the stomach and fixed well so that it will not poke through the anastomotic site. If there is a very small gastric pouch remaining, the tube is placed through the anastomotic site into the efferent loop and fastened in place. Again, following a subtotal gastric resection, all patients are given a barium swallow before starting on food.

END RESULTS EXPECTED

The overall worldwide five-year survival rates for radical subtotal and total gastrectomies for cancer of the stomach are in the range between 8% and 25%. Early diagnosis is the key to cure. Patients with superficial gastric lesions and with no lymph node metastasis do very well and have a higher (close to 40% to 50%) five-year survival rate. However, once the lymph nodes become positive, the rate decreases considerably. Diagnosing the patient's disease in an early stage has been done best by the Japanese through their endoscopic gastric surveys; they are now obtaining good results in early T1 lesions as well. In this country where carcinoma is not so prevalent, such a screening program is not cost-effective. One should observe carefully those patients with constant reflux symptoms, either from duodenal reflux into the stomach or gastric reflux into the lower esophagus. Of the last five gastrectomies

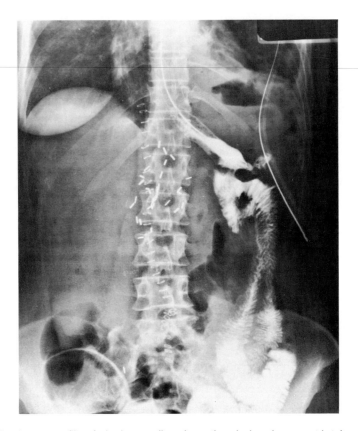

FIG. 1. The above x-ray film of a barium swallow shows the misplaced nasogastric tube penetrating the anastomotic line following a subtotal gastrectomy. Barium and free air with a fluid level can readily be seen. The tube was removed, the subdiaphragmatic space surgically drained, and hyperalimentation continued until the anastomosis healed in about ten days.

performed here in 1980, three patients had a history of long-standing reflux problems.

SUMMARY

Gastric resection, either radical subtotal or total, is the procedure of choice whenever possible for carcinoma of the stomach. Early diagnosis is necessary to accomplish good results. At the present time, the overall worldwide five-year survival rate is between 8% and 25%. However, only approximately one third of the patients seen have resectable lesions. More patients should be surgically explored, and explored early, especially those with long-standing symptoms of indigestion and gastric reflux or ulcer disease. All ulcer patients should be observed carefully for postgastrectomy stump carcinoma occurring at a later date. With the use of hyperalimentation before and after surgery, and in the event of an esophagojejunostomy failure, the morbidity and mortality rate can be reduced. Compared to the mortality rate of 54.4% obtained in the first 257 cases reported in the world literature in the 1880's and 1890's, the mortality now should not be more than 4% to 5%. The two main factors governing the prognosis in gastric cancer are penetration of the primary lesion and lymph node metastasis. This is characteristic of all gastrointestinal cancers; using the TNM classification, one can determine the resectability of the lesion and prognosticate reasonably the survival rate.

REFERENCES

American Joint Committee for Cancer Staging and End Results Reporting. 1978. Manual for Staging of Cancer 1978. Whiting Press, Chicago, p. 73.

Bloss, R. S., T. A. Miller, and E. M. Copeland. 1980. Carcinoma of the stomach in the young adult. Surg. Gynecol. Obstet. 150:883–886.

Herfarth, C., and P. Schlag, eds. 1979. Gastric Cancer. Springer-Verlag, Berlin.

Kajitani, T., and K. Miwa, eds. 1979. Treatment Results of Stomach Carcinoma in Japan, 1963–1966. WHO Collaborating Center for Evaluation of Methods of Diagnosis and Treatment of Stomach Cancer, Tokyo.

McNeer, G., and G. T. Pack. 1967. Neoplasms of the Stomach. J. B. Lippincott Co., Philadelphia, pp. 408–415.

Mountford, R. A., P. Brown, P. R. Salmon, C. Alvarenga, C. S. Neumann, and A. E. Read. 1980. Gastric cancer detection in gastric ulcer disease. Gut 21:9–17.

Ochsner, A., T. E. Weed, and W. R. Nuessle. 1980. Cancer of the stomach. Am. J. Surg. 141(1):10–14.

Papachristou, D. N., and J. G. Fortner. 1980. Adenocarcinoma of the gastric cardia. Ann. Surg. 192(1):58–64.

ReMine, W. H., J. T. Preistley, and J. Berkson. 1964. Cancer of the Stomach. W. B. Saunders Co., Philadelphia, pp. 97–116.

Schonleben, K., P. Langhans, W. Schlake, G. Kautz, and H. Bunte. 1979. Gastric stump carcinoma—Carcinogenic factors and possible preventive measures. Acta Hepato-Gastroenterol. 26:239–247.

Shiu, M. H., D. N. Papachristou, C. Kosloff, and G. Eliopoulos. 1980. Selection of operative procedure for adenocarcinoma of the midstomach. Ann. Surg. 192(6):730–737.

Wangensteen, O. H., and S. D. Wangensteen. 1978. The Rise of Surgery. University of Minnesota Press, Minneapolis, pp. 147–152.

Gastrointestinal Cancer, edited by
John R. Stroehlein and
Marvin M. Romsdahl.
Raven Press, New York © 1981.

Radiotherapy in the Treatment of Carcinoma of the Esophagus

H. T. Barkley, Jr., M.D., David H. Hussey, M.D., Jerrold P. Saxton, M.D., and William J. Spanos, Jr., M.D.

Division of Radiotherapy, The University of Texas System Cancer Center M. D. Anderson Hospital and Tumor Institute, Houston, Texas

THE MAGNITUDE OF THE PROBLEM

It is projected that carcinoma of the esophagus will account for 1.1% of the new cancer cases this year, and 1.9% of the new cancer deaths. It is predominantly a disease of males; 2.5% of the cancer deaths for males will be attributable to this disease as compared with 1.1% for females. The age-adjusted death rate per 100,000 population has shown an almost imperceptible increase since 1930.

Although the onset of this disease may be either insidious or abrupt, progression after diagnosis is most often rapid and fatal. The End Results Group of the National Cancer Institute reported a five-year survival from 1940–1949 of 1% for males and 5% for females, and from 1965–1969 of 2% for males and 6% for females. Esophageal cancer was the only listed type in which survival for those patients diagnosed as having regional disease (5%) was greater than that for those patients having localized disease (4%) (Silverberg 1980). This paradox is due to the clinical inability to evaluate nodal status or local extension of disease.

HISTORICAL RADIOTHERAPY

Although the chronology of surgical successes follows a distinct pattern associated with progressive knowledge of anesthesia and physiology, the beginnings of radiation therapy for esophageal cancer are obscure. Apparently some abortive attempts at external radiation were attempted within a short time after the discovery of the x-ray, but the approach was abandoned due to the lack of penetration of the available beam. In 1904, Einhorn in New York and Exner in Vienna reported the intracavitary treatment of cancer of the thoracic esophagus by radium bromide salt in nine and six patients, respectively. The technique consisted of attaching a hard rubber capsule containing the radium salt to a bougie and inserting it for varying lengths of time and at varying intervals. Both authors were impressed by the quality of palliation achieved.

Over the ensuing years, filtration, direct vision application, occasional use of concomitant external beam therapy, fluoroscopic control with bismuth or barium for positioning of the sources, and treating the entire length of the lesion by varying the number and position of sources improved the method. With these refinements, long-term survivors were reported, proven free of local disease by repeated endoscopies and biopsies.

In Europe, this method was considered as a replacement for gastrostomy because it was better tolerated by the patient and much more satisfactory psychologically. The eventual requirement of a gastrostomy was considered evidence of treatment failure. Conversely, in the United States gastrostomy was advised prior to the first attempt at treatment with radiation. Whatever the refinement of the technique, however, the universal application of endocavitary therapy to all patients with carcinoma of the esophagus resulted in a high percentage of complications, particularly fistulae and hemorrhage. By 1920, Guisez suggested that patients whose esophagus was essentially completely obstructed could not be maintained through radiation treatment, and that patients with recurrent nerve paralysis, hemoptysis, or severe pain should not be treated. With these selection criteria, 61 patients experienced adequate palliation, and three had negative biopies more than five years after treatment.

By the mid-1920's disillusionment with the method was fairly universal, the impression being that endocavitary radium was essentially no better than periodic bougienage. There followed direct implantation of radon seeds, attachment of radioactive seeds to the walls of Souttar and other tubes, and combinations of external beam therapy and radon implantation. By the late 1930's external beam irradiation had almost completely replaced endocavitary therapy. This was the result of improved equipment with greater beam penetration. Either multiple fields or rotation was used, and a considerable improvement in results was noted. However, early on, radiation pneumonitis was responsible for almost as many deaths as esophageal cancer; 44% and 50%, respectively, in the 1941 series of Strandqvist, who used six fixed fields. By reducing the distance between fields and treating each field each day, Smithers (1943) produced no pulmonary fibrosis and reported 44% survival at one year, 16% at more than two years, and 3/32 patients alive with no evidence of disease from four years, nine months to six years, four months after treatment. In addition, 11 patients were found to have no evidence of disease at the primary site at the time of autopsy, although three had distant metastases. Tumor doses of 6,000 to 7,000 R were delivered in five to six weeks with 400 Kv apparatus. With rotation, as reported by Nielsen in 1944, pulmonary fibrosis was reduced to 3/174 (one symptomatic). In this group 68% were completely relieved of their symptoms, 25% survived one year, and 15% survived more than two years. Tumor doses were calculated between 4,000 and 5,000 Roentgens for 20,000—30,000 R in air delivered in 4 to 5 weeks, with 180-200 Kv.

Some results from the literature through 1970 were summarized by Appelqvist (1972). For patients treated by radiation therapy and receiving a minimum of 5,000 R, the five-year survival was 6.4% (91/1,420). The finest achievement by radiation therapy alone has been a five-year survival of 19% (32/169) in selected cases by Pearson (1974) using 50 gray (Gy) in four weeks with megavoltage.

TREATMENT AT M. D. ANDERSON HOSPITAL

From January 1970 through December 1979, 232 patients with squamous carcinoma and 11 with adenocarcinoma of the esophagus received part or all of their treatment with radiation therapy at M. D. Anderson Hospital. Patient characteristics are demonstrated in Table 1. Perhaps the only unusual aspect of the patient population is the relatively small number of black male patients, since there has been a rapidly increasing rate per 100,000 population in this group.

Taking the mean weight loss for all patients as a percentage of the mean admission weight, 10.8% of usual body weight had been lost as a result of anorexia or dysphagia prior to admission. Dysphagia was an almost universal symptom, appearing as the chief complaint in 91% of all patients. This was invariably described in relation to swallowing solids. A few patients had progressed to difficulty with liquids, but only for short periods of time. There was an equal number of patients having no complaints referrable to the esophagus. Pain was a much less frequent complaint and usually not described in relation to swallowing but as substernal or epigastric, occasionally exacerbated by swallowing. The recorded duration of symptoms is directly proportional to the reliability of the patient's medical history. Most patients

Table 1. *Patient Characteristics*

	Black Male	Black Female	White Male	White Female	All
No. Patients	34	8	137	64	243
Mean Age	63.5	67.8	62.3	60.9	62.3
Mean Admission Weight in lbs	132	121	153	122	141
Mean Weight Less in lbs	29	25	16	13	17
Patients with Dysphagia	33	7	123	59	222
Mean Length of Lesion by X-ray in cms	6.9	10.0	7.1	6.2	6.95
Mean Length of Lesion by Endoscopy in cms	6.7	10.0	6.0	6.4	6.4
Mean Duration of Symptoms in Months	5.3	4.5	4.3	3.9	4.3

are apparently unwilling to admit to anything but the most brief experience of difficulty, with the mean being about 4.3 months. The activity status of this group of patients is difficult to assess. Many have multiple unrelated medical complaints which restrict activity to a point where it is difficult to say to what extent the burden of esophageal cancer has contributed. Our best considered assessment was that the average patient was still capable of maintaining himself or herself with little or no assistance.

The anatomical sites of disease were defined by barium swallow and/or endoscopy according to the classification from the Manual of Staging and End Results Reporting of the American Joint Committee. The cervical esophagus extends from the cricopharyngeus to the thoracic inlet or from the cricopharyngeus to 18 cm from the upper dental margin. The upper and middle thoracic esophagus are considered as one site, extending from 18 cm to 31 cm from the upper dental margin or to the lower border of the eight thoracic vertebrae. The lower segment extends from 30 or 31 cm to the esophagogastric junction, usually about 40 cm from the upper dental margin. From available information, there were 24 patients with cervical lesions, 145 with upper and middle thoracic lesions, 59 with lower thoracic lesions, and 14 patients whose site could not be determined.

Unfortunately, the TNM staging system for esophageal cancer is almost completely dependent on surgical exploration for assessment of the N compartment. An exploration of the neck, thorax, and abdomen would be required for complete evaluation, but most of the patients do not have even one of the three. Indirect evidence by diagnostic radiology is not accepted, although the increasing use of CT scanning is providing noninvasive evidence of mediastinal extension and nodal metastasis never before available. As the ability to interpret these findings increases, the staging system will require expansion to include them. With the evidence available, nearly all patients were staged N_x, with the T and M areas being assessed by barium swallow, endoscopy, and diagnostic x-rays or radioactive scans. Pretreatment evaluation of staging is shown in Table 2. It is remarkable how few of the patients were assessed as having distant metastases, prior to treatment.

Varieties of Treatment

Four major plans were available prior to treatment for the 243 patients considered here. They were 1) palliative irradiation, 2) curative irradiation, 3) preoperative irradiation with either esophagogastrectomy or colon interposition and esophagectomy, and 4) irradiation with chemotherapy. In fact, however, 23 separate plans of treatment were used, which simply emphasizes the vagaries of the disease process. A group of 19 miscellaneous combinations is encompassed in the fifth category of Table 3. The table indicates the number of patients planned for each of the four major treatment categories and the number eventually having that proposed treatment, by year, as well as those

Table 2. *Distribution by Stage*

Stage	No. of Patients	% of Total
I	29	12
II	107	44
III	78	32
Unstaged	29	12

who fell into the fifth category. The principal reasons for change in treatment plan were the presence of metastases in either nodes or liver at the time of abdominal exploration, extension of disease through the wall of the esophagus or through the capsule of lymph nodes in the mediastinum, or deterioration of the patient's condition during the initial phase of treatment.

Palliative radiation consisted of a single course of 30 Gy given in 10 fractions. The patients were seen after three to four weeks and offered a similar course, but it became apparent that those who had not responded well to the first course would not be improved by the second. At the same time, if a second course was given, those who had achieved satisfactory palliation from the single course would be placed at risk for complications, but with no increase in survival time.

Curative radiation for the first five years of this period consisted of two courses of 30 Gy in 10 fractions separated by a month. The last five fractions of the second course were given through posterior oblique fields in order to avoid the spinal cord. In the latter half of the decade, continuous fractionation schemes have been utilized giving 55–70 Gy in 5–7 weeks, by means of three field techniques. In curative treatments for the thoracic esophagus an attempt is made to cover the entire organ, reducing the fields at 45 and 50 Gy.

Table 3. *Method of Treatment by Year*

Year	Palliative XRT Alone	Curative XRT Alone	Curative XRT + Surgery	XRT + Chemo	Palliative XRT ± Surgery ± Chemo	Total Treated
1970	2/4*	1/0	1/0	5/5	6	15
1971	1/3	1/1	4/2	11/11	3	20
1972	3/3	3/4	4/4	6/6	2	19
1973	1/3	9/9	4/1	5/5	3	21
1974	4/6	4/4	13/10	0/0	7	27
1975	5/8	5/6	13/5	1/1	6	26
1976	4/6	7/7	13/6	0/0	9	28
1977	0/1	3/3	11/6	1/2	7	19
1978	7/8	8/8	16/11	0/1	7	35
1979	4/4	5/5	17/12	3/5	7	33
Total	31/46	46/47	96/57	32/36	57	243

*Treatment planned/treatment given.

Curative radiation and surgery consists of 30 Gy in 10 fractions given through parallel opposed fields, followed by the selected surgery. A 5-cm margin on either side of the lesion is used. Over the years there has been a progressive shortening of the interval between the completion of irradiation and the surgery. At present when a staged procedure is planned, the interposition is often done the day following completion of radiation therapy. This is followed by the esophagectomy as healing permits.

Combination radiation therapy and chemotherapy consisted of three plans during this 10-year period; in two, the modalities were used concomitantly and in one chemotherapy was given after radiation.

The first of the concomitant plans was the use of hydroxyurea given in divided doses four hours prior to irradiation and again immediately after treatment. Thirty Gy were given in 10 fractions and repeated after one month's rest. Normal tissue reactions were so severe that the radiation dose was reduced to 25 Gy each course. The most popular postradiation combinations included 5-fluorouracil (5-FU), Adriamycin, methotrexate, cyclophosphamide, and MeCCNU. In the last two years an ambitious program of hyperalimentation together with continuous infusion of bleomycin with Adriamycin and cis-platinum, in combination with 25 Gy of irradiation, has been undertaken. The course is repeated after two to three weeks. This program has been applied to a few very advanced cases, and has shown beneficial effects.

Survival by Patient or Disease Characteristics

Since the first successful therapeutic maneuver for carcinoma of the esophagus 103 years ago, a number of disease or patient characteristics have come to be considered of major prognostic significance. Each of these is analyzed in the following section.

1. Sex and race.

Traditionally survival for women is said to be higher than that for men, and survival for whites is higher than that for blacks. Table 4 appears to justify this assumption. In some surgical series (Nakayama 1979) the five-year survival for women is nearly three times as great as that for men. The racial difference is primarily due to the more advanced stage of disease when first seen in the black patients.

Table 4. *Expected Median Survival by Race and Sex*

Characteristic	No. of Patients	Median Survival in Months
Black	42	8
Male	171	9.1
White	201	11.4
Female	72	14.8

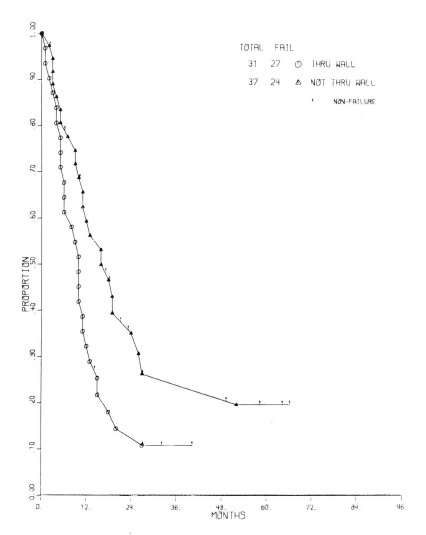

FIG. 1. Survival related to extension through wall.

2. Extension of disease through the wall of the esophagus.

This pathologic feature is considered one of the two most ominous prognostic factors. In its grossest form, as manifested by a tracheoesophageal, bronchoesophageal, or esophagopleural fistula, only treatment to alleviate the symptoms is beneficial. When the manifestation of extension is microscopic in the surgical specimen, it is almost as certainly lethal. Figure 1 compares survival of 31 patients having extraesophageal extension with 37 patients whose disease was confined to the esophageal wall. The respective median expected survivals are 10.4 and 17.9 months. In the surgical experience at

Peking Medical College (Wu and Huang 1979), five-year survival decreased from 33% to 7% when the lesion had infiltrated beyond the esophageal wall.
3. Lymph node metastases.

The occurrence of regional lymph node metastases is the other most ominous prognostic factor. A comparison of survivals for 78 patients with biopsy-proven metastatic lymph nodes at all levels and of 164 patients assumed to be without lymph node metastases revealed the median expected survivals to be less than half a month apart. This indicates the lack of ability to evaluate the N compartment without exploration. When the comparison is limited to those 86 patients who had surgical exploration (Figure 2), positive

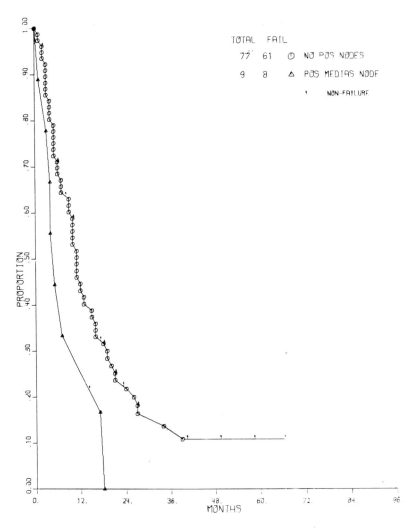

FIG. 2. Survival related to mediastinal node metastasis.

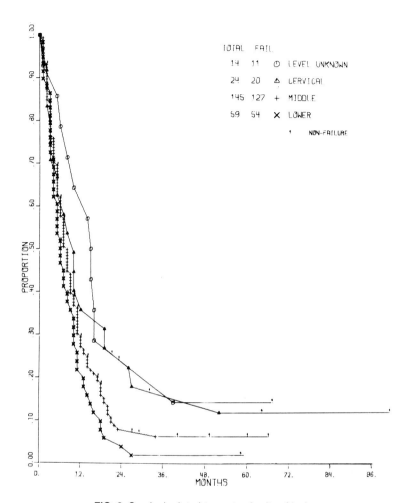

FIG. 3. Survival related to anatomic site of lesion.

node status in the mediastinum (9) versus negative node status (77) reveals median expected survivals of 5.5 and 11.4 months, respectively.

4. Level of lesion.

In most surgical series, survival is best for patients with lesions in the lower third of the esophagus, worst for those with lesions in the middle third, and intermediate for those with lesions in the upper third. With regard to radiation therapy, survival has decreased proportionally with distance from the upper dental margin. In the current series considering all treatment categories, Figure 3 shows conformation to the radiotherapy pattern with expected median survivals of 10.3, 8.1, and 6.5 months for lesions of cervical, upper and middle, and lower esophagus. The 14 patients for whom information is not available had treatment elsewhere prior to referral, grossly abnormal mucosa

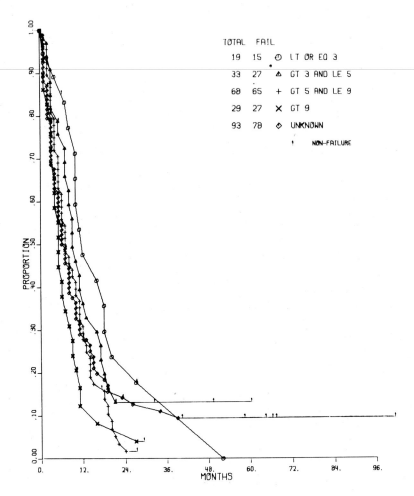

TOTAL	FAIL		
19	15	○	LT OR EQ 3
33	27	△	GT 3 AND LE 5
68	65	+	GT 5 AND LE 9
29	27	×	GT 9
93	78	◇	UNKNOWN
		↑	NON-FAILURE

FIG. 4. Survival related to length of lesion.

throughout the esophagus, or indefinable disease whose diagnosis was established by cytology or blind biopsy.

5. Length of lesion.

Lesions 9 or 10 cm in length have been considered beyond effective therapeutic intervention for at least 50 years. Figure 4 confirms this expectation. Median expected survival for patients with lesions less than 3 cm in length is 13.8 months, whereas it is 5.7 months for those with lesions over 9 cm long. Pair-wise comparisons reveal statistically significant differences in survival for the following: 3 cm and 9 cm, 3 cm and 5–9 cm, 3–5 cm and 9 cm.

6. Circumferentiality and degree of obstruction.

The American Joint Committee staging system gives credence to the importance of this factor, and by it, a T1 lesion can be separated from a T2 lesion without respect to length. Figure 5 demonstrates that those patients with less than 75% obstruction or a lesion identified as not involving the entire circumference have a median expected survival of 10.5 months compared to 6.9 months for those with tumors which exhibit a high degree of obstruction or which are completely circumferential.

RESULTS OF TREATMENT

Curative Radiation Alone (Table 5)

1. Split Course
    Nine patients were given split course irradiation. Two patients received only the first course; one died in the interval between courses with a tracheoesophageal fistula and distant metastases, and one refused further treat-

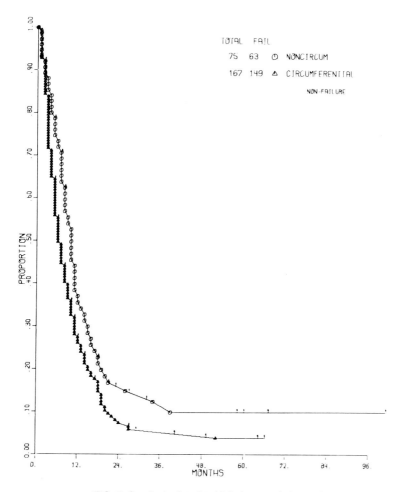

FIG. 5. Survival related to high degree of obstruction.

Table 5. *47 Patients Treated by Curative Radiotherapy*

	Split Course	Continuous	Neutron Only	Neutron + Photon
# Pts	9	17	12	9
Incomplete	2	0	1	1
TEF	3	1	3	3
Hemorrhage	0	1	1	2
Pulm. Fibrosis	0	0	1	0
Stenosis	0	1	2	0
Local Disease	6	2	1	6
Dist. Met	1	8	3	4
Range of Survival in Months	2–18	7–67	2–18	0–19
Alive NED	0	3	0	0

ment after three days of the second course. No patient survived beyond 18 months. Six had progressive local disease, including three with tracheoesophageal fistulae. The anatomic distribution of lesions was two cervical, six upper middle, and one lower. The range of survival was 2–18 months.

2. Continuous Course

Seventeen patients were treated with continuous course radiation. The anatomic distribution of lesions was three cervical, 11 upper middle, and three lower. All planned treatments were completed. There were three complications; one tracheoesophageal fistula, one stenosis and one fatal hemorrhage. There were two patients with proven local recurrence, one following the establishment of distant metastases. Six other patients had documented distant metastasis. Two patients succumbed to second primary cancers. The survival range is 7–67 months, with three patients still alive.

3. Neutrons Only or Mixed Neutrons and Photons

Twelve patients received treatment by neutrons alone and nine with mixed neutron and photon beams. Eight of the latter received their photon irradiation at UT Medical Branch, Galveston. In the neutron-alone group there were one cervical, nine upper middle, and two lower esophageal lesions. In the neutron-photon group there were seven upper middle and two lower esophageal lesions. One patient in each category failed to complete his planned treatment. In the neutron-only group there were three tracheoesophageal fistulae, one associated with persistent local disease and distant metastases. There were one fatal hemorrhage, one severe pulmonary fibrosis, three patients with distant metastasis, one proven case of recurrent local disease, and two stenoses. Range of survival was 2–18 months. In the group receiving mixed-beam therapy, there were one tracheoesphageal fistula, one esophagopleural fistula, five local recurrences, three instances of distant metastases, and one fatal hemorrhage. The range of survival was 0–19 months.

The median expected survival for all patients treated with curative XRT was 8.7 months.

Preoperative Radiation Therapy and Surgery

Eighty-six patients treated by preoperative irradiation underwent thoracotomy, with a resection rate of 88% (76 patients) and a curative resection rate of 66% (57 patients) for 39 upper middle and 18 lower esophageal lesions. The mean tumor length in resected specimens was 3.5 cm compared to the clinical estimate of 6.5 cm before treatment. Of the 57 patients whose tumors were curatively resected, 7 (12%) died postoperatively, 8 (14%) had no histologic evidence of cancer, and 9 (16%) had evidence of mediastinal lymph node metastasis. This finding is at great variance with the experience of others. Giuli and Gignoux found 63% mediastinal lymph node metastases in squamous carcinomas whether or not radiation therapy had been given. Marks et al. found that only 3% of patients had been rendered histologically negative and that the incidence of regional node metastases was 28% after a course of preoperative radiation therapy at least 50% greater than ours. The range of survival for the patients in our group is 0–66+ months, with 14 (25%) alive from 9–66+ months. The median expected survival for all preoperative radiation therapy and surgery patients was 11.6 months.

Radiotherapy and Chemotherapy

The hydroxyurea-radiation program treated 27 patients from 1970–1973. More than one third (10) of the patients experienced a serious complication, five tracheoesophageal or bronchoesophageal fistulae and five stenoses requiring treatment. There were three other documented local recurrences and four distant metastases. The survival range is 0–96 months, with the single patient living past 24 months still alive and apparently free of disease. The median expected survival for these patients was 7.6 months.

Palliative Radiation Therapy Alone

Of the 46 patients thus treated, three survived one year and one is alive at 24+ months. The median expected survival for these patients was 4.8 months.

Palliative Combined Therapy

There is an enormous variation in life expectancy for these 57 patients. (For example, 19 underwent esophagectomy.) Nineteen (one third of the group) were alive at 12 months, eight at 24 months, and two for 60+ months. The median expected survival for all patients in this category was 8.4 months.

Figure 6 shows the comparative survival curves for all treatment categories.

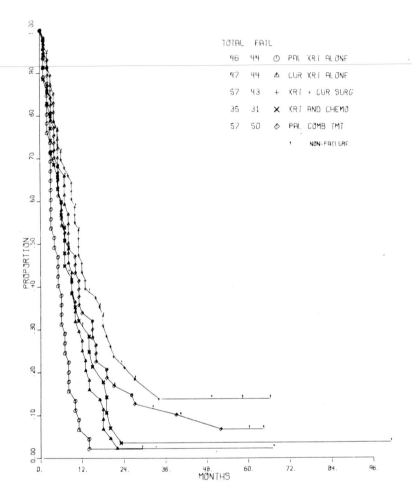

TOTAL	FAIL		
46	44	⊕	PAL XRT ALONE
47	44	△	CUR XRT ALONE
57	43	+	XRT + CUR SURG
35	31	✕	XRT AND CHEMO
57	50	◇	PAL COMB TMT
		'	NON-FAILURE

FIG. 6. Survival related to treatment.

Autopsy Findings

Twenty-four of the 213 patients who died had postmortem examinations. The findings related to the presence of local disease only, local disease and distant metastases, and distant metastases alone according to treatment are seen in Table 6. Twenty of the 24 had persisting or recurrent local disease.

Palliation

It has proved impossible to make an intelligent estimate of the degree or length of palliation in retrospect. In every chart, at the completion of therapy, there is an optimistic statement that deglutition is improved. Although it is

Table 6. *Autopsy Findings in Treated Cases*

Treatment	No. of Patients	Local Disease Only	Local Disease & Distant Metastases	Distant Metastases Only
Pal XRT alone	6	2	4	0
Cur XRT	7	2	3	2
Cur XRT + Surgery	3	0	3	0
XRT + Chemotherapy	4	0	2	2
Palliation XRT ± S ± CT	4	1	3	0
Total	24	5	15	4

obvious that the average patient fails to thrive thereafter, the reason for this is invariably obscure, the emphasis in the chart being on therapeutic maneuvers. Unfortunately, objective evidence is also lacking, since endoscopic and radiographic studies often do not appear to reflect the difficulty that the patient is experiencing. Taking weight maintenance as objective evidence, there is a steady decrease from admission to the last accorded weight; from 141 pounds on admission, to 134 at the end of treatment, to 123 at last recorded value. By treatment category, overall mean weight loss is 10.7 pounds for palliative XRT, 14 for curative XRT, 25.8 for preoperative XRT and surgery, 12 for XRT and chemotherapy, and 21 for palliative combinations. This holds true throughout the decade despite significant efforts at improving nutrition by all means, from supplemental feeding to hyperalimentation. Survival related to the use of hyperalimentation is seen in Figure 7, indicating that in the past, it has probably been reserved for only the most malnourished patients and has not succeeded in altering this condition.

SUMMARY

Seventy percent of these patients were approached with curative intent; 20% were eliminated from curative intent by surgical exploration. Therefore 24% were treated by radiation therapy and surgery, 19% by radiation therapy, and 7% by radiation therapy and chemotherapy. Although there are 19 patients presently alive in these groups, only three were treated prior to 1975, one from each category. In the remaining patients treated by palliative therapy two are alive at more than five years and 11 overall are surviving at present.

Evidence of this nature leads to two conclusions: 1) the ability to assess extent of disease is poor, and therefore the assignment of treatment is often inappropriate, and 2) the best palliation may be the most vigorous treatment the patient is capable of tolerating, assessed by medical rather than disease factors.

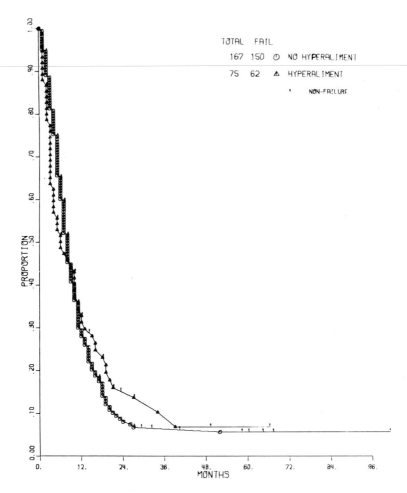

FIG. 7. Survival related to the use of hyperalimentation.

Specific Recommendations for Radiation Therapy

1. The greatest evaluative error made in carcinoma of the esophagus is the failure to systematically assess the tracheobronchial tree in all patients with cervical and upper-middle lesions. Any suggestion of fixation or distortion should be an unavoidable signal to consider exclusion of the esophagus, thus minimizing tracheoesophageal fistulae. Without this maneuver, radiation therapy should be given deliberately by hyperfractionation.

2. Hemoptysis should be considered an absolute contraindication to treatment with radiation.

3. If patients and disease factors are sufficiently ominous to establish short-term palliation as a goal, a short course of radiation therapy, 30 Gy in 10 fractions, will suffice to produce symptomatic relief.

4. If patient factors determine that the patient is not a candidate for surgery but that cure or long-term palliation are the treatment objectives, radiation therapy should be given in a continuous course with daily fraction size of 2 Gy to a total of 60 or 65 Gy. The role of high LET radiation (e.g., neutrons) is not yet established but should be pursued, since its local effectiveness has been shown.

5. When surgery is possible, a combination of radiation therapy and surgery is indicated. Preoperative radiation therapy should be given, followed by colon interposition and esophagectomy or esophagogastrectomy, as indicated by the level of the primary tumor. The optimum dose for preoperative radiation has not been established, although a dose of 30 Gy in 10 fractions appears adequate for the purpose.

6. If the lesion does not meet criteria for resection but the patient is medically able to undergo surgery, total esophageal bypass should be done and curative irradiation administered with the fields arranged to avoid irradiation to the interposed colon segment.

ACKNOWLEDGMENT

This investigation was supported by Grant Number CA 06294, awarded by the National Cancer Institute, Department of Health and Human Services.

REFERENCES

American Joint Committee for Cancer Staging and End Results Reporting. 1977.

Appelqvist, P. 1972. Carcinoma of the oesophagus and gastric cardia: A retrospective study based on statistical and clinical material from Finland. Acta Chir. Scand. (Suppl.) 430:1–86.

Einhorn, M. 1904. Observations on radium. Med. Rec. 66:164–168.

Exner, A. 1904. Ueber die behandlung von oesophagus-karzinomen mit radiumstrahlen. Wein. Klin. Wehnschr. 17:96–97.

Giuli, R., and M. Gignoux. 1980. Treatment of carcinoma of the esophagus: Retrospective study of 2400 patients. Ann. Surg. 192(1):44–52.

Guisez, J. 1920. Traitement du cancer l'esophage et du larynx par les applications locales de radium. Paris Medical 8:392–397.

Marks, R. D. Jr., H. J. Scruggs, and K. M. Wallace. 1976. Preoperative radiation therapy for carcinoma of the esophagus. Cancer 38(1):48–49.

Nakayama, K. 1979. My experience in the management of esophageal cancer. Int. Surg. 64(4):7–11.

Nielsen, J. 1944. Clinical results with rotation therapy in cancer of the esophagus. Acta Radiologica 26:361–391.

Pearson, J. G. 1974. Value of radiation therapy. JAMA 227(2):181–183.

Silverberg, E. 1980. Cancer statistics. Cancer 30(1):23–39.

Smithers, D. W. 1943. The X-ray treatment of carcinoma of the oesophagus. Br. J. Radiol. 16:317–322.

Strandqvist, M. 1941. Transthoracic roentgen treatment of cancer of the esophagus. Acta Radiol. Stockh. 22:172–193.

Wu, Y-K., and K-C. Huang. 1979. Chinese experience in the surgical treatment of carcinoma of the esophagus. Ann. Surg. 190(3):361–364.

Gastrointestinal Cancer, edited by
John R. Stroehlein and
Marvin M. Romsdahl.
Raven Press, New York © 1981.

Chemotherapy for Gastric and Esophageal Cancer

Frederick P. Smith, M.D., Patrick J. Byrne, M.D., Paul V. Woolley, M.D., and Philip S. Schein, M.D.

Division of Medical Oncology, Vincent T. Lombardi Cancer Research Center, Georgetown University School of Medicine, Washington, D.C.

Malignant disease of the gastrointestinal tract has in the past been the leading cause of cancer death in the United States, having only recently been surpassed by cancers of the lung. In spite of the relative importance of gastrointestinal cancer, little effort has been devoted to defining nonoperative modalities of therapy until the past six years. The present resurgence of interest has come from the knowledge that the majority of patients with gastrointestinal cancer will not be cured by surgery alone, as well as the recognition that former preconceptions of nonresponsiveness of these tumors were not entirely justified. For gastric cancer, important studies have been made, and it is now appreciated that this neoplasm is the most responsive site in the gastrointestinal tract. In contrast, the chemotherapeutic management of esophageal cancer remains at a relatively early stage of development. This progress report will provide a review of the current status of nonsurgical management of gastric and esophageal cancer.

GASTRIC CANCER

Gastric cancer is the most responsive of the gastrointestinal adenocarcinomas to chemotherapy (Moertel 1975). While only a few drugs have been adequately evaluated, response rates ranging from 10% to 25% have been established for 5-fluorouracil (5-FU), doxorubicin (Adriamycin), mitomycin-C, and the chloroethyl nitrosoureas BCNU and methyl-CCNU (Woolley et al. 1977). Single-agent therapy, however, produces response of brief duration and there is little impact on patient survival. The most important recent development in the chemotherapy of advanced gastric cancer is the demonstration that Adriamycin-containing drug combinations produce a significant increase in therapeutic activity over single agents.

COMBINATION CHEMOTHERAPY IN ADVANCED DISEASE

The drug regimens that have been used for metastatic gastric carcinoma have all employed 5-FU in combination with either nitrosoureas, Adriamycin and/or mitomycin. Kovach et al. (1974) have reported the results of a randomized trial comparing 5-FU or BCNU as single agents, or in combination (Table). The regimen of 5-FU plus BCNU produced a higher response rate (41%) than either 5-FU or BCNU used alone (29% and 17%, respectively). Survival for patients treated with BCNU alone was inferior to that of the other two treatment groups, and was essentially identical to an untreated historical control. A superior survival rate with the combination was observed at 18 months of follow-up with 25% alive versus 10% with the single drugs. A subsequent study from the Eastern Cooperative Oncology Group (ECOG) reported that the combination of 5-FU and methyl-CCNU was superior to methyl-CCNU alone (Moertel et al. 1976); in addition, the latter drug produced only an 8% response rate in this trial, compared to 40% with the combination.

Table *Combination Chemotherapy for Advanced Gastric Cancer*

Regimen	No. of Patients	Response Rate (CR + PR) %	Reference
5-FU + BCNU	34	41	
vs			
5-FU	28	29	Kovach et al. 1974
vs			
BCNU	23	17	
5-FU + MeCCNU	30	40	
vs			
MeCCNU	37	8	Moertel et al. 1976
Adriamycin	37	22	Moertel and Lavin 1979
vs			
5-FU + MMC	53	32	
vs			
5-FU + MeCCNU	49	24	
5-FU + Mito-C	43	14	Buroker et al. 1979
vs			
5-FU + MeCCNU	54	9	
5-FU + MMC + Ara-C	18	17	Gastrointestinal Tumor Study Group 1979.
vs			
5-FU + Adr + MeCCNU	15	47	
vs			
Adriamycin	17	24	
5-FU + Adr + Mito-C	62	43	Macdonald et al. 1980
5-FU + Adr + Mito-C	11	55	Bitran et al. 1979
5-FU + Adr + BCNU	35	52	Levi et al. 1979

5-FU = 5-fluorouracil; BCNU = 1,3-bis(2-chloroethyl)-1-nitrosourea; MeCCNU = methyl 1-(2-chloroethyl)-3-cyclohexyl-1-nitrosourea; Adr = Adriamycin; Mito-C = mitomycin-C.

Based upon these data the ECOG undertook a three-arm, randomized study, which compared the former regimen of 5-FU and methyl-CCNU with a combination of 5-FU and mitomycin or Adriamycin as a single agent. Patients treated with 5-FU plus mitomycin-C achieved a response rate of 32%, whereas 5-FU and methyl-CCNU produced objective responses in 24%, lower than that previously recorded by this same group (Moertel and Lavin 1979). This modest response rate for the latter combination has been confirmed in a trial conducted by the Gastrointestinal Tumor Study Group (GITSG). In patients who had not received prior chemotherapy, a 22% response rate was obtained with Adriamycin alone.

Buroker et al. (1979) have reported results of the Southwest Oncology Group's (SWOG) randomized trial comparing 5-FU given in a continous 96-hour infusion with either intravenous mitomycin-C or oral methyl-CCNU. Responses were seen in only 6 of 43 (14%) patients treated with 5-FU-mitomycin-C, compared to 5 of 54 (9%) treated with 5-FU plus methyl-CCNU.

Ota et al. in Japan (1972) and DeJager et al. from the Memorial Sloan-Kettering Cancer Center (1976) have conducted trials with the combination of 5-FU, mitomycin-C, and cytosine arabinoside (FMC). In the former trial, a 55% response rate was reported. The GITSG (1979) undertook a comparative study of a similar combination versus Adriamycin alone and the combination of 5-FU, Adriamycin, and methyl-CCNU (FAMe). The FMC regimen employed in this study produced a disappointing 17% response rate in patients with no prior chemotherapy, but the authors note that the dose schedule was different from that employed in the Japanese and Memorial Sloan-Kettering studies. The activity of single agent Adriamycin for gastric cancer was confirmed with objective responses recorded in 24% of patients with advanced measurable tumor. FAMe produced objective responses in 47% of previously untreated cases. Furthermore, patients treated with FAMe had statistically better survival and a longer time to disease progression than did those treated with FMC or with Adriamycin alone.

In 1974 the Division of Medical Oncology at the Vincent T. Lombardi Cancer Research Center initiated a Phase II trial of a combination of the three most active drugs for gastric cancer, 5-fluorouracil, Adriamycin, and mitomycin-C (FAM). In this regimen, 5-FU 600 mg/m^2 was administered i.v. on weeks 1, 2, 5, and 6; Adriamycin 30 mg/m^2 i.v. on weeks 1 and 5; and mitomycin-C 10 mg/m^2 i.v. week 1 only. This schedule for mitomycin-C was chosen in recognition of the delayed and cumulative bone marrow toxicity of this agent, and the cycle was repeated every two months. Objective tumor regression was seen in 43% of 62 patients with advanced measurable disease treated with FAM (Macdonald et al. 1980). Responders evidenced a median survival of 12.5 months compared to 3.5 months for nonresponders, a significant improvement. FAM was well tolerated with mild to moderate myelosuppression as the principal dose-limiting toxicity. Bitran et al. (1979) have presented confirmatory data employing a slightly modified FAM regimen and achieving a 55% response rate with significant survival benefit for responders. The activity of FAM has further been substantiated by a randomized study performed by the Southwest Oncology Group which compared the FAM regimen to a sequential schedule of the same three drugs (Pannettiere and Heilbrun 1979). A total of 123 patients with advanced metastatic disease were evaluated. Responses were recorded in 44% of those treated with the original FAM regimen compared to 27% of those treated sequentially with the same three drugs (Pannettiere, personal communication). For advanced gastric cancer, FAM has become the standard of comparison for advanced stages of disease. Phase III comparative protocols with FAM are now in progress in several cooperative groups, and this regimen is now being evaluated as a surgical adjuvant therapy.

In summary, the introduction of Adriamycin into combination with 5-FU for gastric cancer has resulted in a tangible improvement in patient response. This is supported by the results achieved with the FAM program, as well as with FAMe and the combination of 5-FU, Adriamycin, and BCNU (FAB) which produced a 52% response rate in a recently reported Phase II trial (Levi et al. 1979).

LOCALLY UNRESECTABLE GASTRIC CANCER

This stage of gastric cancer refers to cases in which local tumor extension into lymph nodes or adjacent organs precludes complete en bloc surgical resection. In practical therapeutic terms, the residual cancer can be encompassed within a moderate-sized radiation port. Falkson and Falkson (1969) studied the combined use of radiation therapy and 5-FU for patients with locally unresectable gastric cancer. They reported an objective improvement in 55% of patients treated with the combination, while none were improved with radiation alone and only 17% responded to 5-FU. Subsequently, the Mayo Clinic reported a controlled trial of combined modality therapy for patients with locally unresectable gastric cancer (Moertel et al. 1969). All patients received a radiation dose of 3,500–4,000 rads. By random selection, half of the patients received 5-FU at a daily dose of 15 mg/kg for 3 days. The median survival of patients treated with the combination was approximately 7 months, versus 5 months for irradiation alone. There was, however, a significant increase in *mean* survival of the radiation/5-FU group compared to that of the group receiving radiation alone (13.0 vs 5.9 months, respectively), with three patients (12%) alive at five years.

The Gastrointestinal Tumor Study Group has subsequently undertaken a randomized trial to compare the value of chemotherapy alone to combined radiation and chemotherapy for locally advanced gastric cancer (Schein and Novak 1980). One group received intravenous 5-FU, 325 mg/m² on days 1–5 and 375 mg/m² on days 36–40, combined with methyl-CCNU, 150 mg, orally on day 1, all repeated in 10-week cycles. The combined modality group received irradiation in two courses of 2,500 rads, each given over 3 weeks and separated by a 2-week rest period. This was accompanied by intravenous 5-FU, 500 mg/m², for the first 3 days of each radiation course. The latter group was then placed on maintenance chemotherapy with the same 5-FU plus methyl-CCNU regimen. The initial analysis of this study demonstrated improved survival and patient tolerance for the chemotherapy alone group. In a recent update of this study, median survival for the chemotherapy alone group remains favorable—70 weeks compared to 36 weeks for the combined modality group (Schein and Novak 1980). The difference is accounted for by an increase in early toxicity and hematologic and nutritional complications, as well as tumor-related deaths in the combined modality group. Interestingly, the two arms of the survival curves have now crossed; the study now shows a 20% disease-free survival for patients who received combined modality. In contrast, patients treated with chemotherapy alone have shown a continuing probability for tumor relapse and death from their disease. Palliative resection of the primary tumor was shown to improve survival independent of the form of postoperative treatment. It is likely that this result can be improved by reducing the toxicity of upper abdominal radiation therapy, and in particular with more careful attention to nutrition and the use of a more effective form of chemotherapy such as the FAM regimen.

ADJUVANT THERAPY OF GASTRIC CANCER

The value of adjuvant chemotherapy in high-risk patients having undergone surgical resection of their tumors remains to be demonstrated. The few published studies have consisted largely of short-term single-agent therapy with Thiotepa (a drug without known efficacy for this tumor), mitomycin-C, or 5-fluorodeoxyuridine (VASAG 1965, Hattori et al. 1966, Serlin et al. (1969). Nakajima et al. (1977) have reported a possible benefit of a short course of combination chemotherapy with 5-FU, mitomycin-C, and cytosine arabinoside followed by oral 5-FU or Ftorafur, when compared to a control group. Disease-free survival at 36 months was 71% and 61%, respectively, for the treated groups, compared to 58% for the controls. There was no statistical analysis provided. The GITSG and the ECOG are presently evaluating a randomized trial of 5-FU plus methyl-CCNU compared to controls in the adjuvant setting of gastric cancer. With the demonstration of improved efficacy of the Adriamycin-containing regimens, such as FAM, in advanced gastric cancer, these combinations are now being evaluated in randomized trials by the Central Acute Leukemia Group B (CALGB) and the SWOG as adjuvant therapy for patients with gastric cancer who remain at high risk for relapse because of serosal or lymph node involvement.

ESOPHAGEAL CANCER

Chemotherapy for esophageal squamous cell cancer, in contrast to that for gastric cancer, remains poorly defined. This is in part due to the low incidence of this disease, and also to the difficulty in defining measurable disease which is required to assess tumor responsiveness to treatment. In addition, patients with advanced esophageal cancer are often severely debilitated by their disease, and this poor performance status makes them an unfavorable group of patients in which to evaluate the efficacy of drug treatment. As a result, only a few single agents have undergone adequate study.

Of the drugs with reported activity, 5-fluorouracil, bleomycin, and CCNU have been reported to produce responses in 10%–20% of cases (Smith et al. 1979). Adriamycin has recently been claimed to show activity, with a reported 33% response rate in 18 patients (Kolaric et al. 1977). The Eastern Cooperative Oncology Group (ECOG) randomized patients to receive either Adriamycin, 60 mg/m^2 i.v. q3 weeks; methotrexate, 40 mg/m^2 i.v. q1 week; or 5-fluorouracil, 500 mg/m^2 i.v. x 5 days every 5 weeks (Desai et al. 1979). Responses were seen in 1 of 18 (5%), 2 of 27 (7%), and 4 of 26 (15%) patients, respectively; the median survival was 61 days with Adriamycin, 98 days with methotrexate, and 106 days with 5-fluorouracil. 5-Fluorouracil also proved to be the least hematotoxic in this group of patients.

The Memorial Sloan-Kettering Cancer Center evaluated vindesine, a new vinca alkaloid, in 25 patients with squamous cell esophageal cancer (Kelsen et al. 1979). Fifteen of these cases had received prior chemotherapy. Starting with an initial dose of 3 mg/m^2 and escalating in 0.5 mg/m^2 increments to 4.5 mg/m^2, the drug was initially administered weekly for 7 weeks, then every other week. Twenty-two patients were deemed evaluable and one complete response and two partial responses (14%) were recorded. Whether these responses are meaningful will require longer follow-up to adequately assess their duration and the impact on survival.

Additional single-agent studies in esophageal cancer testing established that antineoplastic agents as well as newly developed drugs are clearly needed. With such meager single-agent information and the discouraging results that have been recorded thus far, it should not be surprising that combination chemotherapy of squamous cell cancer of the esophagus has been little explored.

Memorial Sloan-Kettering Cancer Center had reported their experience with a cis-platinum and bleomycin combination in 47 patients with this disease (Kelsen et al. 1978). The rationale for the use of this combination was the impressive results obtained with cis-platinum and bleomycin in squamous cell carcinoma of the head and neck. A 19% response rate was recorded in 38 evaluable patients. Since many of these patients subsequently underwent surgical resection, an analysis of response duration or survival impact cannot be made.

The combination of cis-diaminedichloroplatinum, bleomycin, and methotrexate has also been tested in a smaller number of patients with metastatic esophageal cancer. Hentek et al. (1979) evaluated the "MBD" regimen based upon the excellent response rate seen with this combination in patients with head and neck cancer; eight patients were treated with 40 mg of methotrexate i.m. on days 1 and 5; 10 units of bleomycin i.v. weekly; and 50 mg/m² cis-platinum i.v. on day 4. This cycle was repeated every three weeks. A complete remission was recorded in one of two patients with lung metastases for six months; responses were also seen in two of two patients with lymph node involvement and one of four patients with a positive esophagogram. Myelosuppression, nausea, and vomiting constituted the major toxicities. Whereas this report suggests encouraging results for the "MBD" combination in managing esophageal cancer, the number of patients and the follow-up time are such that the results must be considered quite preliminary.

A combined modality approach to the management of resectable and unresectable squamous cell esophageal cancer has also been studied. Kolaric et al. (1977) administered Adriamycin, 40 mg/m², for 2 days every 3 weeks in combination with radiation therapy of 4,500 to 5,200 rads; they report a 60% response rate in 15 patients. Franklin et al. (1979) described their results using an infusion of 5-fluorouracil, 1,000 mg/m²/24h x 4 days, with mitomycin-C, 10 mg/m² i.v. on day 1; radiation therapy was administered concurrently at a dose of 3,000 rads for resectable and 5,000 to 6,000 rads for inoperable cases. Of ten patients with resectable tumors, five were deemed to have obtained curative resections following the above combined modality approach. Seven patients were alive from 1 to 13.5 months. The relative contribution of chemotherapy and radiation therapy cannot be distinguished in such a trial, particularly since the activity of the 5-fluorouracil and mitomycin-C combination in esophageal cancer is not adequately defined.

CONCLUSION

Substantial progress has been made in the nonsurgical management of gastric cancer. Stomach cancer is now recognized as the most responsive site to antineoplastic agents of all gastrointestinal sites. Combination regimens containing Adriamycin have made tangible improvements in patient response. Identification of new drugs and the development of combinations of these must continue. Consistent with this philosophy, the Vincent T. Lombardi Center has recently initiated a Phase II trial of a new combination of 5-fluorouracil, Adriamycin, and cis-diaminedichloroplatinum (FAP). The inclusion of cis-platin is based upon the findings of Brugolaris et al. who report objective tumor regression in 5 of 19 patients with advanced gastric cancer who had previously been treated with multiagent therapy (Desai, personal communication). For locally unresectable gastric cancer, combined modality therapy appears to have the best prospect for long-term disease-free survival, after a palliative resection of the primary tumor when technically possible. A reduction of toxicity from upper abdomen irradiation and the use of more effective combination chemotherapy should result in an improvement in the 20% four-year disease-free survival now being achieved. Controlled adjuvant trials with the more active Adriamycin-containing regimens are now in progress, and it is hoped that these will define the role for such an approach.

Continued efforts in the management of esophageal cancer will be needed. But as this review indicates, such work is in progress and the early trials represent encouraging departures from the formerly dismal results in patients with cancer of the esophagus.

REFERENCES

Bitran, J. D., R. K. Desser, M. F. Kozloff, A. A. Billings, and C. M. Shapiro. 1979. Treatment of metastatic pancreatic and gastric adenocarcinomas with 5-fluorouracil, adriamycin, and mitomycin-C (FAM). Cancer Treat. Rep. 63:2049–2051.

Buroker, T., P. N. Kim, C. Groppe, J. McCracken, R. O'Bryan, F. Pannettiere, J. Costanzi, R. Bottomley, G. W. King, J. Bonnet, T. Thigpen, J. Whitecar, C. Hass, V. K. Vaitkevicius, B. Hoogstraten, and L. Heilbrun. 1979. 5-FU infusion with mitomycin-C vs. 5-FU infusion with methyl-CCNU in the treatment of advanced upper gastrointestinal cancer: A Southwest Oncology Group study. Cancer 44:1215–1221.

DeJager, R. L., C. B. Magill, R. B. Golbey, and I. H. Krakoff. 1976. Combination chemotherapy with mitomycin-C, 5-fluorouracil, and cytosine arabinoside in gastrointestinal cancer. Cancer Treat. Rep. 60:1373–1375.

Desai, D., R. Gelber, E. Ezdinli, and G. Falkson. 1979. Chemotherapy of advanced esophageal carcinoma. Proc. Am. Soc. Clin. Oncol. 20:381. No. C-374.

Falkson, G., and H. C. Falkson. 1969. Fluorouracil and radiotherapy in gastrointestinal cancer. Lancet 2:1252–1253.

Franklin, T., T. R. Buroker, G. V. Vaishampayan, and V. K. Vaitkevicius. 1979. Combined therapies in esophageal squamous cell cancer. Proc. Am. Soc. Clin. Oncol. 20:223. No. 902.

Gastrointestinal Tumor Study Group. 1979. Phase II-III chemotherapy studies in advanced gastric cancer. Cancer Treat. Rep. 63:1871–1876.

Hattori, T., I. Ito, H. Katsvr, K. Hirata, T. Iizuka, and K. Abe. 1966. Results of combined treatment in patients with cancer of the stomach: Palliative gastrectomy, large dose mitomycin-C, and bone marrow transplantation. Gann 57:441–451.

Hentek, V., S. E. Vogl, B. H. Kaplan, and E. Greenwald. 1979. Combination chemotherapy of advanced esophageal cancer with methotrexate, bleomycin and diamine-dichloroplatinum. Proc. Am. Soc. Clin. Oncol. 20:400. No. C-449.

Kelsen, D. P., M. Bains, R. Golbey, and T. Woodcock. 1979. Vindesine in the treatment of esophageal carcinoma. Proc. Am. Soc. Clin. Oncol. 20:338. No. C-193.

Kelsen, D. P., E. Cvitkovic, M. Bains, M. Shils, J. Howard, S. Hopfan, and R. B. Golbey. 1978. Cis-dichlorodiamineplatinum (II) and bleomycin in the treatment of esophageal carcinomas. Cancer Treat. Rep. 62:1041–1046.

Kolaric, K., Z. Maricic, A. Roth, and I. Dujmovic. 1977. Adriamycin alone and in combination with radiotherapy in the treatment of inoperable esophageal cancer. Tumori 63:485–491.

Kovach, J. S., C. G. Moertel, A. J. Shutt, R. G. Hahn, and R. J. Reitemeier. 1974. A controlled study of combined 1,3-bis-(2-chloroethyl)-1-nitrosourea and 5-fluorouracil therapy for advanced gastric and pancreatic cancer. Cancer 33:563–567.

Levi, J. A., D. N. Dalley, and R. S. Aroney. 1979. Improved combination chemotherapy in advanced gastric cancer. Br. Med. J. 2:1471–1473.

Macdonald, J. S., P. S. Schein, P. V. Woolley, T. Smythe, W. Ueno, D. Hoth, F. Smith, M. Boiron, C. Gisselbrecht, R. Brunet, and C. Lagarde. 1980. 5-Fluorouracil, doxorubicin, mitomycin (FAM) combination chemotherapy for advanced gastric cancer. Ann. Int. Med. 93:533–536.

Moertel, C. G. 1975. Carcinoma of the stomach, *in* Cancer Therapy; Prognostic Factors and Criteria of Response to Therapy, M. J. Staquet, ed. Raven Press, New York, pp. 229–236.

Moertel, C. G., D. S. Childs, R. Reitemeier, M. Y. Colby, and M. A. Holbrook. 1969. Combined 5-fluorouracll and supervoltage radiation therapy of locally unresectable gastrointestinal cancer. Lancet 2:865–867.

Moertel, C. G., and P. T. Lavin. 1979. Phase II-III chemotherapy studies in advanced gastric cancer. Eastern Cooperative Oncology Group. Cancer Treat. Rep. 63:1863–1869.

Moertel, C. G., J. A. Mittelman, R. F. Bakemeier, P. Engstrom, and J. Hanley. 1976. Sequential and combination chemotherapy of advanced gastric cancer. Cancer 38:678–682.

Nakajima, T., H. Ota, K. Takagi, and T. Kajitani. 1977. Combination of multi-drug therapy (i.v.) and long-term oral chemotherapy as an adjuvant to surgery for gastric cancer. J. Jpn. Soc. Cancer Ther. 226.

Ota, K., S. Kurita, M. Nishimura, M. Ogawa, Y. Kamei, K. Imai, Y. Ariyoshi, K. Kataoka, M. O. Murakami, A. Hoshino, H. Amo, and T. Kato. 1972. Combination therapy with mitomycin-C, 5-fluorouracil and cytosine arabinoside for advanced cancer in man. Cancer Chemother. Rep. 56:373–385.

Pannettiere, F., and L. Heilbrun. 1979. Comparison of two different combinations of adriamycin, mitomycin-C, and 5-FU in the management of gastric carcinoma. A SWOG study. Proc. Am. Soc. Clin. Oncol. 20, No. C-102, p. 315.

Schein, P. S., and J. Novak. (For the Gastrointestinal Study Group.) 1980. Combined modality therapy (XRT-chemo) versus chemotherapy alone for locally unresectable gastric cancer. Proc. Am. Soc. Clin. Oncol. 21:419.

Serlin, O., J. S. Wolkoff, J. M. Amadeo, and R. J. Keehn. 1969. Use of 5-fluoro-deoxyuridine (FUDR) as an adjuvant to the surgical management of carcinoma of the stomach. Cancer 24:223–228.

Smith, F. P., P. J. Byrne, R. C. Cambareri, and P. S. Schein. 1979. Gastrointestinal cancer, *in* Cancer Chemotherapy 1979, H. M. Pinedo, ed. Exerpta Medica, Amsterdam, pp. 292–316.

VASAG—Veteran's Administration Cooperative Surgical Adjuvant Study Group. 1965. Use of thiotepa as a adjuvant to the surgical management of carcinoma of the stomach. Cancer 18:291–297.

Woolley, P. V., J. S. Macdonald, and P. S. Schein. 1977. Chemotherapy of malignancies of the gastrointestinal tract. Prog. Gastroenterol. 3:671–692.

Gastrointestinal Cancer, edited by
John R. Stroehlein and
Marvin M. Romsdahl.
Raven Press, New York © 1981.

Pancreatic Cancer: Introduction and Etiologic Considerations

David A. Karlin, M.D.

*Department of Medicine, The University of Texas System Cancer Center
M. D. Anderson Hospital and Tumor Institute, Houston, Texas*

INCIDENCE

Adenocarcinoma of the pancreas ranks fourth in morbidity and mortality among cancers in the United States. In 1980 there will be an estimated 23,000 new cases and 21,000 deaths (American Cancer Society 1980). For most Western countries its annual incidence is 9-10/100,000 (Morgan and Wormsley 1977).

Because its incidence has been rising in Western or industrial countries, pancreatic cancer, a rare disease in the first half of this century, has become a major health problem in the second half. Since 1930 the annual incidence of pancreatic cancer has tripled in the United States and doubled in England and Wales; in the past 25 years it has doubled in Norway and quadrupled in Japan (Morgan and Wormsley 1977). In the United States pancreatic cancer appears to be increasing at a steady rate of 15% per decade (Mainz and Webster 1974). These rising rates parallel the increases in other "Western diseases" such as colonic cancer, breast cancer, and atherosclerosis (Fraumeni 1975, Wynder et al. 1976, Berg and Connelly 1979).

Pancreatic cancer is rare in individuals under age 25, uncommon under age 45, and frequent over age 75. In the latter group it is eight to ten times more frequent than in the general population, with an incidence up to 100/100,000 (Morgan and Wormsley 1977).

Males outnumber females in almost every country or population group. This is especially apparent in the population under age 50. The incidence of this disease is rising faster in males than females (Wynder et al. 1973, Fraumeni 1975, Morgan and Wormsley 1977). In the United States and most Western countries the ratio is 2:1.

Within the United States pancreatic cancer is more frequent in Negroes than in Caucasians (Wynder et al. 1973). Since the late 1950s its incidence has been rising faster in Negroes (Fraumeni 1975). Other high-risk groups include Jews (especially females), American Indians (especially females), and native Hawaiians (Wynder et al. 1973, Wynder et al. 1976).

Table 1. *Pancreatic Cancer Geographic Distribution**

	1964–65 Age-Adjusted Deaths/100,000†	
Population	Male	Female
U.S.A.: Non-white	10	6
White	8	5
Canada	8	5
England and Wales	7.5	4.5
Israel	7	4.5
Japan	4	2.5
Italy	4	2.5

*Adapted from Wynder et al. 1973 and Wynder et al. 1976.
†Rounded off to nearest 0.5

There is marked variation in the geographic distribution of pancreatic cancer. Within countries there is also variation among subpopulations (Tables 1 and 2). Metropolitan areas of the United States have a higher incidence of pancreatic cancer than rural areas, with the exception of southern Louisiana (Wynder et al. 1973, Fraumeni et al. 1975, Wynder et al. 1976).

Studies of the incidence of pancreatic cancer in migrant populations demonstrate a relationship to environmental factors. Japanese immigrants to the United States probably represent the most thoroughly investigated migrant group. Although they are catching up, native Japanese have a lower risk of pancreatic cancer than Western populations. Japanese immigrants to the United States have a higher incidence than native Japanese. Japanese immigrants also have a greater incidence than Japanese born in the United States. This latter observation might indicate that either pancreatic cancer is underdiagnosed in Japan (i.e. more often called gastric cancer which is extremely

Table 2. *Pancreatic Cancer Geographic Distribution**

	Age-Adjusted Incidence/100,000 World Population†	
Population	Male	Female
New Zealand: Maori	21	7.5
European	9.5	5
Hawaii: Hawaiian	15	14
Japanese	8	5
Israel: All Jews	8	6
Non-Jews	4	1.5
South Africa, Cape Prov.:		
White	6	3.5
Negro	6	2.5
Bantu	2.5	4
India, Bombay	2.0	1

*Adapted from Wynder et al. 1973 and Fraumeni 1975.
†Rounded off to nearest 0.5

common) or the immigrant population is somehow more susceptible to environmental factors than the U.S.-born population (Wynder et al. 1973, Fraumeni et al. 1975, Wynder et al. 1976).

ETIOLOGIC CONSIDERATIONS

Genetics

Hereditary factors account for a small percentage of the annual incidence of adenocarcinoma of the pancreas. The three hereditary predisposing conditions that have been identified are: (1) familial pancreatic cancer, (2) familial pancreatitis, and (3) diabetes.

Only a single pancreatic cancer family has been reported. Within the family there were four adult siblings with adenocarcinoma of the pancreas, but without any other apparent predisposing conditions (MacDermott and Kramer 1973).

Familial pancreatitis is rare. Patients may be divided into two groups, having either: (1) hereditary pancreatitis, or (2) chronic calcifying pancreatitis. The former has a dominant mode of inheritance with incomplete penetrance and a 15%–30% risk of pancreatic cancer. The latter is polygenic with a 6%–25% risk of pancreatic cancer (McConnell 1976).

In discussing the relationship of diabetes and pancreatic cancer it is important to distinguish diabetes from other causes of carbohydrate intolerance. Hyperglycemia after a carbohydrate challenge is present in 50% of patients with pancreatic cancer. Pancreatic cancer (and other cancers) cause cachexia, and carbohydrate intolerance is a common metabolic abnormality in cachexia. Pancreatic cancer by direct invasion or by pancreatitis resulting from pancreatic duct obstruction can cause islet cell destruction. In this situation diabetes is acquired after the development of pancreatic cancer. If only those diabetics are considered in whom diabetes is present for one or more years before the diagnosis of pancreatic cancer, then there appears to be a two-fold risk of pancreatic cancer over the general population. This risk appears to be definite in females but less certain in males. Adding support to this etiologic relationship is the identification of populations with a high incidence of both diabetes and pancreatic cancer. These groups include the New Zealand Maoris, Hawaiians, Negroes, Jews, and American Indians (Wynder et al. 1973, Mainz and Webster 1974, Fraumeni 1975, Morgan and Wormsley 1977).

Negative Associations

Neither obesity nor alcoholism is associated with pancreatic cancer (Wynder 1973, Monson and Lyon 1975, Fraumeni 1975). Acute pancreatitis does not predispose to pancreatic cancer, although pancreatic cancer by causing pancreatic duct obstruction may have its clinical presentation as acute pancreatitis. If pancreatic cancer is not considered as one of the causes of acute pancreatitis, the diagnosis of pancreatic cancer may be delayed (Mainz and Webster 1974, Morgan and Wormsley 1977). There is a possibility that non-familial chronic pancreatitis predisposes to pancreatic cancer, but this is uncertain at present (Mainz and Webster 1974, Fraumeni 1975, Morgan and Wormsley 1977).

Positive Associations

Diet may be an etiologic factor for pancreatic cancer. Studies of its geographic distribution demonstrate a correlation with per capita fat and cholesterol consumption. The rapidly rising rate of pancreatic cancer in Japan since 1950 correlates with the "Westernization" of the Japanese diet. Since that time the Japanese have progressively increased their meat and fat consumption (Wynder et al. 1973, Fraumeni 1975, Morgan and Wormsley 1977).

Cigarette smoking is the strongest etiologic association demonstrated. There is a 2- to 2.5-fold increase in the risk of developing pancreatic cancer in smokers. In addition the median age of onset of pancreatic cancer in smokers is 10–15 years younger than that of nonsmokers. Some data indicate cigarette dose response phenomenon and an increased risk in pipe and cigar smokers also, but the data supporting these observations are limited (Wynder et al. 1973, Mainz and Webster 1974, Fraumeni 1975, Wynder 1976, Morgan and Wormsley 1977, Berg and Connelly 1979).

Cholelithiasis appears to be a positive association with pancreatic cancer in females but not in males. There is an increased risk in females with gall stones or who have had a cholecystectomy (Wynder et al. 1973, Mainz and Webster 1974, Fraumeni 1975).

Industrial or environmental carcinogens also may be associated with an increased risk of developing pancreatic cancer. Industrial exposure to various chemicals (Mainz and Webster 1974, Fraumeni 1975, Morgan and Wormsley 1977), gasoline-associated occupations, and halogenated hydrocarbons (e.g., trichloroethylene used in dry cleaning and decaffeinating coffee) (Lin and Kessler 1979) have been correlated with pancreatic cancer risk.

Hypothesis

Although the etiology for adenocarcinoma of the pancreas is unknown, Wynder has proposed a working hypothesis. Carcinogens may reach the pancreas via the blood or the pancreatic duct. Wynder favors the latter route. This hypothesis requires the following anatomic relationships: (1) the common bile and pancreatic ducts must form a common channel (which occurs in 70% of the population); (2) obstruction of bile flow into the duodenum by gall stones, spasm of the sphincter of Oddi, or edema of the papilla of Vater; and

(3) bile duct pressure exceeds pancreatic duct pressure. If these relationships are present, metabolites of carcinogens (dietary, tobacco, or industrial) excreted in bile may reflux into the pancreatic duct. Cancer would arise in the pancreatic duct, common bile duct, and ampulla of Vater. These tissues must have varied susceptibilities because pancreatic cancers are more common. Of the pancreatic cancers, more would be expected to arise in the head of the pancreas, which is the case (Wynder et al. 1973).

CONCLUSION

Pancreatic cancer is increasing at an alarming rate. Because virtually all patients are diagnosed late, surgical cure is rarely possible, and annual incidence and mortality rates are nearly identical. Probably the only hope for reducing the death rate lies with further research into the etiology of pancreatic cancer. With the etiologic factors clearly identified, efforts can be directed at primary prevention.

REFERENCES

American Cancer Society. 1980. Facts and figures. American Cancer Society, New York.

Berg, J. W. and R. R. Connelly. 1979. Undating the epidemiologic data on pancreatic cancer. Semin. Oncology 6:275–283.

Fraumeni, J. F. 1975. Cancers of the pancreas and biliary tract: Epidemiological considerations. Cancer Res. 35:3437–3446.

Lin, R. S. and I. I. Kessler. 1979. Epidemiologic findings in pancreatic cancer. Joint Meeting of American Pancreatic Association and National Pancreatic Cancer Project, Chicago, Nov. 1, 1979.

MacDermott, R. P. and P. Kramer. 1973. Adenocarcinoma of the pancreas in four siblings. Gastroenterology 65:137–139.

Mainz, D. and P. D. Webster. 1974. Pancreatic carcinoma: A review of etiologic considerations. Dig. Dis. 19:459–464.

McConnell, R. B. 1976. Genetic aspects of gastrointestinal cancer. Clin. Gastroenterol. 5:483–503.

Monson, R. R. and J. L. Lyon. 1975. Proportional mortality among alcoholics. Cancer 36:1077–1079.

Morgan, R. G. H. and K. G. Wormsley. 1977. Progress report: Cancer of the pancreas. Gut 18:580–596.

Wynder, E. L., K. Mabuchi, N. Maruchi, and J. G. Fortner. 1973. Epidemiology of cancer of the pancreas. J. Natl. Cancer Inst. 50:645–667.

Wynder, E. L., B. S. Reddy, G. D. McCoy, J. H. Weisberger, and G. M. Williams. 1976. Diet and gastrointestinal cancer. Clin. Gastroenterol. 5:463–482.

Gastrointestinal Cancer, edited by
John R. Stroehlein and
Marvin M. Romsdahl.
Raven Press, New York © 1981.

Cross-Sectional Imaging of Pancreatic Neoplasms

Michael E. Bernardino, M.D., and John L. Thomas, M.D.

*Department of Diagnostic Radiology, The University of Texas System Cancer Center
M. D. Anderson Hospital and Tumor Institute, Houston, Texas*

Previously the pancreas has been evaluated by barium examinations, angiography, and endoscopic retrograde cholangiopancreatography (ERCP) (Freeny and Ball 1978). These diagnostic modalities have been less than adequate for a number of reasons. The routine upper GI series examination is not very sensitive and is quite nonspecific. The majority of lesions detected by this examination are in the head of the pancreas. The barium examination of the upper gastrointestinal tract can be augmented by inducing hypotonia and introducing air for double contrast effect. This augmented examination, although superior to the routine examination, also has a poor degree of sensitivity. In addition, it is an invasive procedure requiring the passage of a nasogastric tube into the second portion of the duodenum. ERCP is another invasive examination, which requires a significant degree of skill in order to cannulate the common pancreatic duct. It is quite sensitive; however, because of the amount of skill needed to perform this examination, it cannot be used as a screening procedure for pancreatic disease. Angiography is relatively sensitive in detecting pancreatic disease, but some of the angiographic findings are nonspecific for pancreatic carcinoma; these same findings might also be seen in arteriosclerotic disease. Significant technical expertise is needed to perform this examination, and it is not suitable as a screening procedure for pancreatic disease since it is also quite invasive.

With the advent of the two cross-sectional imaging modalities, ultrasound and computed tomography (CT), the pancreas can now be visualized noninvasively. These modalities demonstrate the entire gland and its relationship to the major surrounding vessels and abdominal organs (Filly and London 1979, Lawson 1978, and Simeone et al. 1980). They are more sensitive than most of the older methods for evaluating the pancreas. Also, they allow more than one organ to be visualized during the same examination. Both modalities can be performed much more quickly and with less technical expertise than either angiography or an ERCP (Go and Sheedy 1978).

Ultrasound and computed tomography examinations are extremely easy to reproduce. They may be used to guide percutaneous needle biopsies for histologic diagnosis (Ferrucci et al. 1978). Both modalities can be used not only for the initial diagnosis and staging but also to determine the efficacy of subsequent therapy.

TECHNIQUE—ULTRASOUND

Sonography of the pancreas can be performed with either a B scan or a real time unit. Both transverse and sagittal sections should be obtained through the entire pancreas region, usually at 1 cm intervals or less. The key to obtaining an adequate pancreatic ultrasound scan is identifying the vascular anatomy. The uncinate process is located posterior to the superior mesenteric artery and vein and anterior to the inferior vena cava aorta. The pancreatic head lies anterior to the inferior vena cava and medial to the second portion of the duodenum. The body of the pancreas lies anterior to the superior mesenteric artery and splenic vein. It lies posterior to the left lobe of the liver or gastric antrum. The tail of the pancreas is located anterior to the left kidney. This area is sometimes difficult to evaluate by routine supine scans. Therefore, examinations with the patient in a prone position (Figure 1) using the kidney as an "acoustical window" may be necessary to visualize the tail of the pancreas (Goldstein and Katragadda 1978).

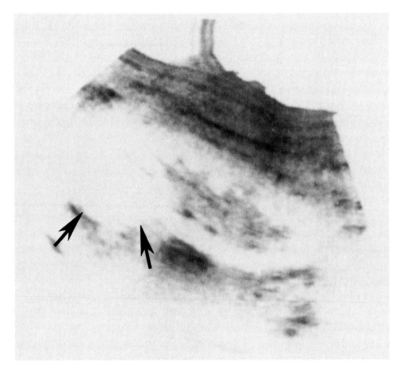

FIG. 1. Prone sagittal sonogram demonstrates a carcinoma of the tail of the pancreas (arrows) anterior to the left kidney.

It is sometimes difficult to obtain a diagnostic study of the body and tail of the pancreas because of interfering intestinal gas. Some authors have advocated placing the patient in the right posterior oblique position and filling his stomach with water. After this has been done, 1 mg of glucagon is given intravenously to produce bowel paralysis. Thus, the fluid remains in the stomach and acts as an acoustical window so that the tail of the pancreas may be visualized.

If real time systems are used, identification of the pancreatic duct and the common duct can be accomplished in almost every patient. This may have significant application in determining the location of the patients' lesions (Weinstein and Weinstein 1979). In some cases, identification of these structures helps to distinguish obstructive jaundice due to a tumor from obstructive jaundice caused by stones.

TECHNIQUE—COMPUTED TOMOGRAPHY

Most CT scans of the pancreas also include other organs of the upper abdomen. These examinations are performed with adjacent or overlapping slices through the area of the pancreas. This means that pancreatic scans are no greater than 10 mm apart. The patient is given 300 cc of diluted oral barium or gastrografin solution 20 to 30 minutes before the examination to opacify the small bowel. Another 200 cc is given within five minutes of the start of the examination. The latter contrast is administered in the hope of delineating both the stomach and all portions of the duodenum. Intravenous contrast medium is administered to the patient through a pedal vein. This increases the amount of iodinated contrast within the inferior vena cava and helps to distinguish the cava from the surrounding soft tissues such as the pancreatic head. Some authors have advocated a bolus of iodinated contrast while scanning through the pancreatic region (Kivisaari et al. 1979, Marchal et al. 1979). This raises the density of the surrounding vessels as well as the density of the pancreas. By raising the inherent density of the organ itself, the pancreatic ducts and surrounding soft tissues can easily be distinguished.

Intravenous glucagon is given to patients who are studied on second-generation or older scanners. This material paralyzes the bowel. Thus, fewer streak artifacts from intestinal motility are seen. However, the rapid injection of 1 mg of glucagon may cause vomiting in a few patients. Glucagon is not needed on third- or fourth-generation scanners because of their extremely rapid scan times.

Diagnosis—Ultrasound

The normal pancreas when imaged by sonography has a homogenous echo pattern. This echo pattern is slightly greater than that of the adjacent liver. It is also minimally coarser than the liver. The gland is rarely greater than 3 cm when measured at the pancreatic head, 2 cm at the body, and 1½ to 2 cm when measured at the pancreatic tail (Arger et al. 1979). Using size as a criterion, any enlargement or distortion of the gland is believed to be the result of disease.

Pancreatic tumors may appear more echogenic than the surrounding parenchyma (echogenic), or less echogenic than the surrounding parenchyma (hypoechoic). There is no specificity of the sonographic findings when compared to the histology of the lesion. Also, a localized increase in the size of the gland may be due to a focal area of pancreatitis. Thus, the sonographic findings are also nonspecific when compared to other forms of nonmalignant pancreatic conditions. A diffusely enlarged pancreas is usually seen in pancreatitis; however, it may also be seen in a patient who has a pancreatic carcinoma in the region of the head of the pancreas with pancreatitis distal to this obstruction lesion.

Using real time sonographic equipment, the common and pancreatic ducts can be seen in more than 80% of the patients in which a technically adequate examination can be obtained. It is important to follow the common duct from its formation by both hepatic ducts to the ampulla of Vater. Again, if the patient has an obstructed biliary tree, it may be the result of something other than malignant disease of the pancreas. The main pancreatic duct can be obstructed in pancreatic carcinomas. By identifying the pancreatic duct, the exact site of the obstruction can be determined. This is important in the case of lesions that are less than 3 cm in size, which are located solely within the gland and cause no distortion of the anatomy.

Although sonography is a sensitive method for evaluating the pancreas, it has one technical drawback. Sound waves are not propagated in air but are dispersed. In patients who have an excessive amount of intestinal gas, a technically inadequate study is thus obtained. Some authors have advocated a repeat examination one week later; however, in our experience these repeat examinations are usually futile. Also, patients who have had previous surgery to relieve biliary obstruction are poor sonographic candidates. The rearrangement of the intestinal tract in such patients makes it extremely difficult to evaluate them by sonography. Other poor sonographic candidates are patients who are extremely obese. In obese patients, the pancreas usually lies deeper than the focal length of the transducer, and therefore the area is inadequately evaluated.

Diagnosis—Computed Tomography

The normal pancreas has a homogenous density. As the patient ages, the pancreatic margins become serrated. This is due to fatty replacement within the gland. The uncinate process usually has a triangular shape. If 1 cm sections are obtained through the gland, the common duct can be seen in at least 50% of the cases, and the pancreatic duct may be seen in 20% to 40% of normal patients. If close adjacent sections are obtained, the pancreatic duct should be visualized in all patients in whom it is obstructed. A key pitfall in CT diagnosis is failure to be aware of the fat plane between the splenic vein and the posterior portion of the pancreas. This fat can mimic a dilated pancreatic duct in a normal individual.

As with sonography, the diagnosis of pancreatic lesions by computed tomography is based on gross distortions of anatomy. These gross distortions of anatomy are nonspecific when compared to the histologic diagnosis of the lesion (Stanley et al. 1977, Sheedy et al. 1977). A small pancreatic carcinoma which causes no distortion of anatomy could be missed by computed tomography. Also, a localized mass can be either a pancreatic carcinoma, a focal area of pancreatitis, or, in rare cases, a normal variant (Figure 2). This latter problem has been particularly noticed in masses which occupy the uncinate process.

The major advantage of computed tomography is that it examines not only the pancreas but the entire retroperitoneum and liver as well. Thus, staging of pancreatic lesions can be performed through one noninvasive examination.

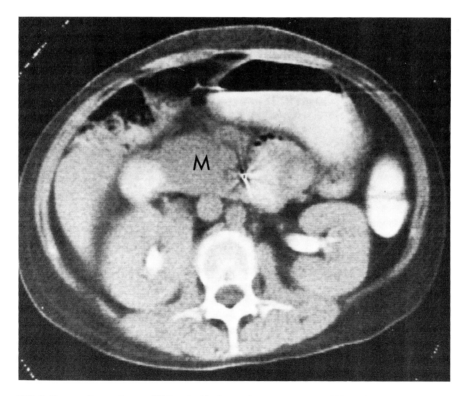

FIG. 2. Pancreatic carcinoma (M) located in the uncinate process would be difficult to distinguish from focal pancreatitis by CT alone.

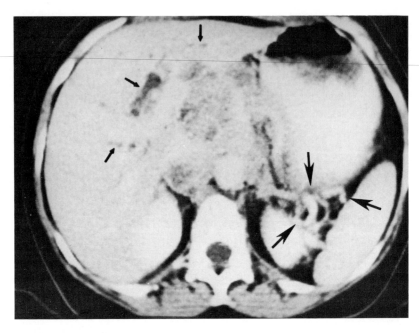

FIG. 3. Large pancreatic carcinoma is obstructing the biliary tree (small arrows) and the splenic vein. Retrogastric collateral veins are seen (large arrows).

Determination of whether a lesion is operable from a single examination is also possible. If the splenic vein is obstructed, retrogastric and retroperitoneal collateral vessels may be noted, serendipitous adrenal metastases can be detected, and retroperitoneal adenopathy can be visualized (Figures 3 and 4). This type of information could be obtained in the past only by other more invasive diagnostic procedures, involving a significantly costly hospital stay.

Correlation of the Two Modalities

In recent reports, CT and ultrasound were compared as to their ability to detect pancreatic tumors (Hessel et al. in press, Lee et al. 1979, and Kamin et al. 1980). Computed tomography was more accurate and consistent in these studies (Table 1). This is quite significant since the reports were both based on studies performed with early CT scanners. These early CT scanners are not as accurate or as sensitive as the equipment now routinely used. The main reason for sonography faring poorly when compared to CT is that roughly 30% of the studies were technically inadequate due to interfering intestinal gas. In those studies where there was a technically adequate study, sonography had an 85% accuracy rate. However, a reliably accurate ultra-

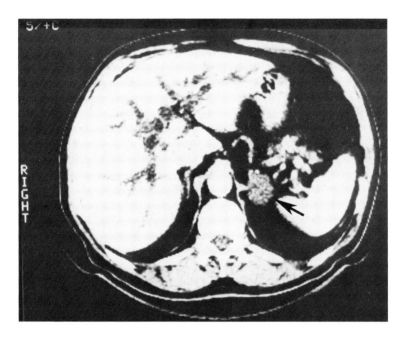

FIG. 4. CT scan through the liver of a patient with pancreatic carcinoma and obstructed biliary radicals detects an unsuspected adrenal metastasis (arrow).

sound examination was obtained in less than 60% of patients (Kamin et al. 1980). Thus, it may be that CT should be the modality of choice in evaluating patients for possible malignant disease of the pancreas because of its reliability and accuracy.

Percutaneous Biopsies

Both cross-sectional imaging modalities can be extremely helpful in guiding percutaneous biopsies (Simeone et al. 1980, Ferrucci et al. 1978). The lesion can be localized by these modalities. Larger lesions can be localized by ultrasound while biopsies of smaller lesions should be guided by computed tomography. The best approach is then selected and the depth to the mass measured. If CT is used, repeated scans over the needle can determine if the

Table 1. *Comparison of Noninvasive Imaging*

Accuracy	Total Patient Population
Ultrasound 54/64 (84%)	54/102 (53%)
Computed Tomography 96/100 (96%)	96/102 (94%)

needle is progressing in the proper direction. The biggest drawbacks to the use of CT in needle biopsies are the size of the scanning gantry, the scanning time, and the time to reconstruct each scan. In older pieces of equipment these prolonged times might add up to several minutes. In newer generation CT equipment, however, the same procedure might take only a few seconds.

REFERENCES

Arger, P. H., C. B. Mulhern, J. A. Bonavita, D. M. Stauffer, and J. Hale. 1979. An analysis of pancreatic sonography in suspected pancreatic disease. J. Clin. Ultrasound 7:91–97.

Ferrucci, J. T., Jr., J. Wittenberg, E. B. Black, R. H. Kirkpatrick, and D. A. Hall. 1978. Computed tomography in chronic pancreatitis. Radiology 130:175.

Filly, R. A., and S. S. London. 1979. The normal pancreas: Acoustic characteristics and frequency of imaging. J. Clin. Ultrasound 7:121–124.

Freeny, R. C., and T. J. Ball. 1978. Rapid diagnosis of pancreatic carcinoma. Radiology 127:627–633.

Go, V. L. W., and P. F. Sheedy. 1978. Ultrasonography, computed tomography, endoscopic retrograde cholangiography and angiography in the diagnosis of pancreatic cancer. Med. Clin. North Am. 62:129–140.

Goldstein, H. M., and O. S. Katragadda. 1978. Prone view ultrasonography for pancreatic tail neoplasms. Am. J. Roentgenol. 131:231–234.

Hessel, S. J., S. S. Seigelman, and D. F. Adams. Prospective analysis of computed tomography and ultrasound in evaluating the pancreas. Radiology (in press).

Kamin, P. D., M. E. Bernardino, S. Wallace, and B.-S. Jing. 1980. Comparison of ultrasound and computed tomography in the detection of pancreatic malignancy. Cancer 46:2410–2412.

Kivisaari, L., M. Kormano, and V. Rantakokko. 1979. Contrast enhancement of the pancreas in computed tomography. J. Comput. Assist. Tomogr. 3:722–726.

Lawson, T. L. 1978. Sensitivity of pancreatic ultrasonography in the detection of pancreatic disease. Radiology 128:733–736.

Lee, J. K. T., R. J. Stanley, G. L. Melson, and S. S. Sagel. 1979. Pancreatic imaging by ultrasound and computed tomography. Radiol. Clin. North Am. 16:105.

Marchal, G., A. L. Baert, and G. Wilms. 1979. Intravenous pancreatiography in computed tomography. J. Comput. Assist. Tomogr. 3:727–732.

Sheedy, P. F., II, D. H. Stephens, R. R. Hattery, R. L. MacCarty, and B. Williamson, Jr. 1977. Computed tomography of the pancreas. Radiol. Clin. North Am. 15:349.

Simeone, J. F., J. Wittenberg, and J. T. Ferrucci. 1980. Modern concepts of imaging of the pancreas. Invest. Radiol. 15:6–18.

Stanley, R. J., S. S. Sagel, and R. G. Levitt. 1977. Computed tomographic evaluation of the pancreas. Radiology 124:715.

Weinstein, D. P., and B. J. Weinstein. 1979. Ultrasonic demonstration of the pancreatic duct: An analysis of 41 cases. Radiology 130:729–734.

Gastrointestinal Cancer, edited by
John R. Stroehlein and
Marvin M. Romsdahl.
Raven Press, New York © 1981.

Pancreatic Cancer—Diagnostic Modalities and Preoperative Evaluation

A. R. Moossa, M.D.

Department of Surgery, University of Chicago, Chicago, Illinois

*The earlier and more curable the tumor
the more difficult it is to achieve a
positive diagnosis, even at laparotomy.*

J. M. Howard and G. L. Jordan, Jr.
(*Current Problems in Cancer*
vol. 2, no. 3, 1977)

INTRODUCTION

The critical issue in the evaluation of diagnostic modalities for the detection of early pancreatic cancer is the careful definition of a clinical and surgical-pathological data base with which one can determine, at the outset, whether a particular diagnostic approach is a feasible option. This data base includes the site and size of the pancreatic cancers, their histologic characteristics, their resectability, and information as to whether potentially curable lesions can be detected with the techniques employed. These parameters were rarely defined in patient populations studied and reported in the literature prior to 1976 (Moossa and Levin 1979).

Thus far, a group of patients at high risk for the development of pancreatic cancer has not been defined epidemiologically. No screening test exists which can be usefully applied to general, asymptomatic populations. Case findings must rely, at present, on the application of available tests to patients believed, on *clinical* grounds, to have a high probability of pancreatic cancer. Predictably, such a group includes multiple clinical subgroups. A majority of the patients will have no pancreatic disease and thus could be subjected to an unnecessarily extensive investigative protocol. A minority will have resectable pancreatic cancer; they will be matched by a third, approximately equal group with nonresectable cancer. Finally, a fourth group of patients, nearly equal in size to the combined resectable and nonresectable pancreatic cancer groups, will have chronic pancreatitis. This clinical base is essential for the formulation of any approach to the diagnosis of pancreatic cancer. It is readily apparent that clinical methods remain the only means for screening a patient population for further diagnostic study. The patient must see the physician while the symptoms are still vague and nonspecific. The physician must have a high index of suspicion and order the appropriate diagnostic investigations, and a team of experienced surgeons must be available who will adequately explore the retroperitoneum and identify and resect small cancers. It is generally agreed (Moossa and Levin 1980) that any technique for detection of early pancreatic cancer must be capable of identifying lesions less than 2 cm in size situated in, but not deforming, the pancreas. Failing that, or in addition, any imaging modality that can identify either a normal pancreas or chronic pancreatitis can also be a valuable aid in the formulation of a useful diagnostic strategy.

SELECTION OF PATIENTS FOR INVESTIGATION

During the past decade, numerous invasive and noninvasive tests have been developed to provide information about the pancreas in general and pancreatic cancer in particular. However, in spite of substantial technical developments, the main problem remains that of the *selection* of patients for investigations of the pancreas, for three main reasons:

1. The early signs and symptoms of pancreatic cancer are usually vague and nonspecific and are often ignored by the patients for several weeks or months. This factor can be referred to as "patient delay."

2. The physician often gains a false sense of security when the results of physical examination, routine laboratory tests, and contrast studies of the gastrointestinal and biliary tracts are all normal. This can be labeled as "physician delay." It cannot be overemphasized that any patient over 40 years old with seemingly genuine abdominal symptoms of recent onset and a negative workup for common benign disorders, such as peptic ulcer, gallstones, hiatal hernia, and diverticular disease of the colon, should be suspected of having a pancreatic cancer until it is proved otherwise. In addition, the presence of any such benign disorders does not necessarily preclude the concomitant presence of a pancreatic cancer.

3. The patient may not have access to diagnostic centers where experience and expertise in the investigation of the pancreas are available.

Table 1. *Noninvasive Tests for the Diagnosis of Pancreatic Cancer*

1. Ultrasonography
2. Computed Tomography
3. Radionuclide Scans (Pancreatic Scintigraphy)
4. Pancreatic Function Tests +
   Duodenal Cytology
5. Tumor Markers

Table 2. *Invasive Tests for the Diagnosis of Pancreatic Cancer*

1. ERCP + Pancreatic Juice Cytology + Brush Cytology
2. Celiac and Superior Mesenteric Angiography
3. Direct Percutaneous Fine Needle Aspiration Cytology of the Pancreas

The available tests which are generally used in various combinations for the diagnosis of pancreatic cancer are outlined in Tables 1 and 2. It is widely agreed that noninvasive tests should be employed as the first line of investigation because of the high rate of patient acceptability, the low complication rate, and limited risk factors, and also because they may provide a guide to further approaches to the individual patient.

NONINVASIVE TESTS FOR THE DIAGNOSIS OF PANCREATIC CANCER

Ultrasonography vs. Computed Tomography vs. Pancreatic Scintigraphy

Much has been written about the three techniques for imaging the pancreatic parenchyma; namely, ultrasonography, computed tomography (CT scan), and radionuclide scanning. Since these three methods of imaging the pancreas are currently the subject of intense investigation at several centers, further technological developments are highly likely in the next decade. It is therefore pertinent to review their current status in some detail and to predict where future developments are likely to lie.

The use of *computed tomography (CT scan)* has been reported by several centers (Haaga et al. 1977, Stanley et al. 1977, Sheedy et al. 1977, Mackie et al. 1979, Bowie and Moossa 1980). These reports demonstrate that it is unlikely that computed tomography (employing first- or second-generation scanners) can meet the criteria that we suggest are essential for the detection of early pancreatic cancer by means of an imaging technique. Haaga et al. reported that intrapancreatic neoplasms produced no change in CT scan attenuation numbers. If there was also no change in the size of the pancreas, then tumors were missed. They further stated that a mass produced by an inflammatory reaction could not be differentiated from a tumor on the basis of the scan. These findings were corroborated by Stanley et al. (1977) in a retrospective study of 352 cases—"Early (theoretically curable) carcinoma of the pancreas will go unrecognized on a CT scan, based on our present experience." The above authors also indicated that the quality of CT scans was less than optimal or unacceptable in 15% of the studies; that is, one in six studies was deemed less than satisfactory.

A comparison between computed tomography and *ultrasonography* is offered in two of these reports, involving 19 patients and 59 patients, respectively (Haaga et al. 1977, Stanley et al. 1977). In both series, ultrasonography gave less favorable results than CT scan. Neither article specified the site or size of the confirmed cancers. In the comparative study by Haaga et al., only seven patients had cancer. At the University of Chicago, a prospective study on 238 patients who underwent investigations for pancreatic cancer over a seven-year period demonstrated that ultrasonography, when performed by an experienced investigator, is better than CT scan on several counts. In this study, 102 patients had pancreatic cancer, 44 had chronic pancreatitis, and 33 had other cancers, including ampullary, common bile duct, and duodenal cancers and lymphomas. The sensitivity for the diagnosis of resectable as opposed to unresectable pancreatic cancer is shown in Figure 1 for each of five investigations. The information is based on an analysis of 39 resectable cancers and 63 unresectable ones. The fact that ultrasonography was slightly better in the detection of resectable than of unresectable cancers seems paradoxical, but can easily be explained by the fact that virtually all resectable cancers are located in the head of the pancreas. Ultrasonography is best at visualizing this area of the gland where tumors tend to obstruct both the

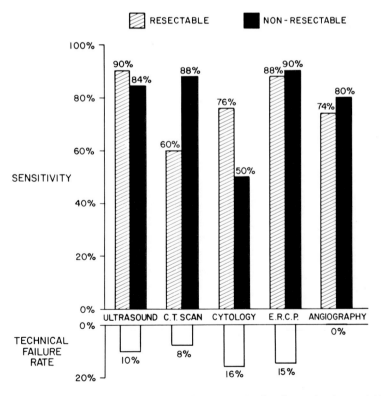

FIG. 1. Sensitivity and technical failure rate of five tests in the diagnosis of resectable and unresectable pancreatic cancer.

common bile duct and the pancreatic duct and thus facilitate localization of the lesion. An experienced ultrasonographer can gain a reliable *subjective* appreciation of alterations in the echo pattern in the presence of a small tumor of the head of the pancreas. Lesions of the body and tail, however, are not well visualized by ultrasonography unless they are extremely large. Conversely, computed tomography is highly sensitive for lesions that cause a recognizable alteration in the size or contour of the pancreas. Therefore, it often fails to diagnose small tumors that are usually located in the head. Dr. J. Bowie at Duke University (Bowie and Moossa 1980) has analyzed some 200 pancreatic sonograms and identified a number of internal echo patterns that could be correlated with the ultimate clinical diagnosis. Five such subjective patterns have been identified and have proved to be useful in determining the presence and nature of disease in the pancreas, even when the gland has a normal size or contour. However, the fact that these are subjective assessments of background pattern prevents this technique from becoming more widely accepted and employed. Dr. Rubin at the University of Chicago is attempting to show that computer texture recognition programs can be developed to detect pattern abnormalities and provide an objective basis for analysis of B-mode background patterns. In the past, the emphasis in ultrasound imaging has been on detectability of a single target in a known background. Little study has been directed towards detection of background alterations. Yet, these alterations contain the information which may permit detection of small tumors or diffuse infiltrating conditions. The use of the computer may facilitate an objective assessment of these background alterations, the subjective recognition of which has already made it possible, in our institution, to detect pancreatic tumors as small as $1.2 \times 0.6 \times 0.5$ cm. Thus detection of altered background patterns permits identification of tumors before they are large enough to distort the contour of the pancreas.

One major difference between the two techniques of imaging the pancreas is the frequency with which the entire gland may be visualized. The conventional technique of ultrasonography has a nonvisualization rate of about 20%. When ascites or extreme obesity is present, often all or a portion of the pancreas cannot be seen on ultrasonography. The patient with a past history of multiple upper abdominal operations, especially if surgical hemoclips were employed, also has a high rate of pancreatic nonvisualization by ultrasonography. In these instances CT scan is superior.

Currently, CT examinations are about three times more expensive than ultrasonography. And, if multiple serial studies are required, the accumulated surface radiation dose may be as high as 10 rads per study. In contrast, ultrasound exposure carries no detectable radiation hazard and the test may be repeated more frequently. Further, when the patient cannot suspend respiration or remain motionless during scanning, the CT study is usually inadequate, while ultrasonography may still produce valuable diagnostic information. Finally, it is important to emphasize that most reported studies have employed first- or second-generation CT scanners. As fourth-generation equipment becomes more widely available it is likely that the value of computed tomography in the diagnosis of pancreatic cancer will have to be reappraised.

The *standard pancreatic scintigraphy* using ^{75}Se-selenomethionine has proved to be of no value in the diagnosis of pancreatic cancer (Hall et al. 1977, Cooper and Harper 1980). However, when single-photon longitudinal multiplane emission tomography (LMET) is used, the diagnostic accuracy is improved markedly. The development of radiopharmaceuticals and instruments is progressing rapidly in this field. In the past, the only possibilities of substantial gain in accuracy in pancreatic imaging appeared to be in the development of agents with improved tissue specificity. Radiopharmaceuticals and agents with substantial localization in adjacent organs (liver, kidneys, spleen) were considered undesirable. It has now been shown that the tomographic approach can effectively separate the image of the pancreas from images of adjacent organs. Hence, other agents, hitherto considered impractical, may become effective with the tomographic approach (Cooper and Harper 1980). The dilemma of distinguishing pancreatitis from pancreatic cancer is, however, still unresolved.

Positron tomography in its various forms is not new. The longitudinal approach was originally introduced by Anger; since then, a variety of configurations for transverse axial tomography (Ter-Pogassian et al. 1975, Derenzo et al. 1975, Muehllehner 1975) related to computer-assisted X-ray tomography have appeared. Even the early beginnings of this approach antedated the mathematical developments which make the CT scan an everyday procedure. Positron emission tomography as opposed to photon tomography has several advantages. The absence of mechanical collimation requirements frees this approach from the compromise between sensitivity and resolution. The resolution does not become degraded as the object is moved away from the detector face, and the distortions introduced by attenuation may, in principle, be eliminated because of the depth independence of the detection probability for a positron annihilation event. The main problem with positron tomography is the choice of the radionuclide label. There is no known positron emitter which can be used for pancreatic imaging which does not require on-site production facilities. Furthermore, since positron emitters emit much of their energy as nonpenetrating radiation, this imposes the requirement of short half life if substantial quantities of the nuclide are to be administered while radiation doses are kept within reasonable limits. Although the requirement of on-site production makes positron tomography in community hospitals impossible, it is quite feasible in a university medical research setting. The label of choice must be a positron emitter that can be readily produced and can be easily incorporated into a compound with known pancreatic uptake. Carbon-11 is currently our choice as the optimal label for pilot studies for the following reasons:

1. adequate quantities of carbon-11 can be produced routinely by a cyclotron;
2. it can be incorporated into organic compounds by established methods, with minimal alteration of physiologic behavior (it is a "native" label);
3. its half life of 20.4 minutes is longer than those of other native labels, allowing more time for multistep synthetic approaches and for both localization and data collection after it is administered to the patient; and
4. its positrons are of moderate energy, so that imaging problems due to positron range are minimized.

Two carbon-11-labeled amino acids, carbon-11-tryptophan and carbon-11-valine, have been synthesized and have also been shown to localize in the pancreas. Preliminary data at the University of Chicago (Cooper and Harper 1980) are highly encouraging. Thus, pancreatic scintigraphy in its various forms is an important research tool, but at the moment it cannot be recommended for widespread clinical use.

Pancreatic Function Tests

Pancreatic function tests are based on the direct quantification of one or several components of pancreatic secretion following stimulation by hormones (secretin or cholecystokinin) or a test meal. Alteration of pancreatic secretory function has been demonstrated in patients with ductal adenocarcinoma of the pancreas. The exact method of performing the tests varies from institution to institution. In brief, the duodenum is intubated under fluoroscopic control, and the duodenal juices collected are analyzed for volume, pH, bicarbonate, and pancreatic enzymes. In addition, the material obtained is centrifuged, and the sediment provides material for cytologic examination. The Mayo Clinic group (Go et al. 1970) has demonstrated that only 32% to 40% of the secreted duodenal juice can be recovered at the ligament of Treitz under standard conditions. They have developed a continuous perfusion technique using nonabsorbable markers. This allows accurate quantification of the defects of the simple test, although their technique is considerably more complex and time-consuming. Further, the simpler standard test, as performed at the University of Chicago (Cooper et al. 1978), provides positive cytologic findings in about 66% of patients with cancer of the pancreas, compared to a much lower yield (23%) of positive cytologic findings produced by the Mayo Clinic technique (DiMagno et al. 1977). The main disadvantage of pancreatic function tests is they cannot differentiate between inflammatory and neoplastic causes of pancreatic disease. Thus if patients with chronic pancreatitis are included in a group of patients studied, the specificity of the test will be appreciably lowered. The Mayo Clinic group (DiMagno et al. 1979) has compared pancreatic enzyme outputs with the length of the main duct, measured from the ampulla of Vater to the point of the neoplastic obstruction, and has shown that a detectable decrease in enzyme output occurs only with obstruction at less than 6 cm. These data support the notion that most of the secretory acinar mass is located in the head of the pancreas and explain why cancers of the body and tail often escape detection by pancreatic function tests.

To conclude, tests of pancreatic exocrine function may approximate about 90% sensitivity and 90% specificity for the diagnosis of pancreatic disease. They do not, however, differentiate between pancreatic cancer and pancreatitis unless a positive cytologic specimen is obtained from the duodenal aspirate.

Tumor Markers as an Aid to the Diagnosis of Pancreatic Cancer

Since the pancreas is difficult to visualize and examine directly, any blood test that is highly sensitive and specific for early pancreatic cancer would be exceedingly helpful. We have prospectively investigated the value of measuring various peptide hormones (gastrin, calcitonin, parathormone, insulin, C-peptide, proinsulin, glucagon, human chorionic gonadotrophin), various enzymes (amylase, alkaline phosphatase, leucine aminopeptidase, ribonuclease), and oncofetal antigens (alphafetoprotein, carcinoembryonic antigen, and pancreatic oncofetal antigen). Apart from the last two mentioned tumor-associated antigens, none of the tumor markers has proved to be of any value in diagnosis, staging, or monitoring of the disease (Mackie et al. 1980a, Moossa et al. 1980). Plasma carcinoembryonic antigen (CEA) is not cost-effective in diagnosis or screening of pancreatic cancer in a group of patients selected at random. A highly elevated CEA level (> 10 ng/ml) usually indicates metastatic disease. Although pancreatic oncofetal antigen (POA) levels above normal are found in about 20% or more of sera from patients with various nonpancreatic benign and malignant diseases, the greatest elevation and the highest frequency of POA elevation (47%) is found in sera of patients with pancreatic cancer. A normal POA level is of no diagnostic significance. A POA level greater than 20 is usually associated with metastatic disease. If POA (or CEA) is elevated in a patient with pancreatic cancer, serial plasma determinations are useful in monitoring the completeness of surgical excision and the response to adjuvant therapy, and in the diagnosis of recurrence (Gelder et al. 1979, Cooper et al. 1978).

INVASIVE TESTS IN THE DIAGNOSIS OF PANCREATIC CANCER

Endoscopic Retrograde Cholangiopancreatography

Endoscopic retrograde cholangiopancreatography (ERCP) combines the advantages of endoscopic, radiologic, and cytologic techniques. The duodenum and papilla of Vater can be directly visualized, and any obvious tumor invasion or deformity can be seen and a direct-vision biopsy for histology or a brush specimen for cytology taken. The retrograde pancreatogram and/or cholangiogram measure varying degrees of blockage or stenosis of the main ducts. It may occasionally be difficult to distinguish pancreatitis from carcinoma on the basis of the pancreatogram and/or cholangiogram alone. Direct aspiration of pancreatic juice for cytologic examination is a very useful adjunct. ERCP is an invasive, time-consuming, and somewhat unpleasant procedure. It requires an expert endoscopist and radiologist as well as sophisticated and expensive equipment. Even when performed by an expert, it has a rather high technical failure rate (as high as 15%) and carries a small but definite risk of inducing complications. It should not be undertaken by the occasional endoscopist in a small community hospital without adequate backup facilities.

As currently employed, ERCP with standard iodinated contrast pancreatography-cholangiography is highly accurate and specific for the diagnosis of pancreatic cancer in more than 90% of cases in which it can be technically performed. In the other 10%, technically feasible conventional pancreatography-cholangiography either fails to differentiate pancreatic cancer from chronic pancreatitis or to diagnose tumors located in a juxta-ductal position which do not compress the main ducts. Conventionally performed endoscopic pancreatography does not opacify ductal structures beyond the main duct and its major side branches, as attempts to provide parenchymal detail have been associated with an unacceptable incidence of pancreatitis (Blackstone 1980). Preliminary work in our laboratory by Dr. Michael Blackstone has demonstrated that technetium-99m microspheres can be injected endoscopically directly into the pancreatic duct of dogs to obtain a scan which gives a far better image of the pancreas than that which can be obtained by the conventional pancreatogram. If this technique can be developed, more precise delineation of pancreatic cancers may be forthcoming, with possible parenchymal outline of the tumor mass itself. Further, an imaging pattern may emerge which could distinguish pancreatitis from carcinoma, and which, when combined with the standard pancreatogram, may increase the diagnostic yield of ERCP in patients with pancreatic diseases.

Abdominal Angiography

Recent improvements in angiographic techniques have resulted in claims of a "92% diagnostic accuracy rate and a capability to diagnose lesions as small as 1.5 cm in diameter" (MacGregor and Hawkins 1973). These authors employed high-pressure selective injections in conjunction with intra-arterially administered epinephrine and tolazoline, catheters with side holes, magnification radiography, and the Valsalva maneuver. They did not, however, mention the stages of all tumors diagnosed or the resectability rate in their series.

Prospective studies performed at the University of Chicago (Mackie et al. 1980b) and other centers (DiMagno et al. 1977) have failed to confirm that such selective pharmacodynamic angiography is really "the single most effective tool presently available for the diagnosis of cancer of the pancreas" (MacGregor and Hawkins 1973). Pancreatic cancer is usually avascular and spreads locally by invasion rather than by expansion. The angiographic manifestations are usually subtle and elusive in the early stage of the disease. The single most useful and reliable angiographic sign of pancreatic cancer is arterial encasement. Large-vessel (splenic, hepatic, or superior mesenteric artery) encasement usually indicates unresectability (Figure 2). Similarly, major venous (portal, splenic, or superior mesenteric vein) occlusion due to involvement by tumor is also highly suggestive of a nonresectable cancer (Figure 3). A further difficulty lies in the fact that all of these angiographic signs of pancreatic cancer may also be present in patients with chronic pancreatitis. Occasionally, an angiogram may disclose the presence of hepatic metastases, thus indicating the malignant nature or incurability of a pancreatic lesion. The main value of preoperative angiography is not in the diagnosis of pancreatic cancer, but in the planning of pancreatic resections by delineating major anatomic variations of the foregut vasculature (Figure 4).

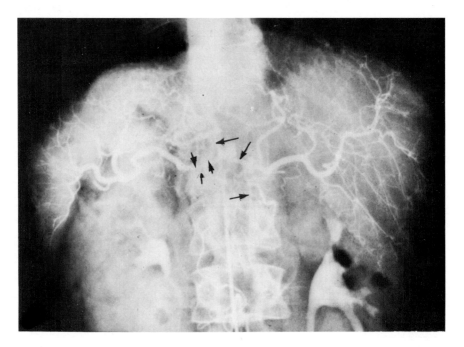

FIG. 2. Celiac angiogram showing major (hepatic, splenic, left gastric) arterial encasement, indicating unresectability of cancer of the body of the pancreas.

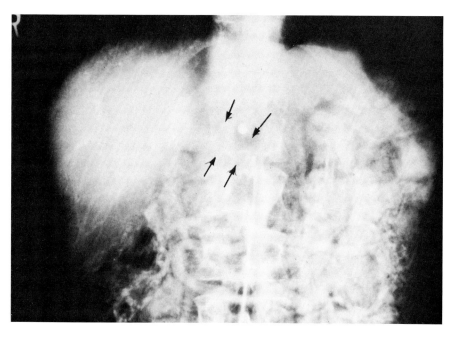

FIG. 3. Venous phase of superior mesenteric angiogram in same patient as seen in Figure 2. Major venous (portal and superior mesenteric veins) occlusion indicates unresectability of the cancer.

Direct Percutaneous Aspiration of the Pancreas for the Cytologic Diagnosis of Pancreatic Cancer

Percutaneous fine needle aspiration of pancreatic masses with ultra-sonography, CT scan, angiography, or ERCP used as a guide in localization has now been undertaken in several centers. Another alternative is to perform direct needle aspiration of the pancreas at laparoscopy (Cuschieri et al. 1978). These techniques are often wrongly labeled with the term "biopsy" —the aspirated material is used for "cytologic" *not* "histologic" examination. Between 1972 and 1978, eight studies reporting some 263 cases have supported the feasibility and diagnostic value of fine needle aspiration of pancreatic masses for cytologic examination (Beazley 1979). The reported sensitivity for the diagnosis of malignant disease of the pancreas ranged from 50% to 100%. These techniques, to date, are relatively free of complications. More experience is necessary, however, before judgment is passed on their safety. There is always the theoretical risk of tumor implantation or dissemination and of damage to hollow viscus and major vessels. The need for a skilled cytopathologist to accurately interpret the aspirated material is self-evident.

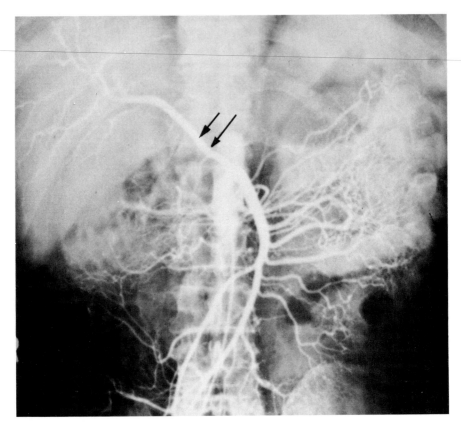

FIG. 4. Superior mesenteric angiogram showing a common anomaly of the foregut arterial tree. The right hepatic artery originates from the superior mesenteric artery and can be damaged during pancreatoduodenal resections.

The author knows of two recent instances when a malignant lymphoma was wrongly diagnosed as pancreatic cancer, and inappropriately treated. In both instances the patients and their relatives were given a much worse prognosis than necessary on the basis of aspiration cytology alone. It must also be emphasized that a negative cytologic diagnosis does not exclude the presence of a cancer. Thus, these techniques should not be attempted and, indeed, would have an exceedingly high failure rate for patients with suspected "early" cancer of the pancreas. However, they have a very important place in avoiding laparotomy in the frail, elderly, debilitated patient with a cancer of the body or tail of the pancreas who is unfit for laparotomy and in whom palliation is not indicated. Nevertheless, the jaundiced patient, unless he is in a moribund state, should not be denied the benefits of a laparotomy for internal biliary decompression and possible duodenal bypass.

THE DIAGNOSIS OF EARLY PANCREATIC CANCER

On the basis of prospective studies conducted at the University of Chicago, we recommend that ultrasonography be used as the initial investigation for any patient suspected of having pancreatic cancer. The CT scan should be reserved for cases where ultrasonography fails or is inconclusive. When ultrasonography shows a definite pancreatic abnormality, CT scan is unlikely to improve on the result. However, ultrasonography often fails to delineate clearly the anatomy of the body and tail of the pancreas. Hence, the CT scan and ultrasonography can be considered as complementary techniques. When any pancreatic abnormality is demonstrated by either of these two noninvasive tests, ERCP and cytologic examination should be performed, since these tests are most likely to provide a definitive diagnosis. At our institution we employ pancreatic function tests only to obtain material for cytologic examination when ERCP has failed to do so for technical reasons. An angiogram is recommended prior to laparotomy to delineate an anomalous arterial blood supply to the foregut structures, to predict unresectability, and to warn the surgeon about subclinical portal hypertension due to splenic and/or portal vein occlusion which may intensify intraoperative hemorrhage.

Moossa and Levin (1981) have reviewed 64 resected pancreatic cancers and found that only 17 of them satisfied the criteria for early cancer, as defined by the following parameters:

1. Tumor diameter of 2 cm or less.
2. No histologic evidence of capsular invasion.
3. Absence of distant metastases at laparotomy.
4. Absence of histological findings of lymph node involvement following careful examination of the resected specimen.

One of these 17 patients died of metastatic pancreatic cancer three years after diagnosis due to microscopic metastases undetected at the time of resection. Only 13 of the 17 cancers were diagnosed by a combination of ultrasonography, ERCP, cytologic studies, angiography, and CT scan. The remaining four patients underwent pancreatectomy for chronic pancreatitis, and the cancers were found incidentally at histologic examination.

It has become clear that patient survival following pancreatic resection for ductal adenocarcinoma varies with the pathological stage of the disease at the time of operation. We (Mackie et al. 1979) have emphasized that survival is adversely affected by late development of symptoms, by delay in seeking medical advice, and by delay in diagnosis. We have subdivided pancreatic cancers into two groups with different prognostic implications:

1. Those with favorable pathologic features
   (a) are located in the head of pancreas;
   (b) cause "early specific" symptoms, e.g., obstructive jaundice, acute pancreatitis;

      (c) remain localized in the gland for a long time;

      (d) have no tendency to early dissemination.

2. Those with unfavorable pathologic features

      (a) are located distally—in the body or tail of the pancreas;

      (b) cause "late vague nonspecific" symptoms, e.g., anorexia, weight loss, dyspepsia;

      (c) infiltrate diffusely in the gland;

      (d) have a tendency to early dissemination.

PREOPERATIVE PREPARATION OF THE PATIENT

Patients with pancreatic cancer are often undernourished and have numerous nutritional deficiencies. In addition, oral intake may be curtailed for several days while the patient is undergoing various investigations. Occasionally, however, the patient is already in optimum condition and little is gained by exhaustive preparations. Attention should be paid to the following aspects of patient care in the preoperative period:

1. Hydration and nutrition.

For at least one week prior to operation, the patient must take by mouth only an elemental diet (Vivonex, Precision, or Ensure) with multi-vitamin supplements. Additional intravenous fluids must be given to insure good hydration. Since renal failure due to hypovolemia is a tremendous hazard in the jaundiced patient, continuous diuresis must be insured at all times. In selected grossly malnourished individuals, a period of parenteral alimentation both before and after operation may be of additional benefit.

2. Correction of blood and fluid deficiencies.

Accurate blood studies, especially red cell mass, serum protein levels, and electrolytes, must be monitored. Anemia is corrected by blood transfusion as required. Since hemorrhage is the most common single complication of total pancreatectomy, especially in the jaundiced patient, we insist on a preoperative hematocrit of around 40%. All jaundiced patients receive daily injections of vitamin K intramuscularly, preferably for five days prior to operation, whether or not the prothrombin index is normal. Six units of fresh-frozen plasma, six units of platelets, and at least six units of blood are made available in the operating room.

3. Cardiopulmonary function.

This is assessed carefully by pulmonary function tests, chest X-ray examination, and electrocardiogram. Intensive pulmonary physiotherapy, active mobilization, and leg exercises are strongly encouraged. Smoking is prohibited. The question of prophylactic digitalization and of diuretic therapy is considered in individual cases, so that maximal cardiovascular compensation is achieved.

4. Bowel preparation.

The elemental diet and clear liquid diet are supplemented by appropriate doses of laxatives and by saline enemas which provide the maximum mechanical bowel preparation over a period of four to five days. Oral kanamycin is also given for two days. A well-prepared colon obviates the need for colostomy in case the transverse colon needs to be removed following devascularization by excision of the transverse mesocolon with the pancreas.

5. Prophylactic systemic antibiotics.

All patients with biliary tract obstruction and those in whom the surgeon suspects that operative contamination may occur are given broad-spectrum antibiotics such as penicillin and chloromycetin intravenously for four days, starting six hours prior to operation.

6. Preoperative biliary decompression.

External biliary decompression via the percutaneous transhepatic route should always be considered for any patient who has a highly elevated bilirubin (greater than 20 mg percent), or for patients regarded as relatively unfit for laparotomy because of associated and potentially reversible disease such as biliary sepsis, hepato-renal failure, or cardiopulmonary disease. It is the general clinical impression that the mortality due to major pancreatic resection can be lowered appreciably if a period of preliminary biliary decompression is recommended under such circumstances.

CONCLUSIONS

Numerous diagnostic tests are currently available for the diagnosis of pancreatic cancer. We have found the sequence of tests recommended to be the most effective one when performed in our institution and with our patient population. The physician must consider the relative advantages and disadvantages of each test and the degree of experience and expertise for performing these tests in each institution. In general, the procedure with the fewest risks and the greatest proven accuracy in a given institution should be used as a first line of investigation. If the levels of expertise for all diagnostic procedures are similar, then the sensitivity, specificity, predictive values, diagnostic accuracy, risk to patients, and cost-benefit ratio have to be taken into account.

The state of the art in pancreatic cancer diagnosis has been summarized by Moossa and Levin (1981) as follows:

Under the most favorable circumstances,

1. About one-third of all pancreatic cancers diagnosed are resectable.
2. About one-third of all resected cancers, that is, one-ninth of the total, are in an early stage.
3. Early diagnosis of cancer of the body and tail of the pancreas cannot be achieved in a symptomatic population.

Thus 10% to 11% of patients with pancreatic cancer at our institution have potentially curable tumors. Because of the complexities of the investigations described, the preoperative preparation, and the surgical procedures themselves, such patients are best studied and treated in referral centers where the necessary interest and expertise are available.

REFERENCES

Beazley, R. M. 1979. Percutaneous needle biopsy for diagnosis of pancreatic cancer. Semin. Oncol. 6:344–346.

Blackstone, M. O. 1980. Endoscopic retrograde cholangiopancreatography in the diagnosis and treatment of pancreatic tumors, *in* Tumors of the Pancreas, A. R. Moossa, ed. Williams & Wilkins, Baltimore, pp. 307–353.

Bowie, J., and A. R. Moossa. 1980. Ultrasonography and computed tomography in the diagnosis of pancreatic neoplasms, *in* Tumors of the Pancreas, A. R. Moossa, ed. Williams & Wilkins, Baltimore, pp. 259–306.

Cooper, M., and P. V. Harper. 1980. Radionuclide scintigraphy of the pancreas: Perspectives in its role in the diagnosis of pancreatic neoplasms, *in* Tumors of the Pancreas, A. R. Moossa, ed. Williams & Wilkins, Baltimore, pp. 245–257.

Cooper, M. J., D. E. Moossa, L. Cockerham, T. J. Hall, B. Levin, and A. R. Moossa. 1978. The place of duodenal drainage studies in the diagnosis of pancreatic disease. Surgery 84:457–464.

Cuschieri, A., A. W. Hall, and J. Clark. 1978. The value of laparoscopy in the diagnosis and management of pancreatic carcinoma. Gut 19:672.

Derenzo, S., H. Zaklad, and T. F. Bidinger. 1975. Analytical study of a high-resolution positron ring detector system for transaxial reconstruction tomography. J. Nucl. Med. 16:653–657.

DiMagno, E. P., J. R. Malagelada, W. F. Taylor, and V. L. W. Go. 1977. A prospective comparison on current diagnostic tests for pancreatic cancer. N. Engl. J. Med. 297:737–742.

DiMagno, E. P., J. R. Malagelada, and V. L. W. Go. 1979. The relationships between pancreatic ductal obstruction and pancreatic secretion in man. Mayo Clin. Proc. 54:157–160.

Gelder, F. B., C. Reese, A. R. Moossa, and R. Hunter. 1979. Studies on a pancreatic oncofetal antigen, POA. Cancer 42:1635–1645.

Go, V. L. W., A. F. Hofmann, and W. H. Summerskill. 1970. Simultaneous measurements of total pancreatic, biliary and gastric output in man using a perfusion technique. Gastroenterology 58:321–324.

Haaga, J. R., R. J. Alfidi, and T. R. Havrilla. 1977. Definitive role of CT scanning of the pancreas. Radiology 124:723–730.

Hall, T. J., M. Cooper, R. G. Hughes, B. Levin, D. B. Skinner, and A. R. Moossa. 1977. Pancreatic cancer screening—analysis of the problem and the role of radionuclide imaging. Am. J. Surg. 134:544–548.

MacGregor, A. M. C., and I. F. Hawkins, Jr. 1973. Selective pharmacodynamic angiography in the diagnosis of carcinoma of the pancreas. Surg. Gynecol. Obstet. 137:917–921.

Mackie, C. R., J. Dhorajiwala, M. O. Blackstone, J. Bowie, and A. R. Moossa. 1979. Value of new diagnostic aids in relation to the disease process in pancreatic cancer. Lancet 2:385–389.

Mackie, C. R., A. R. Moossa, V. L. W. Go, G. Noble, G. Sizemore, R. A. B. Wood, A. W. Hall, T. Waldman, F. Gelder, and A. H. Rubenstein. 1980a. Prospective evaluation of some candidate tumor markers in the diagnosis of pancreatic cancer. Dig. Dis. Sci. 25:161–172.

Mackie, C. R., A. R. Moossa, and P. H. Frank. 1980b. The place of angiography in the diagnosis and management of pancreatic tumors, *in* Tumors of the Pancreas, A. R. Moossa, ed. Williams & Wilkins, Baltimore, pp. 354–380.

Moossa, A. R. and B. Levin. 1979. Collaborative studies in the diagnosis of pancreatic cancer. Seminars in Oncology 6:298–308.

Moossa, A. R. and B. Levin. 1981. The diagnosis of "early" pancreatic cancer—The University of Chicago experience. Cancer (suppl.) 47:1688–1697.

Moossa, A. R., C. R. Mackie, F. B. Gelder, and J. M. Dhorajiwala. 1980. The value of tumor markers in the diagnosis and management of nonendocrine tumors of the pancreas, *in* Tumors of the Pancreas, A. R. Moossa, ed. Williams & Wilkins, Baltimore, pp. 397–414.

Muehllehner, G. 1975. Positron camera with extended counting rate capability. J. Nucl. Med. 16:653–657.

Sheedy, P. F., II, D. H. Stephens, and R. R. Hattery. 1977. Computed tomography in the evaluation of patients with suspected carcinoma of the pancreas. Radiology 124:723–730.

Stanley, R. J., S. S. Sagel, and R. G. Levitt. 1977. Computed tomographic evaluation of the pancreas. Radiology 124:715–722.

Ter-Pogossian, M., M. Phelps, E. J. Hoffman, and N. A. Mullani. 1975. A positron-emission transaxial tomography for nuclear imaging. Radiology 114:89–98.

Gastrointestinal Cancer, edited by
John R. Stroehlein and
Marvin M. Romsdahl.
Raven Press, New York © 1981.

Surgical Management of Pancreatic Cancer

George L. Jordan, Jr., M.D.

*Cora and Webb Mading Department of Surgery, Baylor College of Medicine,
Houston, Texas*

Pancreatic resection was first performed almost a hundred years ago in 1884 by Billroth, who resected a malignant tumor. In 1898 Codivilla performed a pancreatoduodenectomy for a cancer of the head of the gland. His patient, unfortunately, died. By 1910 Finney was able to collect only 17 cases in which pancreatic resection had been attempted, including one of his own. Forty years after Billroth's operation, Moynihan stated, "Removal of the pancreas, in whole or in part, for neoplasms has rarely been undertaken. . . . I fear there is little chance of their proving very helpful in the future" (Moynihan 1926).

There are three different types of carcinomas of the pancreas. They include adenocarcinomas arising from ductal or acinar cells, cystadenocarcinomas, and carcinomas arising from the islet cells. These must be discussed separately.

ADENOCARCINOMA

Treatment and prognosis is different for lesions in the head of the pancreas than for those in the body or tail, and will be discussed accordingly.

Cancer of the Head of the Pancreas

Successful removal of the head of the pancreas and the entire duodenum was first accomplished by Whipple in 1935 (Howard and Jordan 1960). This operation was performed for carcinoma of the ampulla of Vater, but it demonstrated that the entire duodenum and head of the pancreas could be removed and the patient survive. This was particularly significant, because in the original technique the pancreatic remnant was not anastomosed to the intestinal tract, and therefore there was complete exclusion of the external pancreatic secretion. Pancreatoduodenectomy, now commonly referred to as the Whipple procedure, soon became the operation of choice for all malignant tumors in the region of the head of the pancreas, including those of the pancreas itself, the ampulla of Vater, the duodenum, and the distal common bile duct. Many variations in technique have been employed to lower the operative mortality rate and to provide a better functional result. Even today, there is not a consensus concerning the exact technique of reconstruction; however, certain principles are generally agreed upon:

(1) The pancreatic remnant should be reanastomosed to the gastrointestinal tract.

(2) The common bile duct, rather than the gallbladder, should be utilized for the anastomosis. This is considered important for several reasons. When the gallbladder was used for the anastomosis, the closure of the transected bile duct often leaked, resulting in a biliary fistula. Furthermore, use of the gallbladder required very limited resection of the common bile duct. A more adequate resection, including removal of nodes in the porta hepatis, is accomplished when the common duct is transected above the entrance of the cystic duct. Lastly, the common duct anastomosis functions better than an anastomosis to the gallbladder.

(3) The gastrojejunostomy should be placed sufficiently distal to the pancreatojejunostomy and the choledochojejunostomy to prevent reflux of food into the areas of these anastomoses. The gastrojejunostomy, therefore, should be done 18 inches distal to the pancreatic and biliary anastomoses.

(4) The technique must be one which minimizes the possibility of marginal ulcer as a late complication. This first led to the modification of including partial gastrectomy to decrease the incidence of this complication. Today there are those who advocate vagotomy in addition. In my opinion, a significant factor related to the incidence of marginal ulcer is the technique of reconstruction of the gastrointestinal tract. An afferent loop should be created to produce the same physiological effect as a Billroth II gastrectomy. Bile and pancreatic juice should flow over the gastrointestinal anastomosis. It is difficult to understand the marked differences in the incidence of marginal ulcer reported. Scott et al. from Vanderbilt (1980) have reported a 41% incidence of marginal ulcer following the Whipple procedure, while Grant and Van Heerden from the Mayo Clinic (1979) report only 6%. In my experience, the incidence is only 1%. Braasch and Gray (1977) have also reported a low incidence, further stating that the addition of vagotomy had no influence upon this complication.

Despite the modifications and improvements of the technique of this operation during the 45 years since Whipple's first success, there is no general agreement concerning the place of the operation in the treatment of carcinoma of the pancreas. There are still those who maintain that only palliative procedures should be utilized. One problem is the mortality rate. In earlier days, mortality rates as high as 40% to 50% were reported, with an overall mortality rate averaging approximately 20%. In more recent years many experienced surgeons have recorded decreasing mortality rates. Factors which are believed to be important include improvement in nutrition prior to operation, percutaneous decompression of the biliary tree to relieve obstructive jaundice prior to resection, improved techniques of dissection and repair of major vessels, and attention to specific technical details such as decompression of the afferent loop and specific drainage of the pancreatic duct (Pollack et al. 1979). These, of course, are in addition to improvements in the general supportive care which applies to all patients; e.g., better understanding of fluid and electrolyte problems, antibiotics, and the support of respiratory and cardiovascular systems in intensive care units. Of equal importance, however, has been concern about the low cure rate. The best five-year survival rate reported in the literature was 14.3%, and so far as I can determine from review of the literature no one else has accomplished a five-year survival rate this high in any group of patients large enough to warrant an expression of survival rate (ReMine 1979). Because of this low survival rate, two other procedures have been advocated in recent years.

The first is total pancreatectomy. This procedure was first attempted almost a hundred years ago and has been used sporadically since that time. Twenty years age, the author reviewed the world literature and at that time found that the mortality rate for total pancreatectomy was 36%. No patient had survived five years with adenocarcinoma of the pancreas of either the ductal or acinar type. In more recent years, the theoretic advantages of total pancreatectomy have been stated repeatedly, and have been championed particularly by Brooks and Culebras (1976) and by ReMine (1979). There are basically four factors of importance. The first is that there is no pancreatic anastomosis and, thus, the possibility of pancreatic fistula is eliminated. It has been implied that total pancreatectomy can be performed with a lower mortality rate than pancreatoduodenectomy, as pancreatic fistula was one of the common causes of death in the past. Most surgeons interested in pancreatic disease, however, do not believe that this will change the mortality rate significantly, because at the present time pancreatic fistula is rarely a fatal complication. The second concept is prevention of local seeding of malignant cells which may be floating in the pancreatic ductal system. Cells have been demonstrated in pancreatic juice at the time of pancreatoduodenectomy. Whether or not these cells are viable, however, and how often they may give rise to recurrence is not known. Nevertheless, this is a theoretic point in favor of total pancreatectomy.

Additional evidence supporting the concept of total pancreatectomy includes studies which indicate that pancreatic carcinoma may be multicentric and, thus, tumor may be left if partial resection is performed. Lastly, it is believed that a better dissection of the lymphatic drainage system can be performed with total pancreatectomy.

Total pancreatectomy has major disadvantages, however. It produces not only total exocrine insufficiency uniformly, but also total endocrine insufficiency. While both Brooks and Culebras (1976) and ReMine (1979) state that the diabetic state created by total pancreatectomy does not create a problem in their experience, many other authors have noted significant difficulty with this problem, and deaths from severe hypoglycemia have been reported (Ihse et al. 1977). Following total pancreatectomy, there is a total absence of pancreatic insulin and glucagon, and hypoglycemia may result from very small doses of insulin.

An even more radical en bloc resection has been reported by Fortner, who removes not only the entire pancreas and the spleen, but also portions of the superior mesenteric and portal veins as well as the superior mesenteric artery when indicated. Fortner has reported this procedure in 11 patients with adenocarcinoma of the pancreas (Fortner et al. 1977). This must be considered an experimental approach at the present time and cannot be considered for general utilization.

To assess the present state of pancreatic resection for cancer, I have collected 1,101 cases from the literature published in the past five years, including our own experience. There were 898 pancreatoduodenectomies and 203 total pancreatectomies. Almost all of the series of total pancreatectomies were small, with only two series totalling more than 50 cases. The mortality rates for both procedures vary tremendously from one author to another, and most series are so small that the operative mortality rates have little meaning, since only one or two additional deaths would change the values significantly. The data collected indicate that total pancreatectomy can be accomplished with a mortality rate not significantly different from that for pancreato-duodenectomy. Even in the recent reports the mortality rate was 21% for pancreatoduodenectomy and 18% for total pancreatectomy (Baden and Sorensen 1979, Balasegaram 1976, Brooks and Culebras 1976, Child et al. 1978, Forrest and Longmire 1979, Hoffmann and Donegan 1975, Ihse et al. 1977, Knight et al. 1978, Nakase et al. 1977, Reed et al. 1979, ReMine 1979, Sato et al. 1978, Shapiro 1975, Smith 1978, Stephenson et al. 1977, Warren et al. 1975).

The important consideration, therefore, is whether or not total pancreatectomy will increase the long-term survival rate. Among the 898 patients with the Whipple procedure, there were 41 five-year survivals reported (4.5%). There were 14 five-year survivals in the 203 patients treated by total pancreatectomy (6.8%). If one excludes the operative deaths, the five-year survival rates are increased to 6.5% and 8.2%, respectively. These figures are not completely accurate because in both the total pancreatectomy group and the pancreatoduodenectomy group some reports included patients who were still alive at periods of less than five years. The survival rates in both groups will probably increase slightly with time, but the number of cases is so small that the change will not be of great significance. Thus, at the present, I am unable to conclude that total pancreatectomy has any significant advantage over pancreatoduodenectomy. A national randomized series will be necessary if one wishes to settle this point because there is no single institution at which resection is performed in a large enough number of patients with pancreatic carcinoma to allow sufficient definitive data to be collected.

Unfortunately, most patients with carcinoma of the head of the pancreas have disease which has spread locally and distally beyond the point of resection when first seen. Thus, only 10% to 15% of patients can be treated by resection. The majority of abdominal operations in patients with carcinoma of the pancreas are simple biopsy for the documentation of the disease process, or the performance of a palliative procedure. The most common procedures are those designed to relieve obstructive jaundice, thereby decreasing the significant symptom of itching and eliminating death from the complications of biliary tract obstruction, including ascending cholangitis and pyohepatosis. The survival time following such operations is so short that the technique of operation is not of great importance so long as it does decompress the biliary tract. Thus, if one uses the gallbladder for decompression it must be assured that the tumor has not involved the cystic duct and that there is good communication between the gallbladder and the common duct so that relief of the obstructive jaundice is obtained. The only specific procedure that the author condemns is cholecystogastrostomy, as this may result in inflammation in the gallbladder.

The second procedure for palliation is gastrojejunostomy, when necessary, to alleviate duodenal obstruction. In our experience, duodenal obstruction occurs in approximately 20% of patients with carcinoma of the head of the pancreas, although others have reported a higher incidence. There are those who have advocated gastrojejunostomy as a routine procedure when palliative surgery is undertaken, but I believe that this is not necessary when there is no radiographic evidence of obstruction preoperatively and no evidence of duodenal involvement with tumor at the time of operation. Thus, gastrojejunostomy should be used selectively based upon preoperative and operative indications rather than because of fear of future difficulty caused by duodenal obstruction.

In my opinion at the present, resection of carcinoma of the head of the pancreas should be undertaken whenever possible. Although the salvage rate is low, the reports published in the last five years record five-year survivals only in patients subjected to resective therapy. In a careful review of the world literature undertaken some 20 years ago, only six long-term survivors were identified in the absence of resection (Howard and Jordan 1960). It is apparent that these are so rare that they all represent medical curiosities rather than success of a specific type of therapy.

As indicated previously, it cannot be documented that the long-term results of resection are different when one compares pancreatoduodenectomy with total pancreatectomy. Either procedure can be performed satisfactorily in a center where there is adequate experience with pancreatic surgery and competence in the treatment of patients who have difficult problems with insulin deficient diabetes. I continue to use pancreatoduodenectomy in the majority of patients and still reserve total pancreatectomy for the occasional patient with extensive but localized disease.

Adenocarcinoma of the Body and Tail of the Pancreas

Although the treatment of carcinoma of the head of the pancreas is not associated with many long-term survivals, the results are considerably better than those following treatment with subtotal pancreatectomy of patients with carcinoma of the body and tail of the pancreas. Despite the fact that we are now able to diagnose the lesion more readily than in the past by use of computerized axial tomography and retrograde pancreatography, the number of patients suitable for resective therapy are few. Of more importance is the fact that as of this time, there is no reported five-year survival following resection of adenocarcinoma of the body or tail of the pancreas in the United States. In fact, the only five-year survival reported in the literature which can be identified by this author was reported by Gordon-Taylor in 1934.

CYSTADENOCARCINOMA

Cystadenocarcinoma of the pancreas is perhaps the rarest type of carcinoma. A recent report from the Mayo Clinic revealed only 21 patients treated over a 46-year period (Hodgkinson et al. 1978). The five-year survival rate was 64%. However, an accurate five-year survival rate cannot be calculated as there are not enough patients for review. Nevertheless, it can be stated that the results are much better than those following treatment of adenocarcinoma of the pancreas, because virtually all reports include patients who have survived five years or longer and many of these appear to be completely cured. Our longest survival at the present time is 17 years, and this patient has no evidence of recurrence of disease.

ISLET CELL CARCINOMA

The last class of carcinomas are those arising from the islet cells. Some of these are nonfunctional tumors while others secrete hormones. It is beyond the scope of this presentation to describe in detail all of the syndromes associated with these tumors. The most common malignant islet cell tumor identified today is that associated with the Zollinger-Ellison syndrome. Although this tumor was not described until 1955, there have been more islet cell carcinomas associated with abnormal gastrin secretion than with all other types. The incidence of malignancy in this group of patients varies from 50% to 75% in different reports. In contradistinction to this type of tumor, the insulinomas are usually benign, and malignant tumors are reported in only 5% to 10% of patients (Hsien-chiu et al. 1980, Van Heerden et al. 1979). The glucagonoma is a rare tumor, although now more than 60 cases have been reported and the incidence of malignancy is over 70% (Montenegro et al. 1980). Lastly, tumors causing watery diarrhea and which may secrete VIP or perhaps secretin are also rare islet cell tumors. The exact incidence of malignancy is not known.

Despite the type of islet cell tumor, growth is often slow and it may be possible to obtain a complete cure with removal of all gross tumor, even though metastatic disease has occurred. Thus, an aggressive surgical approach is justified. Even debulking of large masses of tumor may be valuable in hormone-secreting lesions (Montenegro et al. 1980, Murray et al. 1978).

REFERENCES

Baden, H., and T. I. A. Sorensen. 1979. Whipple's operation in 37 patients with periampullary carcinoma. Am. J. Surg. 137:624–628.

Balasegaram, M. 1976. Carcinoma of the periampullary region: A review of a personal series of 87 patients. Br. J. Surg. 63:532–537.

Braasch, J. W., and B. N. Gray. 1977. Considerations that lower pancreatoduodenectomy mortality. Am. J. Surg. 133:480–484.

Brooks, J. R., and J. M. Culebras. 1976. Cancer of the pancreas: Palliative operation, Whipple procedure, or total pancreatectomy? Am. J. Surg. 131:516–520.

Child, C. G., D. L. Hinerman, and G. L. Kauffman. 1978. Pancreaticoduodenectomy. Surg. Gynecol. Obstet. 147:529–533.

Forrest, J. F., and W. P. Longmire. 1979. Carcinoma of the pancreas and periampullary region: A study of 279 patients. Ann. Surg. 189:129–138.

Fortner, J. G., D. K. Kim, A. Cubilla, A. Turnbull, L. D. Pahnke, and M. E. Shils. 1977. Regional pancreatectomy: En bloc pancreatic, portal vein and lymph node resection. Ann. Surg. 186:42–50.

Gordon-Taylor, G. 1934. The radical surgery of cancer of the pancreas. Ann. Surg. 100:206–214.

Grant, C. S., and J. A. Van Heerden. 1979. Anastomotic ulceration following subtotal and total pancreatectomy. Ann. Surg. 190:1–5.

Hodgkinson, D. J., W. H. ReMine, and L. H. Weiland. 1978. A clinicopathologic study of 21 cases of pancreatic cystadenocarcinoma. Ann. Surg. 188:679–684.

Hoffmann, R. E., and W. L. Donegan. 1975. Experience with pancreatoduodenectomy in a cancer hospital. Am. J. Surg. 129:292–297.

Howard, J. M., and G. L. Jordan, Jr. 1960. Surgical Disease of the Pancreas. J. B. Lippincott & Co., Philadelphia, 607 pp.

Hsien-chiu, T., W. Wei-jan, C. Yu, and L. Tung-lua. 1980. Insulinoma. Arch. Surg. 115:647–649.

Ihse, I., B. Lilja, B. Arnesjo, and S. Bengmark. 1977. Total pancreatectomy for cancer: An appraisal of 65 cases. Ann. Surg. 186:675–680.

Knight, R. W., J. P. Scarborough, and J. C. Goss. 1978. Adenocarcinoma of the pancreas: A ten-year experience. Arch. Surg. 113:1401–1404.

Miyata, M., M. Hamaji, T. Yamamoto, K. Nakao, H. Sakaguchi, and T. Sakamoto. 1980. An appraisal of radical pancreatoduodenectomy based on glucagon secretion. Ann. Surg. 191:282–286.

Montenegro, F., G. D. Lawrence, W. Macon, and C. Pass. 1980. Metastatic glucagonoma. Am. J. Surg. 139:424–427.

Moossa, A. R., M. H. Lewis, and C. R. Mackie. 1979. Surgical treatment of pancreatic cancer. Mayo Clin. Proc. 54:468–474.

Moynihan, B. 1926. Abdominal Operations. W. B. Saunders, Co., Philadelphia and London, 2,240 pp.

Murray, F. T., A. F. Nakhooda, P. Rae, B. Langer, U. Ambus, and E. B. Marliss. 1978. Remission of hypoglycemia after partial resection of a metastatic islet cell tumor. Am. J. Surg. 135:846–852.

Nakase, A., Y. Matsumoto, K. Uchida, and I. Honjo. 1977. Surgical treatment of cancer of the pancreas and the periampullary region: Cumulative results in 57 institutions in Japan. Ann. Surg. 185:52–57.

Pollock, T. W., E. R. Ring, J. A. Oleaga, D. B. Freiman, J. L. Mullen, and E. F. Rosato. 1979. Percutaneous decompression of benign and malignant biliary obstruction. Arch. Surg. 114:148–151.

Reed, K., P. C. Vose, and B. S. Jarstfer. 1979. Pancreatic cancer: 30 year review (1947 to 1977). Am. J. Surg. 138:929–933.

ReMine, W. H. 1979. The surgical management of malignant lesions of the pancreas. Jpn. J. Surg. 9:271–278.

Sato, T., Y. Saitoh, N. Noto, and S. Matsuno. 1978. Factors influencing the late results of operation for carcinoma of the pancreas. Am. J. Surg. 136:582–586.

Scott, H. W., Jr., R. H. Dean, T. Parker, and G. Avant. 1980. The role of vagotomy in pancreaticoduodenectomy. Ann. Surg. 191:688–696.

Shapiro, T. M. 1975. Adenocarcinoma of the pancreas: A statistical analysis of biliary bypass vs. Whipple resection in good risk patients. Am. J. Surg. 182:715–721.

Smith, R. 1978. Cancer of the pancreas. J. R. Coll. Surg. Edinb. 23:133–150.

Stephenson, L. W., E. H. Blackstone, and J. S. Aldrete. 1977. Radical resection for periampullary carcinomas. Arch. Surg. 112:245–249.

Van Heerden, J. A., A. J. Edis, and F. J. Service. 1979. The surgical aspects of insulinomas. Ann. Surg. 189:677–682.

Warren, K. W., D. S. Choe, J. Plaza, and M. Relihan. 1975. Results of radical resection for periampullary cancer. Ann. Surg. 181:534–540.

Gastrointestinal Cancer, edited by
John R. Stroehlein and
Marvin M. Romsdahl.
Raven Press, New York © 1981.

The Role of Radiation Therapy in the Management of Carcinoma of the Pancreas and Extrahepatic Biliary Tract

B. B. Borgelt, M.D., Ph.D., J. Kong, M.D., D. H. Hussey, M.D., and J. P. Saxton, M.D.

*Division of Radiotherapy, The University of Texas System Cancer Center
M. D. Anderson Hospital and Tumor Institute, Houston, Texas*

INTRODUCTION

Carcinoma of the pancreas and the extrahepatic biliary tract is a relatively rare disease. However, pancreatic carcinoma is the fourth leading cause of cancer deaths (CA 1980). Carcinomas of the gallbladder and extrahepatic bile ducts occur less frequently; yet, like pancreatic carcinoma, definitive surgery fails to control localized disease, even in the majority of early cases (Tepper et al. 1976, Kopelson et al. 1977).

Approximately 40% to 50% of patients will present with disease limited to local structures and/or regional nodes (Tepper et al. 1976, Hart et al. 1972, Kopelson et al. 1977). At best, only one half of these will be candidates for definitive surgical treatment. In the remainder, only palliative procedures such as enteric by-pass or T-tube placement can be done.

The past eight years have seen a renewed interest in the use of irradiation for the definitive treatment of patients with localized, unresectable pancreatic adenocarcinoma (Dobelbower 1979, Moossa 1980, Cohn in press). Unfortunately, very few reports concerning irradiation of patients with carcinomas of the gallbladder and extrahepatic bile ducts exist in the literature (Table 8, Hudgins and Meoz 1976, Smoron 1977, Whelton et al. 1969, Vaittinen 1970).

This communication will present some of the M. D. Anderson Hospital (MDAH) experience in the radiotherapeutic treatment of patients with carcinomas of the pancreas, gallbladder, and extrahepatic bile ducts and will review the more recent literature. Its purpose is not to conduct an exhaustive review, and the reader is referred to more definitive treatises on the subject (Dobelbower 1979, Cohn in press, Moossa 1980, Vaittinen 1970, Kopelson et al. 1977).

METHODS AND MATERIALS

Pancreatic Carcinoma

Neutron Beam Irradiation

Between September, 1973, and March, 1980, 23 patients with unresectable pancreatic adenocarcinoma received combined high energy photon (60%) and fast neutron (40%) mixed beam irradiation. Two additional patients were treated with neutrons only. The photon portion of the treatment was delivered at either M. D. Anderson Hospital or The University of Texas Medical Branch at Galveston. Twelve patients received continuous course irradiation, 6,000 rad$\eta\gamma$/6½-7 weeks (range, 4,900 to 6,200 rad$\eta\gamma$), and 13 patients received split course treatment, 6,000 rad$\eta\gamma$/10 weeks (range, 5,800 to 6,900 rad$\eta\gamma$). Details of the treatment have been previously reported (Borgelt in press, Al-Abdulla et al. 1981, Hussey et al. 1980).

Gold Grain Implant

Between December, 1964, and September, 1973, 24 patients with adenocarcinoma of the pancreas were treated with radioactive gold grain implants. The mean dose was 10,000 rads (range, 3,500 to 16,000 rad). In 22 of these patients, the implant was the only radiation treatment utilized. The other two patients also received supplemental low dose external beam irradiation. Patient characteristics and details of treatment have been previously reported (Borgelt in press).

Extrahepatic Biliary Tract

Between March, 1957, and May, 1980, 17 patients with carcinoma of the extrahepatic biliary tract received external beam irradiation at MDAH, with either palliative or curative intent. The distribution of primary sites is shown in Table 9. There were seven males and 10 females, with a mean age of 56 years (range, 32 to 76 years). Three patients had distant metastases at the time of treatment. Photon beam irradiation was given to 14 patients (range, 2,000 rad/2 weeks to 6,500 rad/7 weeks). Two patients received mixed photon/neutron beam irradiation (4,400 rad$\eta\gamma$/4 weeks and 6,000 rad$\eta\gamma$/10 weeks) and one patient was treated with neutrons alone (5,100 rad$\eta\gamma$/5 weeks).

RESULTS AND DISCUSSION

Pancreatic Carcinoma

Definitive Photon Beam Irradiation

Haslam et al. (1973) were the first to report the use of high dose external beam irradiation as a definitive treatment for patients with unresectable pancreatic carcinoma (Table 1). They reported a median survival of 7.5

Table 1. *Carcinoma of the Pancreas: Survival*

Reference	No. Patients	Median Survival Post Diagnosis (Months)		
		Overall	Radiation Alone	Radiation + Chemotherapy
Dobelbower et al., 1980.	40	12	12	16
Haslam et al., 1973.	23	7.5	8	10
Tepper et al., 1976. (Localized, resected)	31	10.5	—	—
Moertel and Reitermeier, 1969. (Regional, unresectable)				
Palliative Surgery	67	6.0	—	—
XRT ± Chemotherapy	64	—	6.3	10.4

months for patients treated to a maximum tumor dose of 6,000 rad/10 weeks by a double split course technique. This represented a modest increase over the median survival of six months reported by Moertel and Reitermeier (1969) for patients with comparably staged disease treated by palliative surgery alone. In 1975, Dobelbower et al. postulated that still higher doses delivered by precision techniques would result in improved local tumor control and patient survival. Their premise was supported by early reports (Borgelt et al. 1978, Dobelbower et al. 1978) in which patients with unresectable disease treated to minimum tumor doses of 6,000 to 6,700 rad/7 to 7½ weeks by three- or four-field high energy photon/electron beam techniques had a median survival of 12 months, comparable to that seen following radical surgery for less advanced disease (Tepper et al. 1976). A recent update of that series, now totaling 40 patients (Dobelbower et al. 1980), continues to show a median survival of one year. In spite of the high doses, however, 40% of these patients failed, with locally persistent or recurrent disease.

In both the Duke series (Haslam et al. 1973) and the Thomas Jefferson University Hospital series (Dobelbower et al. 1980), some patients received adjuvant chemotherapy on an unrandomized basis (Table 1). In both series, patients who received adjuvant chemotherapy had a prolonged survival compared to those who received irradiation alone.

In 1969, Moertel and Reitermeier published the results of a randomized study comparing external beam irradiation alone (4,000 rad/6 weeks by split course technique) and external beam irradiation plus adjuvant 5-FU (500 mg/m^2, days 1–3 each course). Survival was significantly longer for patients receiving adjuvant chemotherapy (Table 1).

The Gastrointestinal Tumor Study Group (GITSG) (1979) conducted a three-arm randomized study comparing 4,000 and 6,000 rad split course irradiation plus 5-FU against 6,000 rad split course irradiation alone (Table 2). Both median times to progression and survival were significantly better for the adjuvant chemotherapy groups compared to the irradiation-alone control

Table 2. *Pancreatic Carcinoma**

| | Treatment | | |
	4,000r + 5FU†	6,000r + 5FU†	6,000r
No. Patients	29	32	28
Median Time to Progression (weeks)	28	34	14
Median Survival (weeks)	33	39	23
One-Year Survival	38%	36%	11%

*Gastrointestinal Tumor Study Group, 1979.
†5FU 500 mg/m² iv d 1–3 each split course plus weekly maintenance.

group. However, the one-year survival of the irradiation-alone control group of the GITSG (Table 2) was less than one third of the one-year survival originally reported from Duke for the same treatment regimen (Haslam et al. 1973), and only about one-fifth that reported by Dobelbower et al. (1980) for continuous course precision high dose irradiation alone (Table 1).

The Southwest Oncology Group (SWOG) recently reported a randomized study comparing 6,000 rad/10 weeks plus 5-FU and methyl-CCNU to 6,000 rad plus 5-FU, methyl-CCNU, and spirolactone in patients with unresectable pancreatic carcinoma (McCracken et al. 1980). There was no significant difference between the two groups. The overall one-year survival was 24%, one half of that reported by Dobelbower et al. (1980) for patients receiving precision high dose external beam irradiation alone.

Interstitial Implant With or Without External Beam Irradiation

It has been postulated that the cause of local recurrence following high dose conventional photon beam irradiation is regrowth from areas of persisting radioresistant hypoxic tumor cells. Current definitive radiotherapeutic efforts have been directed toward this problem.

One approach has been to implant the primary tumor with either radioactive gold (Borgelt in press) or iodine seeds (Shipley et al. 1980, Whittington et al. in press) at the time of laparotomy (Table 3). The high incidence of local recurrences (68%) in the 16 patients who failed treatment with implant alone in the M. D. Anderson Hospital (MDAH) series suggests that the dose to involved regional nodes was inadequate to control disease. Investigators at Thomas Jefferson University Hospital (TJUH) and Massachusetts General Hospital (MGH) have combined radioactive iodine implants with external beam irradiation in an attempt to improve local control. Although survival has not improved over that seen with precision high dose irradiation alone, local recurrence rates for those patients who failed have been decreased to 12% in the TJUH series and to 33% in the MGH series. A corresponding increase in

Table 3. *Pancreatic Carcinoma: Implant ± External Beam*

	MDAH*	TJUH†	MGH‡
No. Patients	24	12	12
Treatment	[198]Au Implant Only (10,000r)	[125]I Implant (12,000r) + External (6,000r)	[125]I Implant (16,000r) + External (4,000–4,500r)
Median Survival (months)	9	12	11
Failure:			
Total	16(67%)	8(67%)	9(75%)
Local-Regional Only	2(12%)	1(12%)	2(22%)
Distant Only	3(19%)	4(50%)	4(45%)
Both	9(56%)	0	1(11%)
Surgical Wound	2(12%)	3(38%)§	2(22%)§

*Borgelt in press.
†Whittington et al. in press.
‡Shipley et al. 1980.
§All patients with simultaneous distant metastases.

the incidence of distant metastases (78% to 88%) has been observed. Improved survival may thus be anticipated as more effective systemic treatments become available for use as adjuvant therapy.

Neutron Beam Irradiation

The results of the MDAH/Galveston series are shown in Table 4 and Figure 1. The overall median survival after diagnosis was 11 months. There was no difference in survival between patients treated with a continuous course (6,000 rad$\eta\gamma$/6.5-7 weeks) and those treated with a double split course regimen (6,000 rad$\eta\gamma$/10 weeks). Eleven patients received adjuvant chemotherapy on an elective, nonrandomized basis. Both the median and mean survivals were longer than those of patients who did not receive chemother-

Table 4. *Mixed Beam Radiotherapy* * for Unresectable Pancreatic Carcinoma (MDAH: Analysis 10-1-80)*

		Survival (Months After Diagnosis)	
Treatment	No. Patients	Median	Mean
Continuous Course	12	10	16
Split Course	13	11	18
Chemotherapy	11	12	23
No Chemotherapy	14	7	11
Overall	25	11	17

*60% high energy photons, 40% neutrons. Two patients neutrons only.

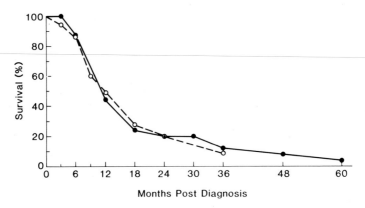

FIG. 1. Comparison of survival of 25 patients with unresectable pancreatic cancer treated at MDAH with mixed neutron/photon beam irradiation (●—●) and 40 patients treated at TJUH with precision high dose photon beam irradiation (○- -○).

apy, suggesting, as have other nonrandomized studies (Haslam et al. 1973, Dobelbower et al. 1980), that the addition of chemotherapy may be beneficial. Although the total doses given by mixed neutron/photon beam irradiation (6,000 rad$\eta\gamma$/6.5 to 10 weeks) were generally lower than those delivered by precision high dose photon techniques (6,000 to 6,900 rad/6.5 to 8 weeks), survival rates of the two series are comparable (Figure 1).

Carcinoma of the Extrahepatic Biliary Tract

Although 75% to 85% of patients with carcinoma of the gallbladder or extrahepatic bile ducts are operable (Kopelson et al. 1977), only one fourth to one third of these prove to have localized disease amenable to curative surgery (Beltz and Condon 1974, Hart et al. 1972, Kopelson et al. 1977). Median or mean survival rates of one year or more have been observed only in patients with limited disease who have curative surgery (Tables 5 and 6).

Table 5. *Carcinoma of the Gallbladder: Survival**

Extent of Disease	Survival		
	1 Year (%)	5 Year (%)	Median (Months)
Localized	50	33	13
Regional Spread	2	0	2.8
Liver Involvement	5	0	1.7
Generalized	1	0	<1

*Hart et al., 1972. 334 patients: 25% curative surgery, 12% palliative surgery, 35% exploration only.

Table 6. *Carcinoma of the Extrahepatic Biliary Tract: Survival**

	Mean Survival (Months Post Surgery)	
Treatment	Gallbladder	Extrahepatic Ducts
Curative Surgery	13†	16.9
Palliative Surgery	4.6	9.3
Untreated or Biopsy Only	1.1	2.7

*Kopelson et al., 1977; collected series.
†Hart et al., 1972. (median survival).

Overall five-year survival following surgery alone is less than 10%, a figure as dismal as that for carcinoma of the pancreas. The majority of these patients die with locally persistent or recurrent disease (Table 7).

There is a potential role for irradiation of patients with localized, unresectable carcinoma of the biliary tract; however, very little data exist in the literature (Table 8). None of these series is large. The doses given vary widely and, in most cases, can only be considered as palliative. Therefore, to draw conclusions from them, other than the conclusion that external beam irradiation can provide effective palliation of symptoms, is unwarranted.

A breakdown by primary disease site of the 17 patients treated at MDAH is shown in Table 9. All patients were referred for irradiation with either unresectable or recurrent disease. Three patients had distant metastases at the time they were treated. Four patients received <3,000 rad; all have died. Three of these were evaluable for the cause of death and all three died with local disease. Seven patients received 3,000 to 5,000 rad. Three died with local disease, two died with distant metastases, and one died with both local and distant disease. One patient is alive with distant metastases at eight months. Six patients received >5,000 rad. Two have died with local disease, and one is alive free of disease at 7.5 months. Three additional patients are living, two

Table 7. *Carcinoma of the Biliary Tract: Effectiveness of "Curative" Surgery**

	Local Recurrence	
Site	Early (< 5 years)	Late (> 5 years)
Gallbladder:		
Simple Cholecystectomy	95/110† (86%)	11/23 (48%)
Radical Surgery	12/16 (75%)	—
Extrahepatic Ducts	18/70 (26%)	—

*Kopelson et al., 1977; collected series.
†Denominator = No. patients not surviving.

Table 8. *Carcinoma of the Biliary Tract: Radiotherapy* ± *Surgery*

| | Gallbladder | | Extrahepatic Ducts* | |
| | Survival (months) | | Survival (months) | |
Reference	No. Patients	Mean (Range)	No. Patients	Mean (Range)
Kopelson et al., 1977.	3	9 (4–16)	7	17 (3–54)
Green et al., 1973.			4	12 (7–17)
Ariel and Pack, 1960.†	3‡	4 (?)	7	7 (?)
Moossa et al., 1975.	1§	—(30)		
M.D.A.H., current series.	4	10 (4–15)	11	9 (4–20)

*Excluding intrapancreatic.
†^{131}I rose bengal.
‡Two additional patients alive at one and nine months.
§One additional patient alive NED at 24 months (pathologic diagnosis).

with distant metastases, both at 13 months, and one with probable local disease at 33 months (Figure 2). Mean survivals for the three groups are 8, 9, and 14 months, respectively.

COMMENTS

The recent application of more aggressive radiotherapeutic techniques in the treatment of patients with localized, unresectable carcinoma of the pancreas appears to be resulting in improved local control. However, overall survival has not improved because of a corresponding increase in the incidence of distant metastases. Several studies suggest that survival may be increased by the addition of adjuvant chemotherapy.

Review of the literature reveals a high rate of local failure in patients undergoing surgery for carcinomas of the extrahepatic biliary tract. The basis,

Table 9. *Unresectable Carcinoma of the Extrahepatic Biliary Tract (MDAH Analysis: 10-15-80)*

| Site | No. Patients | Survival (Months Post-diagnosis) | |
		Mean	(Range)
Hepatic, Common Hepatic	5	9.0	(4–20)*
Cystic	1	—	(6)
Common Duct	5	9.2	(8–13)†
Gallbladder	4	9.5	(4–15)‡
Ampulla	2	20	(7–33)§
Overall	17	10.3	(4–33)

*One patient alive free of disease at 7.5 months.
†Two patients alive with distant metastases at 8 and 13 months.
‡One patient alive with distant metastases at 13 months.
§One patient alive with possible local disease at 33 months.

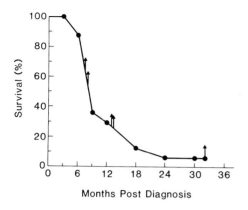

FIG. 2. Survival of 17 patients with unresectable or recurrent carcinoma of the extrahepatic biliary tract treated at MDAH. ↑ = alive.

therefore, exists for the application of more aggressive radiotherapeutic measures in this group of patients, along the same lines as those being utilized for pancreatic carcinoma.

ACKNOWLEDGMENTS

This work was supported in part by Grant Numbers CA06294 and CA12542, awarded by the National Cancer Institute, Department of Health and Human Services.

REFERENCES

Al-Abdulla, S., D. H. Hussey, M. H. Olson, and A. E. Wright. 1981. Experience with fast neutron therapy for unresectable carcinoma of the pancreas. Int. J. Radiat. Oncol. Biol. Phys. 7:165–172.

Ariel, I. M., and G. T. Pack. 1960. The treatment of inoperable cancer of the biliary system with radioactive (I^{131}) rose bengal. A. J. R. 83:474–490.

Beltz, W. R., and R. E. Condon. 1974. Primary carcinoma of the gallbladder. Ann. Surg. 180:180–184.

Borgelt, B. B. (in press). Radiation therapy with either gold grain implant or neutron beam for unresectable adenocarcinoma of the pancreas, *in* Pancreatic Cancer. New Directions in Therapeutic Management, I. Cohn, ed. Masson Publishing Co., New York.

Borgelt, B. B., R. R. Dobelbower, Jr., and K. A. Strubler. 1978. Betatron therapy for unresectable pancreatic cancer. A preliminary report. Am. J. Surg. 135:76–80.

CA—A Cancer Journal for Clinicians. 1980. Cancer Statistics, 1980. 30:23–38.

Cohn, I., ed. (in press). Pancreatic Cancer. New Directions in Therapeutic Management. Masson Publishing Co., New York.

Dobelbower, R. R., Jr. 1979. The radiotherapy of pancreatic cancer. Sem. Oncol. 6:378–389.

Dobelbower, R. R., Jr., B. B. Borgelt, K. A. Strubler, G. J. Kutcher, and N. Suntharalingam. 1980. Precision radiotherapy for cancer of the pancreas: technique and results. Int. J. Radiat. Oncol. Biol. Phys. 6:1127–1133.

Dobelbower, R. R., Jr., B. B. Borgelt, N. Suntharalingam, and K. A. Strubler. 1978. Pancreatic carcinoma treated with high-dose, small-volume irradiation. Cancer 41:1087–1092.

Dobelbower, R. R., Jr., K. A. Strubler, and N. Suntharalingam. 1975. Treatment of cancer of the pancreas with high-energy photons and electrons. Int. J. Radiat. Oncol. Biol. Phys. 1:141–146.

Gastrointestinal Tumor Study Group. 1979. A multi-institutional comparative trial of radiation therapy alone and in combination with 5-fluorouracil for locally unresectable pancreatic carcinoma. Ann. Surg. 189:205–208.

Green, N., W. P. Mikkelson, and J. A. Kernen. 1973. Cancer of the common hepatic bile ducts—palliative radiotherapy. Radiology 109:687–689.

Hart, J., B. Modan, and T. Hashomer. 1972. Factors affecting survival of patients with gallbladder neoplasms. Arch. Intern. Med. 129:931–934.

Haslam, J. B., P. J. Cavanaugh, and S. L. Stroup. 1973. Radiation therapy in the treatment of irresectable adenocarcinoma of the pancreas. Cancer 32:1341–1345.

Hudgins, P. T., and R. T. Meoz. 1976. Radiation therapy for obstructive jaundice secondary to tumor malignancy. Int. J. Radiat. Oncol. Biol. Phys. 1:1195–1198.

Hussey, D. H., C. A. Gleiser, J. H. Jardine, G. L. Raulston, and H. R. Withers. 1980. Acute and late normal tissue effects of 50 MeV$_{d \to Be}$ neutrons, in Radiation Biology in Cancer Research, R. E. Meyn and H. R. Withers, eds. Raven Press, New York, pp. 471–488.

Kopelson, G., L. Harisiadis, P. Tretter, and C. H. Chang. 1977. The role of radiation therapy in cancer of the extra-hepatic biliary system: an analysis of thirteen patients and a review of the literature of the effectiveness of surgery, chemotherapy and radiotherapy. Int. J. Radiat. Oncol. Biol. Phys. 2:883–894.

McCracken, J. D., R. Pranab, L. K. Heilbrun, V. K. Vaitkevicius, J. H. Saiki, S. E. Rivkin, A. H. Rossof, and T. N. Moore. 1980. 5-Fluorouracil, methyl-CCNU, and radiotherapy with or without testolactone for localized adenocarcinoma of the exocrine pancreas. A Southwest Oncology Group Study. Cancer 46:1518–1522.

Moertel, C. G., and R. J. Reitermeier. 1969. Advanced Gastrointestinal Cancer—Clinical Management and Chemotherapy. Harper and Row, New York, pp. 192–204.

Moossa, A. R., ed. 1980. Tumors of the Pancreas. Williams & Wilkins, Baltimore, pp. 521–531.

Moossa, A. R., M. Anagnost, A. W. Hall, A. Moraldi, and D. B. Skinner. 1975. The continuing challenge of gallbladder cancer. Survey of thirty years' experience at the University of Chicago. Am. J. Surg. 130:57–62.

Shipley, W. U., G. L. Nardi, A. M. Cohen, and C. C. Ling. 1980. Iodine -125 implant and external beam irradiation in patients with localized pancreatic carcinoma. A comparative study to surgical resection. Cancer 45:709–714.

Smoron, G. L. 1977. Radiation therapy of carcinoma of gallbladder and biliary tract. Cancer 40:1422–1424.

Tepper, J., G. Nardi, and H. Suit. 1976. Carcinoma of the pancreas: review of the MGH experience from 1963 to 1973. Cancer 37:1519–1524.

Vaittinen, E. 1970. Carcinoma of the gallbladder. A study of 390 cases diagnosed in Finland 1953–1967. Ann. Chir. Gynaecol. Fenn. 168(suppl.):7–81.

Whelton, M. J., M. Petrelli, P. George, W. B. Young, and S. Sherlock. 1969. Carcinoma at the junction of the main hepatic ducts. Q. J. Med., New Series 38:211–230.

Whittington, R., R. R. Dobelbower, Jr., B. Borgelt, F. E. Rosato, K. A. Strubler, and F. B. Gelder. (in press). Combined [125]iodine implantation and precision high dose radiotherapy in the treatment of unresectable pancreatic carcinoma, in Pancreatic Cancer. New Directions in Therapeutic Management, I. Cohn, ed. Masson Publishing Co., New York.

Hepatobiliary and Large Bowel Cancer

Gastrointestinal Cancer, edited by
John R. Stroehlein and
Marvin M. Romsdahl.
Raven Press, New York © 1981.

Etiologic Considerations and Diagnosis of Extrahepatic Biliary Cancer

Josef K. Korinek, M.D., Ph.D.

*Department of Medicine, The University of Texas System Cancer Center
M. D. Anderson Hospital and Tumor Institute, Houston, Texas*

The progress in our understanding of carcinomas of the extrahepatic biliary system has been slow partly because these tumors remain uncommon and their prognosis dismal. Although the first case of primary carcinoma of the common bile duct was reported in 1840 by Fardel and the first successful resection of a primary bile duct carcinoma was performed in 1903 by W. J. Mayo, their diagnosis even now is often delayed and radical, curative surgery is the exception rather than the rule.

TUMORS OF THE EXTRAHEPATIC BILE DUCTS

The gross appearance and histology of some adenocarcinomas of the bile ducts suggest their origin from benign tumors. However, there are only a few reported cases of benign papillomas containing foci of malignant cells in their mucosal lining (Braasch et al. 1967). Several histologic types of benign tumors of the biliary ductal system, such as adenomas, papillomas, leiomyomas, and neurilemmomas, have been documented in the literature, but these benign tumors are extremely rare. Since they are usually clinically indistinguishable from malignant lesions, they require a firm histological confirmation.

The malignant tumors of the extrahepatic bile ducts are approximately 33% as common as carcinomas of the gallbladder, and together with them have been responsible for about 4,500 deaths a year in the United States since 1958 (Fraumeni 1975). These two forms of biliary tumors are epidemiologically (and therefore probably etiologically) different (Bismuth and Malt 1979). Sixty percent of patients with bile duct cancers are men, while 67% of gallbladder cancer patients are women (Fraumeni 1975). The malignant tumors of the extrahepatic bile ducts are adenocarcinomas that can be further histologically subdivided into three types: papillary, nodular, and diffuse. This typing has clinical significance in the differential diagnosis of malignant lesions from benign strictures and sclerosing cholangitis. The distribution of these carcinomas has limited importance for surgical treatment; the predominant location is in the lower end of the common bile duct and in the hepatic duct and its branches (Braasch et al. 1967, van Heerden et al. 1967).

TUMORS OF THE GALLBLADDER

The benign tumors of the gallbladder, which include papillomas, adenomas, fibromas, neurofibromas, leiomyomas, and lipomas, have been the subject of occasional case reports. There is little evidence for malignant transformation of these benign lesions. The malignant tumors of the gallbladder are mostly well-differentiated adenocarcinomas (90%), while a few are squamous cell (5%) or anaplastic carcinomas. They represent almost 20% of all gastrointestinal tumors. These malignant lesions tend to occur most commonly in the fundus and neck of the gallbladder. Preoperative diagnosis is uncommon, although a calcified gallbladder on X-ray examination may indicate carcinoma.

ETIOLOGIC CONSIDERATIONS IN CARCINOMAS OF EXTRAHEPATIC BILE DUCTS

The majority of patients with extrahepatic cholangiocarcinomas have no indication of any etiologic factor. The link of these malignant tumors to calculi, in contrast to gallbladder carcinomas, is unconvincing. According to some statistics only a small percentage of these patients (20%) have cholelithiasis (Braasch et al. 1967).

A recognized relationship, however, exists between cholangiocarcinomas and some underlying gastrointestinal diseases. It has been suggested from retrospective studies that bile duct carcinomas may be 10 times more frequent in patients with chronic ulcerative colitis than in the general population (Ritchie et al. 1974). Furthermore, these carcinomas have an onset approximately three decades earlier than bile duct carcinomas in patients without ulcerative colitis (Akwari et al. 1975). The speculation that some biliary carcinogens are released into the portal circulation from the inflamed colon seems unlikely since the surgical removal of the diseased colon, the extent of the disease, or its medical management have no relationship to the subsequent development of carcinoma. It is of interest that a recent review of cholangiographic findings in 20 patients with inflammatory bowel diseases demonstrated abnormalities of intrahepatic bile ducts in all patients and abnormal changes in extrahepatic ducts in 75% of these patients (Rohrmann et al. 1978).

Studies from the Orient indicate a possible relationship between liver fluke infections and bile duct carcinomas. These parasitic diseases are caused in the most populous countries of Asia by *Clonorchis sinensis* and *Opisthorchis felineus* and in west Malaysia and northeastern Thailand by *Opisthorchis viverrini*. It is believed that these flukes incite an inflammatory reaction in the bile ducts and potentiate the action of carcinogens excreted in the bile. Experimental studies from Thailand demonstrated that all Syrian golden hamsters infected with *Opisthorchis viverrini* and fed with dimethylnitrosamine developed cholangiocarcinomas and cholangiofibrosis

(Thamavit et al. 1978). A similar mechanism probably operates in humans, since the diet of the northeastern Thais is rich in a fermented fish product that contains the components necessary for the formation of nitrosamines.

Recently, it has been shown that another population of patients might be at a risk of developing bile duct carcinomas. There are several reports on cholangiocarcinomas arising in the congenital cysts of the biliary tract (Kagawa et al. 1978, Todani et al. 1979). Although the incidence of malignant complications appears to be relatively small—4% in choledochal cysts (Bloustein 1977)—it could be preventable when possible by surgical excision of the cysts. Such association of carcinomas with congenital biliary cysts may result from a combination of chronic inflammation caused by long-standing cholangitis (Donaldson and Guillou 1979) and frequent formation of stones in cysts with excretion of carcinogenic substances in the bile.

There have been very few documented cases of patients with sclerosing cholangitis and cholangiocarcinomas (Wiesner and LaRusso 1980). However, whether this is purely a coincidence or whether sclerosing cholangitis predisposes to bile duct carcinoma remains to be seen.

Review of Tumor Registry in California between 1955 and 1969 identified 1,808 cases of gallbladder and extrahepatic bile duct carcinomas. Further epidemiologic studies linked the high number of these malignant tumors to workers in rubber and automotive plants and some cases of cholangiocarcinomas to workers in aircraft, chemical, and wood-finishing industries as well (Krain 1972). However, the specific biliary tract carcinogens in the industry and our environment are yet to be identified. A large number of chemicals are being reported to be hepatocarcinogenic in animals but there is no conclusive evidence of their carcinogenicity in human beings (Popper 1979).

ETIOLOGIC CONSIDERATIONS IN GALLBLADDER CARCINOMAS

Gallstones are the major known cause of gallbladder carcinoma. The epidemiological studies indicate that whatever causes cholelithiasis also predisposes to cholecystocarcinoma (Fraumeni 1975, Maram et al. 1979): female sex, age over 55 years, parity, estrogens, obesity, ileal disease and bypass, and abnormalities of bile and lipoprotein metabolism. Some of these characteristics are particularly expressed among American Indians and Latin American populations. The reduction of lithogenicity of bile as well as prophylactic cholecystectomy in patients with calcified (porcelain) gallbladders who are at high risk of malignant transformation should reduce the incidence of cholecystocarcinomas.

Retrospective studies from the Typhoid Carrier Registry of New York City singled out another group of patients with a significantly increased incidence of hepatobiliary cancer. Chronic typhoid carriers died from hepatobiliary tumors, particularly those of the gallbladder, six times more frequently than did matched controls (Welton et al. 1979). Thus, the chronic bacterial infection of the gallbladder, perhaps by causing stone formation, would also predispose to malignancy.

DIAGNOSIS OF EXTRAHEPATIC BILIARY CANCER

Ultrasonography is the most sensitive noninvasive technique that can discriminate between obstructive jaundice and parenchymal liver icterus. The accuracy for identification of dilated bile ducts is 96% (Behan and Kazam 1978) and complications are nil.

Percutaneous transhepatic cholangiography with the Chiba needle demonstrates the site of obstruction with a complication rate of approximately 2%. This method can be further supplemented with guided fine-needle aspiration biopsy (Evander et al. 1978).

Endoscopic retrograde cholangiopancretography is another invasive technique for demonstration of the specific anatomic lesion with complications related to endoscopy, medication, cannulation, and injection of contrast material. Such complications, particularly elevation in the serum amylase, have been reported in as many as 15% to 20% of patients, with the overall mortality less than 0.2%. The successful opacification of the bile ducts is achieved in 87% of cases (Siegel 1978). This method can also be used for brush cytology (Osnes et al. 1975).

Arteriography is useful in delineating the extent of intrahepatic and vascular invasion if the resection of a neoplasm is contemplated. Many angiographic features of cholangiocarcinoma, such as encasement of arteries and arterio-arterial collaterals, have been described (Walter et al. 1976).

Some of the other modern diagnostic methods like computerized tomography, radionuclide liver scan, and liver biopsy can be used as adjuncts to the above diagnostic procedures, but they seldom help in the primary evaluation of a patient with extrahepatic biliary carcinoma.

Intraoperative choledochoscopy may be required to identify multifocal or radiologically inapparent neoplasms.

There are a number of papers, especially in the Japanese literature, that bring new improvements to the current diagnostic methods; these could increase the yield of positive tissue diagnoses and help differentiate early malignant lesions from benign abnormalities. It is hoped that such diagnostic improvements will help more patients to achieve a curative resection.

SUMMARY

Although our knowledge of the epidemiology and etiology of extrahepatic biliary tract cancers is limited, some of the predisposing factors and associated diseases have been already identified.

Since the cancers of the bile ducts are epidemiologically distinct from malignant tumors of the gallbladder, it is most likely that the etiologies of these tumors are different.

The diagnosis of extrahepatic biliary tumors is best established by a combination of noninvasive ultrasonography with one of the invasive techniques like percutaneous transhepatic cholangiography or endoscopic retrograde cholangiopancreatography.

REFERENCES

Akwari, O. E., J. A. van Heerden, W. T. Foulk, and A. H. Baggenstoss. 1975. Cancer of the bile ducts associated with ulcerative colitis. Ann. Surg. 181:303–309.

Behan, M., and E. Kazam. 1978. Sonography of the common bile duct: Value of the right anterior oblique view. A. J. R. 130:701–709.

Bismuth, H., and R. A. Malt. 1979. Carcinoma of the biliary tract. N. Engl. J. Med. 301:704–706.

Bloustein, P. A. 1977. Association of carcinoma with congenital cystic conditions of the liver and bile ducts. Am. J. Gastroenterol. 67:40–46.

Braasch, J. W., K. W. Warren, and G. A. Kune. 1967. Malignant neoplasms of the bile ducts. Surg. Clin. North Am. 47:627–638.

Donaldson, D. R., and P. J. Guillou. 1979. Extrahepatic cholangiocarcinoma in association with long-standing cholangitis. Brit. J. Clin. Pract. 33:297–300.

Evander, A., I. Ihse, A. Lunderquist, U. Tylen, and M. Akerman. 1978. Percutaneous cytodiagnosis of carcinoma of the pancreas and bile duct. Ann. Surg. 188:90–92.

Fraumeni, J. F. 1975. Cancers of the pancreas and biliary tract: Epidemiological considerations. Cancer Res. 35:3437–3446.

Kagawa, Y., S. Kashihara, S. Kuramoto, and S. Maetani. 1978. Carcinoma arising in a congenitally dilated biliary tract. Gastroenterology 74:1286–1294.

Krain, L. S. 1972. Gallbladder and extrahepatic bile duct carcinoma. Geriatrics 27:111–117.

Maram, E. S., J. Ludwig, L. T. Kurland, and D. D. Brian. 1979. Carcinoma of the gallbladder and extrahepatic biliary ducts in Rochester, Minnesota, 1935–1971. Am. J. Epidemiol. 109:152–157.

Osnes, M., A. Serck-Hanssen, and J. Myren. 1975. Endoscopic retrograde brush cytology (ERBC) of the biliary and pancreatic ducts. Scand. J. Gastroenterol. 10:829–831.

Popper, H. 1979. Hepatic cancers in man: Quantitative perspectives. Environ. Res. 19:482–494.

Ritchie, J. K., R. N. Allan, J. Macartney, H. Thompson, P. R. Hawley, and W. T. Cooke. 1974. Biliary tract carcinoma associated with ulcerative colitis. Q. J. Med. 170:263–279.

Rohrmann, C. A., H. J. Ansel, P. C. Freeny, F. E. Silverstein, R. L. Protell, L. F. Fenster, T. Ball, J. A. Vennes, and S. E. Silvis. 1978. Cholangiographic abnormalities in patients with inflammatory bowel disease. Radiology 127:635–641.

Siegel, J. H. 1978. ERCP update: Diagnostic and therapeutic applications. Gastrointest. Radiol. 3:311–318.

Thamavit, W., N. Bhamarapravati, S. Sahaphong, S. Vajrasthira, and S. Angsubhakorn. 1978. Effects of dimethylnitrosamine on induction of cholangiocarcinoma in Opisthorchis viverrini-infected Syrian golden hamsters. Cancer Res. 38:4634–4639.

Todani, T., K. Tabuchi, Y. Watanabe, and T. Kobayashi. 1979. Carcinoma arising in the wall of congenital bile duct cysts. Cancer 44:1134–1141.

van Heerden, J. A., E. S. Judd, and M. B. Dockerty. 1967. Carcinoma of the extrahepatic bile ducts. Am. J. Surg. 113:49–55.

Walter, J. F., J. J. Bookstein, and E. V. Bouffard. 1976. Newer angiographic observations in cholangiocarcinoma. Radiology 118:19–23.

Welton, J. C., J. S. Marr, and S. M. Friedman. 1979. Association between hepatobiliary cancer and typhoid carrier state. Lancet 1:791–794.

Wiesner, R. H., and N. F. LaRusso. 1980. Clinicopathological features of the syndrome of primary sclerosing cholangitis. Gastroenterology 79:200–206.

Gastrointestinal Cancer, edited by
John R. Stroehlein and
Marvin M. Romsdahl.
Raven Press, New York © 1981.

Possible Etiologic Factors for Some Malignant Hepatic Tumors

William M. Christopherson, M.D.

*Department of Pathology, University of Louisville School of Medicine,
Louisville, Kentucky*

Although numerous agents have been shown to be liver carcinogens in animals, evidence that they are operative in man is difficult to interpret. First, primary liver cancer in the Western world is very uncommon; and second, there are so many suspected agents available to man through water, food, food additives, and polluted air that accurate assessment of the role of any single agent is most difficult.

A few of the naturally occurring substances, synthetic compounds, and other agents for which there is some evidence of carcinogenicity are listed in the Table on page 258. There is little evidence that the mycotoxins occur in human food, even though the parent fungi have been detected in foodstuffs (Linsell 1979). Of the group of mycotoxins, aflotoxin has perhaps achieved the greatest attention. Field studies have been carried out in various areas of Africa, and there seems to be some correlation between the degree of contamination of foodstuffs and liver cancer rates (Alpert et al. 1971, Keen and Martin 1971). A major problem with those studies, as noted by investigators, is the reliability of cancer rate data in these developing areas. The studies also have been short-term.

Man also ingests hydrazine mycotoxins when he eats mushrooms. Thus far, 37 hydrazine analogs have been shown to be carcinogenic in animals and the liver is a common site. Although the cultivated mushroom, *Agaricus bisporus,* contains hydrazine compounds, they are most commonly eaten in Europe and North America where primary liver cancer is rare (Toth 1979).

About 30 of some 100 pyrrolizidine alkaloids may have malignant potential in that they are cytotoxic in animals, but there is no evidence for or against liver carcinogenicity in man. There likewise is no evidence of an epidemiological nature that cycasin, safrole, or tannic acid play a role in human carcinogenesis (Linsell 1979).

The nitrosamines and the nitrosamides produce a wide variety of cancers in animals. However, evidence of their relationship to human cancer is scanty although their potential distribution in food is considerable (Linsell 1979).

At least 16 pesticides, herbicides, insecticides, and fungicides are said to be hepatocarcinogenic in animals. Because of their wide use, they obviously would have carcinogenic potential in man (Súgar et al. 1979). However, it would be well to remember that their greatest usage is in the developed countries where hepatocarcinoma is a rare disease, and they are less commonly used in developing countries where liver cancer has a high prevalence.

There is a growing body of evidence from Africa, Asia, and the Mediterranean area that hepatitis B virus is associated with liver cancer. However, it is not entirely clear whether the virus is merely a passenger rather than the driver (Zuckerman 1979). Zuckerman points out that hepatitis B is ubiquitous in areas where macronodular cirrhosis and primary liver cancer are common. Most hepatocellular carcinomas (HCC) arise in cirrhotic livers. It is therefore possible that carcinoma arises from regenerative nodules by mechanisms in which the virus is not involved. This may account for hepatomas that develop in alcoholic cirrhosis where there is no evidence of hepatitis B virus (Zuckerman 1979). It should be noted that the same high association with hepatitis B virus found in developing countries has not been demonstrated in North American and western European countries.

In the United States as many as 80% of the HCC occur in cirrhotic livers (Edmondson and Steiner 1954). The majority of patients with cirrhosis in this country have a long history of excessive ethanol intake. One would thus reason that HCC would be even less common than it is if there were not such widespread use of ethanol. In this respect alcohol might properly be consid-

Table *Potential Hepatocarcinogens in Man*

I. Naturally occurring substances
Mycotoxins
Aflatoxins
Cyclochlorotine
Luteoskyrin
Sterigmatocystin
Pyrrolizidine alkaloids
Cycasin
Safrole
Tannic Acid
II. Synthetic compounds
Nitrosamines and nitrosamides
Chlorinated hydrocarbons
III. Pesticides
IV. Hepatitis B virus
V. Alcohol (?)
VI. Alpha-1-antitrypsin deficiency
VII. Parasitic infestation
VIII. Thorotrast (thorium dioxide)
IX. Vinyl chloride
X. Androgenic anabolic steroids
XI. Oral contraceptives
XII. Hyperestrogen states

ered an important, if indirect, factor in hepatocarcinogenesis in the United States and some European countries. Most investigators believe that it is the presence of the cirrhosis, rather than the alcohol intake, that determines the risk of HCC. In alcoholics with cirrhosis the risk increases with time and is not reduced by discontinuing drinking (Lee 1966). It is claimed that there is no increased risk for HCC in alcoholics without cirrhosis (Anthony 1979). Alcohol has not been found to play a role in HCC occurring in the steroid-related patients in our registry and none had cirrhosis.

Alpha$_1$-antitrypsin (AT) deficiency and its possible relation to HCC is currently being investigated. An unusually high incidence of HCC has been reported in AT deficiency (Erickson and Hägenstrand 1974). Deposits of AT have been found in the tumor cells in patients without the deficiency (Palmer and Wolfe 1976). These deposits are PAS-positive and diastase-resistant, and do, in fact, serve as a tissue tumor marker for both benign and malignant liver tumors in steroid users (Palmer et al. 1977).

Parasitic infestation, such as *Schistosoma japonicum* and *Clonorchis seninsis,* may play a role in cholangiolar carcinoma in Japan and southern China (Gibson and Chan 1972). There is no evidence that it is associated with the more common HCC (Gibson and Chan 1972, Gibson 1971, Nakashima et al. 1975).

Thorotrast is an uncommon, nonetheless interesting, iatrogenic cause of liver cancer. It was widely used between 1930 and 1950 for biliary imaging. The early cases were often angiosarcoma thought to result from the storage by the Kupffer cells of the radioactive thorium dioxide. More recently, epithelial tumors have been reported, and would appear to be at least as frequent as angiosarcoma (Smoron and Battifora 1972, Kiely et al. 1973). Thorotrast has not been used since the early 1950's, and the patients exposed were presumably middle-aged and older. Even though thorium dioxide has a long half-life and negligible excretion, the 30-year span since the discontinuance of its use would imply that this cause of liver cancer will soon vanish. An example of combined hepatocellular carcinoma and cholangiocarcinoma in a male who had received Thorotrast some 20 years earlier is shown in Figure 1.

Although cirrhosis is the basis for most liver cancers in the United States, whatever the oncogenic mechanisms might be, we have been interested in a variety of malignant tumors arising in noncirrhotic livers.

ANGIOSARCOMA

The history of the association of angiosarcoma with vinyl chloride used in the manufacture of the plastic, polyvinylchloride, is particularly interesting since it illustrates the importance of astute clinical observation and serendipity contributing to cancer control. It is of immediate interest since the industrial surgeon who made the initial observation, Dr. John Creech, Jr., is a graduate of the M. D. Anderson Hospital training program in surgical oncol-

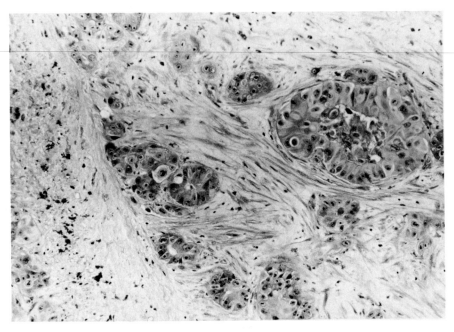

FIG. 1. Combined hepatocellular and cholangiocarcinoma in an elderly male who had received Thorotrast about 20 years earlier. Note the thorium dioxide deposits in the connective tissue to the left and the dense fibrous tissue resulting from ionizing radiation. (H&E ×140.)

ogy. Soon after Dr. Creech returned to Louisville in 1956 he became an industrial surgeon in a large chemical plant. He immediately instigated a system of carefully recording all deaths from cancer that occurred in employees or former employees of the plant. These were obtained from death certificates or from insurance claims. Working with a pathologist, Lazlo Makk, the important observation was made when two workers exposed to vinyl chloride developed angiosarcoma in rapid succession. A retrospective study revealed others with liver problems who had worked at the plant (Creech and Johnson 1974). Through a health screening program three additional cases were discovered among present or past workers. In all, ten workers in the Louisville plant developed angiosarcoma. In 1976, Makk and co-authors reported the clinical-pathological aspects in detail (Makk et al. 1976). All of the patients had worked at the plant over a long period and at a time when exposure could well have been at high levels. All of the victims were actively engaged in the production of vinyl chloride.

The company has instituted rotation of employees away from the areas of exposure and has greatly reduced the exposure level. It seems likely that this occupation-related cancer will, like Thorotrast-related liver tumors, eventually be of only historic interest. No new case has developed in the Louisville plant workers in the past four or five years.

It is interesting to note that Creech was also the first to observe another sequela of the production of plastics at the plant. This complication, acro-osteolysis, seemed to be associated with vinyl acetate. It required rather short exposure, a period of about two years. The problem was resolved by requiring the workers to wear appropriate protective gloves. Since then no new cases have occurred (Wilson et al. 1967).

In the surveillance program and in further epidemiologic studies of the vinyl chloride workers, other possible side effects are being investigated. Although these studies are incomplete, they are being discussed in the lay press. Among them are alleged increases in lung cancer, pancreatic cancer, bowel cancer, and brain tumors.

The presenting symptoms of angiosarcoma in the 15 cases studied by Makk and his co-workers included fatigue, weight loss, anorexia, nausea, abdominal pain, jaundice, and diarrhea. Eleven of the 15 had hepatomegaly on clinical examination. Six, and presumably a seventh patient, had elevated bilirubin. Nine had elevated SGOT, four had elevated LDH, eleven had elevated alkaline phosphatase, three had elevated SGTP, and all three with GGTP determinations had elevated levels. In the latter group none had positive CEA levels and all had negative fetoglobulin determinations (Makk et al. 1976).

The classical gross appearance of angiosarcoma is shown in Figure 2 and the histology is illustrated in Figure 3. The tumors are similar to angiosarcoma of other sites. Although some of the tumors extended to the adjacent organs and tissues, only two of the 15 patients had distant metastases. Death usually occurred soon after diagnosis from local liver destruction. Elsewhere in the liver were areas of subcapsular fibrosis, periportal fibrosis, sinusoidal dilatation, and, at times, marked hyperplasia of the vascular endothelium of the

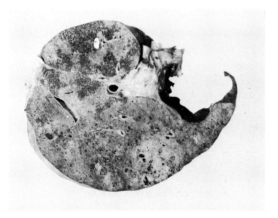

FIG. 2. Gross appearance of an angiosarcoma of the liver in a vinyl chloride worker.

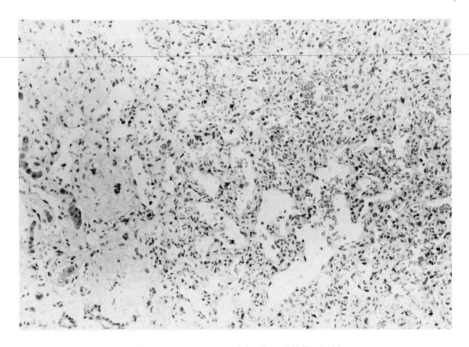

FIG. 3. Angiosarcoma of the liver. (H&E ×140.)

sinusoids. These tumors were also studied at the National Cancer Institute and reported by Thomas and co-workers (Thomas et al. 1975).

STEROID-RELATED ANGIOMAS AND ANGIOSARCOMA

Since the observation of the occurrence of benign liver tumors in oral contraceptive users (Baum et al. 1973), we have maintained a registry of liver tumors at the University of Louisville (Christopherson and Mays 1977). Among the some 250 tumors, both benign and malignant, thus far registered, we have encountered two massive hemangiomas in pill users as well as an angiosarcoma of the liver in a five-year-old girl who had been on steroidal medication for four and one-half years. Peliosis hepatis has been reported in oral contraceptive users (Mays et al. 1974), and at least 25 cases are said to have occurred in patients receiving androgenic anabolic steroids (Westaby et al. 1977).

In 1979 Falk and co-workers reported a retrospective epidemiologic study of deaths from hepatic angiosarcoma in the U.S. There were 168 such cases reported from 1964 through 1974. Thirty-seven were associated with previously identified causes, such as vinyl chloride, Thorotrast, and inorganic arsenic. Four additional cases were associated with the use of androgenic anabolic steroids (Falk et al. 1979). In the single illustration, the histology is indistinguishable from the Thorotrast- and vinyl chloride-related angiosarcomas we have seen. There is also a report of an elderly male treated for 12 years with diethylstilbestrol for prostatic cancer who developed an angiosarcoma of the liver (Hoch-Ligeti 1978).

ANDROGENIC ANABOLIC STEROID-RELATED "HEPATOCELLULAR CARCINOMA"

Since 1965 there have been sporadic publications of hepatocellular carcinoma occurring in patients receiving androgenic anabolic steroids. There are said to be about 25 such cases recorded (Westaby et al. 1977). One such patient is included in our registry. He is living 15 years after biopsy of one of his multiple liver tumors, which we believe to be an adenoma rather than a carcinoma as it was originally diagnosed. It is interesting to note that in only one of the reported androgen-associated tumors has metastasis been claimed. This raises the question of over-diagnosis of these lesions. At the risk of being presumptive, it would seem that at least most "hepatocellular carcinomas" in males ingesting androgenic anabolic steroids will prove to have been benign.

ORAL CONTRACEPTIVES AND HEPATOCELLULAR CARCINOMA

Oral contraceptives have been associated with hepatocellular adenomas, focal nodular hyperplasia (FNH), and lesions that have been classified as liver hamartomas. The latter probably represent the same lesion that others have called focal nodular hyperplasia. Whether or not this is a chance association is difficult to determine since most tumor registries do not include benign tumors, and oral contraceptives have been used or are currently being used by an estimated 50 million women. Be that as it may, benign liver tumors were very rare prior to the introduction of oral contraceptives in the early 1960s.

For those interested in the historical aspects, Sturdevant's publication in 1979 is especially recommended (Sturdevant 1979). He reviews the animal experience and presents a detailed account of the tumors in women. Although he disclaims an all-inclusive review, it seems to be very complete. He provides about 360 citations on the subject. Another review for the interested is that of Klatskin with 107 citations (Klatskin 1977).

Data from two liver tumor registries have been published from time to time (Christopherson and Mays 1977, Christopherson et al. 1978b, Nissen et al. 1976, Nissen et al. 1979). There have been two large surveys (Foster and Berman 1977, Vana et al. 1979). The Foster and Berman survey included 78 hospitals in 48 cities located in 28 states and the District of Columbia. Their monograph is most informative. The American College of Surgeons through its Commission on Cancer surveyed 477 hospitals. They restricted the ages of individuals from 15 to 45, and accessioned 96 adenomas and 58 FNH. In addition, there were 33 tumors classified as hamartomas and 25 other benign tumors. No histologic review of this material has yet been published.

The apparent dependency of at least some benign liver tumors on steroids is of considerable importance. Some have regressed after cessation of the drug, and second tumors have developed when it was continued (Christopherson and Mays 1979, Edmondson et al. 1977).

Among the first 200 registry cases were 20 cases of HCC (Christopherson et al. 1978a). Since then a few more have been added; however, in only 23 do we have sufficient clinical information and follow-up to make a meaningful report (Christopherson et al. in press). The following discussion will deal with these 23 cases.

As previously mentioned all tumors occurred in noncirrhotic livers. Only one patient had jaundice at the time of diagnosis, and in none was there a history of prior hepatitis or excessive use of ethanol.

In 17 of the 23 we could document usage of oral contraceptives. When considering marketing practices in relation to time of diagnosis, no particular preparation could be judged more culpable than another. In 16, the duration of pill usage was known. It averaged 55.4 months. Only one patient had used the pill for less than one year. In the remaining six patients in whom we could not establish oral contraceptive usage, one, our oldest patient, had taken conjugated equine estrogens, 1.25 ml., for 120 months. (It is interesting that we have seen an additional case in a patient outside of the young age range who had used conjugated estrogens for more than 20 years.) Of the remaining five patients, one was pregnant and her tumor was discovered during caesarean section; one was post-partum; in one usage was unknown; and in the remaining two we felt reasonably sure that oral contraceptives had not been taken.

The presenting symptom was pain in 10 patients. Three had hemoperitoneum due to liver rupture. Five patients presented with an abdominal mass. One of these had jaundice. In the remaining patients symptoms consisted of vague abdominal discomfort or vomiting, or were discovered at time of caesarean section.

Four patients had positive alphafetoprotein; in two additional ones the determination was negative. Two patients had positive CEA determinations. Liver scans and/or angiography were frequently helpful in determining the presence of a tumor and in its localization.

The age was known for all patients, and averaged 30.6 years. The average age of the 17 oral contraceptive users was 30.6 years. This was not significantly different from the average age of the benign tumor group.

All 23 cases had a hepatocellular component. In two there was also a mixture of cholangiocellular type. All of the patterns described by Foster and Berman were represented (Foster and Berman 1977). It is of some interest, however, that the type these authors described as "polygonal cell with fibrous stroma" made up only about 6% of their HCC. In our study it accounted for 30%. In addition, there were three tumors with the same type of abundant

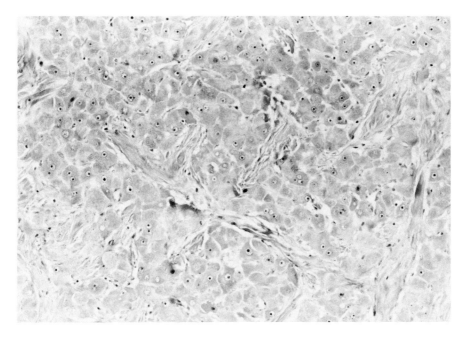

FIG. 4. Eosinophilic glassy cell hepatoma. A minimal amount of hyalin fibrosis can be seen. (H&E ×140.)

glassy eosinophilic cytoplasm which lacked the characteristic pattern of fibrosis (Figure 4). Peters has proposed the term "eosinophilic hepatocellular carcinoma with lamellar fibrosis" for this group of tumors (Peters 1976). He considers them to be an uncommon type, having seen only four cases in his very large autopsy series, and a single case in a 16-year-old boy in a biopsy. The author cites a similar case seen by Edmondson in a 14-year-old girl who is alive and well at 10 years. This tumor type in our series did not appear to have a better prognosis, as has been suggested, since all seven of our patients with the glassy eosinophilic cells and lamellar fibrosis are dead of disease. Also dead are the three with the glassy eosinophilic cells without appreciable fibrosis. The longest survivor of this tumor type in the registry was three years.

A very recent report supports the concept that this subtype of HCC, if resectable, does result in a higher survival rate than other types (Berman et al. 1980). These authors report 12 cases of HCC which they called "polygonal cell type with fibrous stroma." In that series, five of eight patients who underwent resection survived for five years. The median age of their patients was 23 years, although the ages ranged from five to 68 years. None had previously documented cirrhosis, hepatitis, or exposure to hepatotoxins. These authors noted focal nodular hyperplasia adjacent to the HCC in three cases, with one showing an apparent transition to carcinoma. We have seen one case in which we believed that HCC of eosinophilic glassy cell type arose in relation to focal nodular hyperplasia (Christopherson et al. 1977).

Many of the cells contain eosinophilic cytoplasmic inclusions which are readily seen in H&E sections. They are PAS-positive and resistant to diastase digestion (Figure 5). These have been shown to be positive for alpha$_1$-antitrypsin using the immunoperoxidase reaction and are considered to be a protein marker for steroid-related tumors (Palmer et al. 1977).

Electron microscopy was performed on several of the tumors and was of no particular help. The inclusions were seen as granular, electron-dense material within the dilated segments of the rough endoplasmic reticulum.

Twenty of the 23 patients have died, one is terminal, and in two there is no follow-up. All deaths were related to disease or to complications of treatment. Ten patients underwent tumor resection, and of these nine are dead; the status of the other is unknown. Twelve had biopsy only; of these ten are dead, one is terminal, and the status of the other is unknown. The remaining patient, terminal when first seen, was diagnosed at autopsy. This is in marked contrast to the published cases of HCC described in young males receiving anabolic androgenic steroids where metastasis rarely, if ever, occurs. Proven sites of metastasis in the group of women under discussion have included lymph nodes, peritoneum, mesentery, omentum, adrenal gland, spleen, gallbladder, ovary, pleura, lung, and bone.

DISCUSSION

It is generally assumed that the estrogen fraction of oral contraceptives is the agent involved in liver oncogenesis. This belief is reinforced by tumors occurring in the hyperestrogen state of women who do not use oral contraceptives. The examples in our registry include four patients with benign tumors and one with HCC who were long-term users of conjugated equine

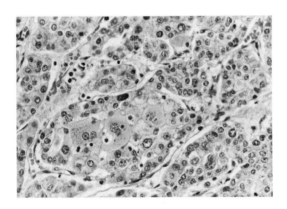

FIG. 5. Hepatocellular carcinoma. Note the cytoplasmic inclusions which stain with PAS and are resistant to diastase digestion. They stain positively by the immunoperoxidase method for alpha-1-antitrypsin. (PAS with diastase ×118).

estrogens. In addition, there was an older woman who, with over 20 years' usage of conjugatd equine estrogens, developed HCC. One patient who had not used oral contraceptives had an estrogen-producing tumor of the ovary. Eight patients had their tumor diagnosed in late pregnancy or early postpartum. Finally, we have seen a benign liver tumor in an elderly male who had taken DES over a prolonged period of time. Another observation that lends support to the steroid relationship is the apparent dependency of some liver tumors on an exogenous source. Regression of both androgenic anabolic steroid-related tumors (Farrell et al. 1975) and the oral contraceptive-related tumors have been observed by us and by others as well, once the exogenous source has been withdrawn (Edmondson et al. 1977, Edmondson et al. 1980). While this does support steroidal dependency, it does not necessarily indict the estrogen fraction of oral contraceptives.

The progestins used in oral contraceptives have a close structural relationship to androgenic anabolic steroids. Nissen et al. in 1976 reported that four patients in their series of benign liver tumors used either medroxyprogesterone acetate or norethinidrone acetate without estrogen. We have seen an HCC in a young woman receiving Provera; however, she also had a history of 18 months' exposure to oral contraceptives.

In conclusion, it should be pointed out that primary carcinoma of the liver is extremely uncommon in the Western world. HCC in the absence of cirrhosis could for all intents and purposes be considered to be rare. Judging from the relatively few oral contraceptive users who have developed HCC, and if the estimate of 50 million exposed women is correct, this possible complication does not present a major public health problem. It does, however, provide provocative material for the understanding of liver oncogenesis.

REFERENCES

Alpert, M. E., M. S. R. Hutt, G. N. Wogan, and C. S. Davidson. 1971. The association between aflatoxin content of food and hepatoma frequency in Uganda. Cancer 28:253–260.

Anthony, P. P. 1979. Precancerous changes in the human liver, *in* Liver Carcinogenesis, K. Lapis, J. V. Johannessen, eds. Hemisphere Publishing, Washington, pp. 131–141.

Baum, J., F. Holtz, J. J. Bookstein, and E. W. Klein. 1973. Possible association between benign hepatomas and oral contraceptives. Lancet 2:926–929.

Berman, M. M., N. P. Libbey, and J. H. Foster. 1980. Hepatocellular carcinoma: Polygonal cell type with fibrous stroma—an atypical variant with a favorable prognosis. Cancer 46:1448–1455.

Christopherson, W. M., and E. T. Mays. 1977. Liver tumors and contraceptive steroids. Experience with the first one hundred registry patients. J. Natl. Cancer Inst. 58:167–172.

Christopherson, W. M., and E. T. Mays. 1979. Relation of steroid to liver oncogenesis. J. Toxicol. Environ. Health 5:207–230.

Christopherson, W. M., E. T. Mays, and G. H. Barrows. 1977. A clinicopathologic study of steroid-related liver tumors. Am. J. Surg. Pathol. 1:31–41.

Christopherson, W. M., E. T. Mays, and G. H. Barrows. 1978a. Hepatocellular carcinoma in young women on oral contraceptives. Lancet 2:38–39.

Christopherson, W. M., E. T. Mays, and G. H. Barrows. 1978b. Liver oncogenesis and steroids, *in* Progress in Clinical Cancer, I. M. Ariel, ed., vol. 7. Grune and Stratton, New York, pp. 153–163.

Christopherson, W. M., E. T. Mays, and G. H. Barrows. (in press). Liver tumors in young women: A clinical pathologic study of 201 cases in the Louisville registry, in Progress in Surgical Pathology, C. M. Fenoglio, M. Wolff, eds., vol. 2. Masson Publishing, New York.

Creech, J. L., Jr., and M. N. Johnson. 1974. Angiosarcoma of the liver in the manufacture of polyvinylchloride. J. Occup. Med. 16:150–151.

Edmondson, H. A., T. B. Reynolds, B. Henderson, and B. Benton. 1977. Regression of liver cell adenomas associated with oral contraceptives. Ann. Intern. Med. 86:180–182.

Edmondson, H. A., and P. E. Steiner. 1954. Primary carcinoma of the liver: An autopsy study of 100 cases among 48,900 necropsies. Cancer 7:462–502.

Edmondson, Q. B., K. L. Nachtnebel, R. R. Penkava, and J. Rothenberg. 1980. Oral-con-traceptive-associated liver tumors. Lancet 1:1251.

Erickson, S., and I. Hägenstrand. 1974. Cirrhosis and malignant hepatoma in alpha-1-antitrypsin deficiency. Acta Med. Scand. 195:451–458.

Falk, H., H. Popper, L. B. Thomas, and K. G. Ishak. 1979. Hepatic angiosarcoma associated with androgenic-anabolic steroids. Lancet 2:1120–1123.

Farrell, G. C., D. E. Joshua, R. F. Uren, P. J. Baird, K. W. Perkins, and H. Kronenberg. 1975. Androgen-induced hepatoma. Lancet 1:430–432.

Foster, J. H., and M. M. Berman. 1977. Solid Liver Tumors. W. B. Saunders Co., Philadelphia, pp. 69–74.

Gibson, J. B. 1971. Parasites, liver disease and liver cancer, in Liver Cancer. IARC Sci. Publ. No. 1, International Agency for Research on Cancer, Lyon, pp. 42–50.

Gibson, J. B., and W. C. Chan. 1972. Primary carcinoma of the liver in Hong Kong: Some possible aetiological factors, in Current Problems in Epidemiology of Cancer and Lymphomas, E. Grundmann, H. Tulinius, eds. Springer-Verlag, Berlin, pp. 107–118.

Hoch-Ligeti, C. 1978. Angiosarcoma of the liver associated with diethylstilbestrol. JAMA 240:1510–1511.

Keen, P., and P. Martin. 1971. The toxicity and fungal infestation of foodstuffs in Swaziland in relation to harvesting and storage. Trop. Geogr. Med. 23:35–43.

Kiely, J. M., J. L. Titus, and A. L. Orvis. 1973. Thorotrast-induced hepatoma presenting as hyperparathyroidism. Cancer 31:1312–1314.

Klatskin, G. 1977. Hepatic tumors: Possible relationship to use of oral contraceptives. Gastroen-terology 73:386–394.

Lee, F. I. 1966. Cirrhosis and hepatoma in alcoholics. Gut 7:77–85.

Linsell, C. A. 1979. Environmental chemical carcinogens and liver cancer, in Liver Car-cinogenesis, K. Lapis, J. V. Johannessen, eds. Hemisphere Publishing, Washington, pp. 173–181.

Makk, L., F. Delorme, J. L. Creech, Jr., L. L. Ogden, E. H. Fadell, C. L. Songster, J. Clanton, M. N. Johnson, and W. M. Christopherson. 1976. Clinical and morphological features of hepatic angiosarcoma in vinyl chloride workers. Cancer 37:149–163.

Mays, E. T., W. M. Christopherson, and G. H. Barrows. 1974. Focal nodular hyperplasia of liver: Possible relationship to oral contraceptives. Am. J. Clin. Pathol. 61:735–746.

Nakashima, T., K. Okuda, M. Kojiro, K. Sakamoto, Y. Kubo, and Y. Shimokawa. 1975. Primary liver cancer coincident with Schistosomiasis japonica. A study of 24 necropsies. Cancer 36:1483–1489.

Nissen, E. D., D. R. Kent, and S. E. Nissen. 1976. Liver tumors and the pill: Analyzing the data. Contrib. Gynecol. Obstet. 8:103–111.

Nissen, E. D., D. R. Kent, and S. E. Nissen. 1979. Role of oral contraceptive agents in the pathologenesis of liver tumors, in Liver Carcinogenesis, K. Lapis, J. V. Johannessen, eds. Hemisphere Publishing, Washington, pp. 61–84.

Palmer, P. E., W. M. Christopherson, and H. J. Wolfe. 1977. Alpha-1-antitrypsin, protein marker in oral contraceptive-associated hepatic tumors. Am. J. Clin. Pathol. 68:736–739.

Palmer, P. E., and H. J. Wolfe. 1976. Alpha-1-antitrypsin deposition in primary hepatic car-cinomas. Arch. Pathol. Lab. Med. 100:232–236.

Peters, R. L. 1976. Pathology of hepatocellular carcinoma, in Hepatocellular Carcinoma, K. Okuda, R. L. Peters, eds. John Wiley and Sons, New York, pp. 107–168.

Smoron, G. L., and H. A. Battifora. 1972. Thorotrast-induced hepatoma. Cancer 30:1252–1259.

Sturdevant, F. M. 1979. Oral contraceptives and liver tumors, in Controversies in Contraception, K. S. Moghissi, ed. Williams and Wilkins, Baltimore, pp. 93–150.

Súgar, J., K. Tóth, O. Csuka, E. Gáti, and S. Somfai-Relle. 1979. Role of pesticides in hepatocarcinogenesis, *in* Liver Carcinogenesis, K. Lapis, J. V. Johannessen, eds. Hemisphere Publishing, Washington, pp. 183-191.

Thomas, L. B., H. Popper, P. D. Berk, T. Selikoff, and H. Falk. 1975. Vinyl chloride-induced liver disease. N. Engl. J. Med. 292:17-22.

Toth, B. 1979. Hepatocarcinogenesis by hydrazine mycotoxins of edible mushrooms, *in* Liver Carcinogenesis, K. Lapis, J. V. Johannessen, eds. Hemisphere Publishing, Washington, pp. 23-32.

Vana, J., G. P. Murphy, B. L. Aronoff, and H. V. Baker. 1979. Survey of primary liver tumors and oral contraceptive use, *in* Liver Carcinogenesis, K. Lapis, J. V. Johannessen, eds. Hemisphere Publishing, Washington, pp. 85-103.

Westaby, D., S. J. Ogle, F. J. Paradinas, J. B. Randell, and I. M. Murray-Lyon. 1977. Liver damage from long-term methyltestosterone. Lancet 2:261-263.

Wilson, R. H., W. E. McCormick, C. F. Tatum, and J. L. Creech, Jr. 1967. Occupational acroosteolysis—Report of 31 cases. JAMA 201:577-581.

Zuckerman, A. J. 1979. Role of hepatitis B virus in primary liver cancer, *in* Liver Carcinogenesis, K. Lapis, J. V. Johannessen, eds. Hemisphere Publishing, Washington, pp. 105-110.

Gastrointestinal Cancer, edited by
John R. Stroehlein and
Marvin M. Romsdahl.
Raven Press, New York © 1981.

Diagnosis and Surgical Management of Primary Malignant Hepatic Tumors

Charles M. McBride, M.D.

Department of Surgery, The University of Texas System Cancer Center
M. D. Anderson Hospital and Tumor Institute, Houston, Texas

The general problem of primary malignant hepatic tumors can be stated by the fact that the average patient survival following diagnosis of such is four months for those patients with primary carcinomas of the liver and 5.7 months for those with metastatic carcinoma in the liver (Bengmark and Hafström 1969). Since the liver is the largest visceral organ in the human body it has been of interest to man for a long time. The ancients inspected the liver in an attempt to predict the future, and hence liver tumors have probably been observed for many millennia. Rokitansky (1849) described the difference between primary and secondary cancers in the liver; this appears to be the first time that such a distinction was clearly appreciated.

Primary malignant tumors in the liver may be of liver cell origin, bile duct origin, or of mixed origin combining both of these previous elements; or they may be sarcomas arising from nonepithelial structures in the liver. Primary carcinoma of the liver is rare in the Western world; only about 2,600 deaths from hepatoma occur annually in the United States; however, it is the most common visceral cancer in males in many regions of Africa and the Orient. In a large autopsy series from this country (Edmondson and Stetner 1954), the observed incidence of primary carcinoma of the liver was 0.21%, 75% of which were liver cell carcinomas.

PATIENT DATA

During the 35 years from 1944 to 1979, 274 patients with primary carcinoma of the liver were seen at The University of Texas System Cancer Center M. D. Anderson Hospital and Tumor Institute. Of these patients, 71% had hepatomas, 21% had cholangiocarcinomas and 8% had the mixed variety. The male-to-female ratio was 2:1; however, females predominated in the child-bearing years from 10 to 39 years of age. The distribution of patients by age, sex and type of primary liver cancer is similar to that previously published (McBride 1979) with the highest incidences in patients in the sixth and seventh decades of life. When treatment results are being reported, it is necessary to use some form of staging to permit a comparison of similar cases. The staging system for primary malignant hepatic tumors used at the U.T. M. D. Anderson Hospital is the one suggested by Almersjö et al. (1972). An estimation of the amount of liver replaced by cancer is a very gross measurement; however, the division of the patients into three groups by staging is a useful clinical tool. Of the 274 patients reported here, 7% were either Stage I, or unstaged in that an exploratory laparotomy was not done to permit staging; 68% were Stage II; and 25% were Stage III. In this study, just over 25% of the patients were known to have cirrhosis. Because the patients with Stage I disease were usually unstaged or had lesions found at autopsy, they were not included in a treatment analysis. The patients with Stage III liver tumors were not usually amenable to surgical therapy and as the small number of primary sarcomas were in this group, they were not analyzed further. The remainder of this investigation deals primarily with the Stage II patients—those with from 20% to 70% of the liver parenchyma replaced by tumor.

RESULTS

The median age of the 186 patients with Stage II liver cancer was 29.5 years, with a range of from 1 to 84 years. Nine percent of these patients survived for more than two years. There were no statistically significant differences in the survival rates for the different cellular types of primary hepatic carcinomas in patients with Stage II or Stage III disease, as reported previously (McBride 1976). For this reason all of the patients with Stage II primary carcinoma of the liver were further analyzed based on the type of treatment regimen employed. Figure 1 shows the survival curves for the patients with Stage II liver cancer according to treatment regimen. Since this retrospective study covered a period of 35 years, 41 patients with Stage II disease were seen during the early years when no form of therapy was recommended. This group of patients was observed only and hence provides a baseline for comparison of the survival rates according to the treatment regimens. The curve for these patients is the standard exponential decay curve which is seen in most biological systems. The survival for the patients treated by systemic chemotherapy (most often 5-fluorouracil) is significantly better than that for the observation group until approximately eight months. Beyond that time, however, the curves are essentially the same. The survival rates for patients undergoing hepatic resection or hepatic dearterialization were significantly better (p = 0.002) at all time intervals than for those who were only observed and the survival rate is better than that for patients treated by regional or systemic chemotherapy at time intervals beyond the eight-month period. The types of hepatic resections performed on this patient group are listed in Table 1. The specimen removed from one patient having a central hepatectomy is shown in Figure 2. Three patients in the resection group (9%) died within 30 days either because of mesenteric or caval thrombosis; however, this surgical mortality compares

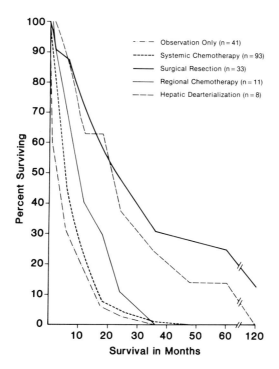

FIG. 1. Stage II liver cancer. Graph demonstrating the usual median survival of four months for untreated patients and significantly better survivals for patients treated by dearterialization or hepatic resection. The small number of cures were in the latter group.

favorably with the 6% of patients with Stage III disease known to have died following percutaneous liver biopsies. Two patients having hepatic resections died beyond the 30-day period as a result of liver failure. An additional two patients who had right hepatic lobectomies were known not to be free of disease when the resections were completed.

The presenting symptoms for the patients with Stage II liver cancer are given in Table 2. As in other series (Inouye and Whelan 1979), pain was the main complaint voiced by most patients. More than 50% of each of the groups of patients with similar presenting symptoms were treated by systemic chemotherapy. Of interest was the fact that more than 20% of the groups of

Table 1. *Surgical Resection for Stage II Primary Carcinoma of the Liver (33 Patients)*

Right Hepatic Lobectomy	13
Extended Right Hepatic Lobectomy	1
Left Hepatic Lobectomy	8
Central Hepatectomy	2
Wedge Resection of Liver	9

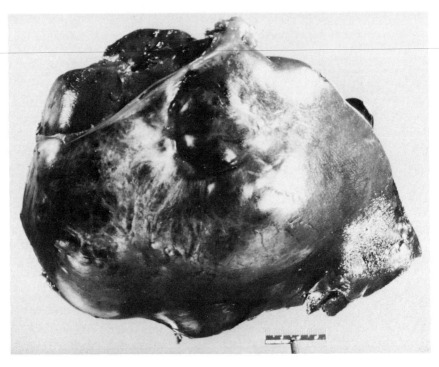

FIG. 2. Hepatic cell carcinoma weighing 1,500 grams resected from a patient undergoing a central hepatectomy (note gallbladder at upper right of illustration).

patients presenting either with pain or with "fever and vomiting" were treated by surgical resections, this percentage being considerably higher than in the other groups. This may suggest that in some patients these latter symptoms occur with localized disease and that localized disease may be less likely with the other presenting symptoms. The median duration of symptoms in patients prior to surgical resection was two months, with a range from one to nine months. In the overall series many patients were symptomatic for over two years; in fact, one Stage II patient had known of her abdominal mass for 20 years. For the patients with Stage II cancer, the absolute rate of cirrhosis was probably much higher than the known 25%. Only 12% of these patients had α-fetoprotein determinations on admission, but of these, 62% of the values were greater than 10 ng/ml.

DISCUSSION

Primary carcinoma of the liver has long been looked upon as a neoplasm with a hopeless prognosis (Alpert et al. 1974), but many of the patients reported in this series were symptomatic for years before the diagnosis was

Table 2. *Presenting Symptoms for Patients with Primary Cancer of the Liver (Stage II)*

Pain	50%
Abdominal Mass	14%
Abdominal Distention	13%
Fatigue and Weight Loss	12%
Fever and Vomiting	8%
Hematemesis	1%
Itching without Jaundice	1%
Asymptomatic	1%

made. This suggests that there is a great deal of room for improvement in the early diagnosis of hepatic cancers. It would be hoped that with earlier diagnosis, the resection rate would be higher than the 18% accomplished in this series and that with earlier exploration, the median survival of two years for this group could be exceeded. At the present, this is not much better than the survival reported from our institution for patients having a mixed group of malignant tumors who underwent various resections involving the right lobe of the liver (McBride and Wallace 1972) and the survivals for all groups are not significantly better than those reported earlier by Chan (1967). Although a majority of the long-term survivors in this series were in the group of patients with liver cell carcinomas, some authors have suggested that patients with cholangiocarcinomas may be the group most likely to present with localized disease which permits resection (Alpert et al. 1974).

Theoretically, all Stage I primary hepatic cancers should be resectable. Because of the high ratio of liver mass to tumor volume, however, these patients' tumors are rarely diagnosed except at autopsy, as an occasional finding at laparotomy, or during workup for another disease condition. Pain was the most common presenting symptom in this and other series (Inouye and Whelan 1979), but may have been present for a long time before the diagnosis was made. The abdominal pain was frequently vague and poorly localized and hence not a symptom for which most clinicians would order a liver scan. The cost/benefit ratio of such a practice would be very low. Some investigators (Lehmann and Wegener 1979) are using serial α-fetoprotein determinations in high risk patients and there is a suggestion that this may lead to earlier diagnosis. As most high risk groups of patients tend to have cirrhosis, however, earlier diagnosis in these patients may not lead to more cures. Major resections are possible in patients without cirrhosis, however, and there has not been any mortality associated with left-sided hepatic resections at this institution, nor with any of the major hepatic resections done for benign disease.

It has been suggested that when patients present with malignant hepatic tumors which are unresectable because of their maldistribution in liver, repeated dearterializations may provide a small chance for a cure (Bengmark et al. 1974). The eight patients in this series who underwent hepatic dearterialization demonstrated good objective responses when checked by isotope scanning and by repeat arteriography. Following dearterialization, there is a variable amount of viable tumor tissue left at the periphery of each tumor nodule. More recently, therefore, repeated dearterializations have been used to try to increase the total tumor kill. These dearterializations are alternated between those done by laparotomy in the operating room and those done percutaneously in the Radiology Department. Both methods seem to be equally effective.

When regional chemotherapy by intra-arterial infusion was used, a permanently indwelling Teflon catheter was usually placed at laparotomy and low-dose continuous drug therapy (most often 5-FU) was administered for at least three months. Some patients, however, had a percutaneous catheter placement. Although the group of patients reported here is too small to show statistically significant results, there has been improvement in survivals for patients treated by intra-arterial infusion (McBride 1975) over survivals for those given systemic chemotherapy. No significant complications related to infusions were seen in the eleven patients reported here.

Although primary carcinoma of the liver is relatively rare in this country, all physicians should be suspicious when there is vague abdominal pain, unexplained anorexia, or a low-grade fever, since many patients may be symptomatic for years before a malignant hepatic tumor is diagnosed. If the disease is discovered while still at a localized stage, it may be resected with some expectation of cure. The exception is when it is associated with significant cirrhosis; in these patients the function of the residual liver tissue may not be adequate to support life. There does not seem to be any predictable difference between the response rates of the various cellular types of primary carcinoma of the liver. Hence, if the disease is unresectable, the patient should be considered for multiple dearterializations, regional chemotherapy by infusion, or systemic chemotherapy, in most cases in that order of priority. For the patients with more than 70% of the liver replaced by cancer (Stage III), only symptomatic treatment is recommended, as few significant responses to any form of therapy have been observed to date and they are easily tipped into hepato-renal failure by any outside manipulation.

REFERENCES

Almersjö, O., S. Bengmark, C. M. Rudenstam, L. Hafström, and L. A. J. Nilsson. 1972. Evaluation of hepatic dearterialization in primary and secondary cancer of the liver. Am. J. Surg. 124:5–8.

Alpert, L. I., F. G. Zak, S. Werthamer, and J. F. Bochetto. 1974. Cholangiocarcinoma: A clinicopathologic study of five cases with ultrastructural observations. Hum. Pathol. 5:709–728.

Bengmark, S., P. Fredlund, L. Hafström, and J. Vang. 1974. Present experiences with hepatic dearterialization in liver neoplasm. Prog. Surg. 13:141–166.

Bengmark, S., and L. Hafström. 1969. The natural history of primary and secondary malignant tumors of the liver. Cancer 23:198–202.

Chan, K. T. 1967. The management of primary liver carcinoma. Ann. R. Coll. Surg. Engl. 41:253–282.

Edmondson, H. A., and P. E. Steiner. 1954. Primary carcinoma of the liver: A study of 100 cases among 48,900 necropsies. Cancer 7:462–503.

Inouye, A. A., and T. J. Whelan. 1979. Primary liver cancer: A review of 205 cases in Hawaii. Am. J. Surg. 138:53–61.

Lehmann, F. G., and T. Wegener. 1979. Etiology of human liver cancer: Controlled prospective study in liver cirrhosis. J. Toxicol. Environ. Health 5(2–3):281–300.

McBride, C. M. 1975. Regional chemotherapy, *in* Cancer Chemotherapy—Fundamental Concepts and Recent Advances (Proceedings of The University of Texas System Cancer Center M. D. Anderson Hospital and Tumor Institute Annual Clinical Conference). Chicago, Illinois, Year Book Medical Publishers, Inc., pp. 369–384.

McBride, C. M. 1976. Primary carcinoma of the liver. Surgery 80:323–327.

McBride, C. M. 1979. Limitations of current treatment methods for primary carcinoma of the liver. J. Toxicol. Environ. Health 5(2–3):387–393.

McBride, C. M., and S. Wallace. 1972. Cancer of the right lobe of the liver: A variety of surgical procedures. Arch. Surg. 105:289–296.

Rokitansky, C. A. 1849. Manual of pathological anatomy. Edwards, London.

Gastrointestinal Cancer, edited by
John R. Stroehlein and
Marvin M. Romsdahl.
Raven Press, New York © 1981.

Chemotherapeutic Management of Hepatobiliary and Pancreatic Cancer

Gerald P. Bodey, M.D., Agop Y. Bedikian, M.D.,
Manuel Valdivieso, M.D., Eugene M. McKelvey, M.D.,
and Yehuda Z. Patt, M.D.

Department of Developmental Therapeutics,
The University of Texas System Cancer Center
M. D. Anderson Hospital and Tumor Institute, Houston, Texas

Malignant tumors of the pancreas, liver, gallbladder, and bile ducts have received little attention from chemotherapists in the past. Recently, it has been recognized that pancreatic carcinoma deserves more extensive investigation because it is the ninth most frequent carcinoma in the United States. It is estimated that 22,000 new cases are diagnosed each year and it appears to be increasing in frequency. Since 95% of cases terminate fatally, pancreatic carcinoma ranks as the fourth leading cause of death among malignant diseases. Only 10% to 15% of cases are considered resectable and the median survival from operation in patients with unresectable tumors is only 3.5 months (Moertel 1974a). The median survival for all patients from onset of symptoms is only 10.5 months and the five-year survival following curative surgery is only 6%.

In the past, pancreatic carcinoma was included with other carcinomas of the gastrointestinal tract in chemotherapy trials and only a few patients were treated with any regimen. Accurate evaluation of the activity of chemotherapeutic agents in the management of pancreatic carcinoma has been hampered by the difficulty in obtaining repeated measurements of tumor masses. Early studies used duration of survival as the parameter for response to antitumor agents. Since less than 50% of patients with pancreatic carcinoma respond to any chemotherapeutic regimen, the median duration of survival does not accurately indicate antitumor activity. Hence, using this measurement as the parameter of response can lead to erroneous conclusions. Likewise, relief of symptoms is an unreliable indicator of response because it is a subjective measurement and can be influenced by the placebo effect or the attitude of the physician. The introduction of computerized tomography and sonography has greatly facilitated evaluation of antitumor activity in pancreatic carcinoma and permitted the use of objective criteria of response.

5-Fluorouracil (5-FU) is the antitumor agent which has been evaluated most extensively in pancreatic carcinoma. In a collated series of 212 cases in which a variety of schedules were utilized, the response rate was 28% (Carter and Comis 1975). However, response rates with 5-FU in individual studies have varied from 0% to 67%. Davis and co-workers reviewed the experience of 129 patients treated with fluoropyrimidines and found the median survival to be only four months (Davis et al. 1974). However, a few patients with metastatic disease involving the liver or peritoneum remained alive for more than one year. The extreme differences in response rates probably can be attributed to patient selection, criteria for response, and variations in drug dosage and schedule. For example, the route of administration appears to affect response to 5-FU (Stolinsky et al. 1975). A comparison of 5-FU 15 mg/kg once weekly given orally or the same dosage schedule given intravenously produced response rates of 0% and 21% (p = .04). Subsequently, pharmacological studies have shown that absorption of 5-FU from the gastrointestinal tract is variable, which most likely explains this difference in response. Schedule of drug administration may also be of importance. In a collated series, 125 patients received 15 mg/kg/d for 4–5 days, followed by 7.5 mg/kg every other day, and 27% responded. In a single report of 50 selected patients who received 15 mg/kg/d in five-day courses every 4–6 weeks, the response rate was 40% (Carter and Comis 1975).

Moertel and his colleagues conducted a randomized trial of radiotherapy alone or combined with 5-FU in patients with unresectable gastrointestinal carcinomas (Moertel et al. 1969). Radiation was administered at a total tumor dose of 3,500–4,000 rads and 5-FU (15 mg/kg/day) was administered on the first three days of radiotherapy only. Despite the modest dose of 5-FU, the mean survival was 6.3 months for patients receiving radiotherapy compared to 10.4 months for patients receiving radiotherapy plus chemotherapy (p < .05). Subsequently, the Gastrointestinal Tumor Study Group conducted a study comparing 6,000 rads radiotherapy alone; 4,000 rads radiotherapy plus 5-FU; or 6,000 rads radiotherapy plus 5-FU (Gastrointestinal Tumor Study Group 1979). Radiotherapy was administered in split courses of 2,000 rads over two weeks at two-week intervals. 5-FU was administered at a dose of 500 mg/m^2/day for the first three days of each course of radiotherapy and weekly thereafter. The median survival was 18 weeks for 25 patients receiving radiotherapy alone compared to 35 weeks for 154 patients receiving radiotherapy plus chemotheraphy. The higher dose of radiotheraphy also improved initial survival (median 39 weeks vs. 31 weeks, p < .09) but this improvement was not sustained for patients surviving beyond one year. Although survival was the parameter used for response in these studies, they have demonstrated that 5-FU shows activity in the management of pancreatic carcinoma.

A variety of other single agents have been tested in pancreatic carcinoma and collated results from the literature are presented in Table 1. However, most studies have involved only a few patients with pancreatic carcinoma in a

Table 1. *Single-Agent Chemotherapy of Pancreatic Carcinoma*

Agent	Patients	% Response	References
5-Fluorouracil	212	28	Carter and Comis 1975
BCNU	55	5	Moertel et al. 1976
Methyl CCNU	76	9	Moertel et al. 1976
			Engstrom et al. 1976
Streptozotocin	49	22	Carter and Comis 1975
			Smith and Schein 1979
Mitomycin C	53	22	Bedikian et al. 1981
Adriamycin	25	8	Schein et al. 1978
Actinomycin D	28	4	Schein et al. 1978
Methotrexate	25	4	Schein et al. 1978
Galactitol	20	5	Smith and Schein 1979
βTGdR	26	4	Kaplan 1978
Neocarzinostatin	92	12	McKelvey, Personal
			Communication
AAFC	6	50	Alberto et al. 1978

larger series of patients with a variety of gastrointestinal tumors. Mitomycin C, an antitumor antibiotic, has activity similar to that of 5-FU but it causes serious myelosuppression which is cumulative and limits its usefulness. The use of intermittent schedules has somewhat reduced the problem of myelosuppression. Adriamycin, methotrexate, and actinomycin D have been evaluated in a randomized trial. None of these agents had substantial activity in pancreatic carcinoma. Neocarzinostatin has been evaluated extensively in Japan but shows little activity. However, three patients achieved complete remissions lasting more than one year. Anhydro-ara-5-fluorocytidine (2,2'-anhydro-arabino-5-fluorocytidine) is a derivative of cytosar which is more resistant to deamination. In two phase II studies, this drug has produced three responses in six patients with pancreatic çarcinoma, a result which deserves further evaluation (Alberto et al. 1977, Alberto et al. 1978).

The nitrosoureas have been evaluated in managing pancreatic carcinoma and neither BCNU or methyl CCNU have had any substantial activity. Moertel and his associates have treated 68 evaluable patients with methyl CCNU 200 mg/m² at seven-week intervals (Moertel et al. 1976). Only one patient achieved a complete remission lasting 22 months. Three patients achieved partial remissions lasting 7 to 21 weeks, and the disease stabilized temporarily in 14 patients. The median survival was only eight weeks (range, 3 days to 33.5 months); hence, many patients received only a single dose of therapy.

Streptozotocin is a newer nitrosourea which is an antibiotic derived from *Streptomyces achromogenes*. It is a specific β islet cell toxin causing mitochondrial swelling, degranulation, and eventually necrosis of the β cells, resulting in a permanent diabetic state. The response rate of 22% with this drug alone appears to be better than that obtained with other nitrosoureas

Table 2. *Combination Chemotherapy for Pancreatic Carcinoma*

Regimen	Patients	% Response	References
5-FU + Mitomycin C	63	25	Buroker et al. 1979 Krauss et al. 1979 Vaitkevicius et al. 1974
5-FU + BCNU	52	31	Bedikian et al. 1981 Stephens et al. 1978
5-FU + Methyl CCNU	76	11	Bedikian et al. 1981 Buroker et al. 1979
5-FU + Streptozotocin	81	19	Bedikian et al. 1981
Cytoxan + Streptozotocin	51	12	Moertel et al. 1977
Mitomycin C + Streptozotocin	46	35	Bedikian et al. 1981
5-FU + Mitomycin + Cytosar	9	0	De Jager et al. 1976
Ftorafur + BCNU + Adriamycin	26	19	Hall et al. 1979
5-FU + Adriamycin + Mitomycin	40	40	Smith et al. 1979 Bitran et al. 1979
5-FU + Mitomycin C + Streptozotocin	39	38	Abderhalden et al. 1977 Wiggans et al. 1978
5-FU + Adriamycin + Mitomycin C + Streptozotocin	18	33	Schacter et al. 1979
5-FU + Streptozotocin + Tubercidin	39	8	Awrich et al. 1979

(Smith and Schein 1979). Streptozotocin causes only mild myelosuppression but nausea and vomiting is usually severe, and prolonged use is associated with nephrotoxicity.

In recent years, combination chemotheraphy has been evaluated in pancreatic carcinoma (Table 2). Most studies have evaluated combinations of 5-FU plus a nitrosourea and have reported response rates of less than 20%. In general, results with three-drug combinations have been superior to those with two-drug combinations. Although the number of patients in most of these studies is not very large, the best results have been obtained with 5-FU and mitomycin C plus either Adriamycin or streptozotocin. Bitran et al. (1979) obtained one complete remission and five partial remissions in 15 patients treated with 5-FU 500 mg/m^2 weekly, mitomycin C 10 mg/m^2 every six weeks, and Adriamycin 30 mg/m^2 every three weeks. The median survival was greater than 13 months (projected) for responding patients compared to 2.8 months for nonresponders (p = .001). Wiggans et al. (1978) treated 23 patients with 5-FU 600 mg/m^2 and streptozotocin 1 gm/m^2 once weekly on weeks 1, 2, 5, and 6 and mitomycin C 10 mg/m^2 every nine weeks. One patient achieved a complete remission, nine achieved partial remissions, and five had stabilized disease. The median duration of response was 7+ months, and four patients remained alive and in remission for 7–23 months. The median survival was 7.5+ months for responders compared to three months for nonresponders.

Several chemotherapeutic regimens have been subjected to randomized comparative trials. 5-FU 13.5 mg/kg/day × 5 days was compared to BCNU 50 mg/m²/day × 5 days and 5-FU 10 mg/kg/day plus BCNU 40 mg/m²/day, both for five days (Kovach et al. 1974). Objective responses were observed in 16% of 31 patients who received 5-FU, none of 21 who received BCNU, and 33% of 30 patients who received the combination. There did not appear to be any survival advantage associated with the combination regimen, although no data were provided for responding patients only. 5-FU alone has been compared to 5-FU plus tubercidin and streptozotocin in 105 patients, of whom only 73 were evaluable (Awrich et al. 1979). Partial responses were obtained in 21% of the 34 patients who received 5-FU and 8% of the 39 patients who received the combination. The patients who received 5-FU fared slightly better with respect to time to progression and duration of survival.

The combination of 5-FU with testolactone or spironolactone was reported to cause remarkable improvement in patients with pancreatic carcinoma and led to three comparative studies (Waddell 1973). Stephens and associates compared 5-FU and BCNU to 5-FU and BCNU plus spironolactone (Stephens et al. 1978). Three of 18 patients achieved partial remission with the former regimen compared to two of 20 patients with the latter regimen. One-year survivals were 11% and 20%, respectively. Moertel and his colleagues compared 5-FU alone to 5-FU plus spironolactone, 5-FU plus streptozotocin, or all three drugs (Moertel et al. 1979). Only survival was evaluated in this study, but no difference existed between any of the regimens. McCracken et al. (1980) compared 5-FU, methyl CCNU, and radiotherapy to the same regimen plus testonolactone. Only survival was measured, but the median was 30 weeks with testonolactone compared to 38 weeks without testonolactone. Of the total 62 eligible patients, 15 survived one year. Six patients suffered significant gastrointestinal hemorrhage which resulted in the deaths of two patients. All of these studies fail to suggest any role for testonolactone or spironolactone in pancreatic carcinoma. Although the combination of 5-FU with radiotherapy has improved survival, the addition of methyl CCNU may increase the risk of serious complications, at least among patients receiving 6,000 rads radiotherapy.

The combination of 5-FU and mitomycin C has been compared to 5-FU and methyl CCNU in a randomized trial (Buroker et al. 1979). The response rate was 22% among the 45 patients who received the former regimen, and two patients achieved a complete remission. The response rate was only 5% among the 43 patients who received the latter regimen. The median duration of response for all responding patients was 13 weeks with a range of four to 61 weeks. The median survival was 31 weeks for responders compared to 11 weeks for nonresponders. Neither of these regimens offered any substantial improvement in therapy although a few patients had meaningful responses. The Eastern Cooperative Oncology Group compared streptozotocin plus cyclophosphamide to streptozotocin plus 5-FU (Moertel et al. 1977). Among the 51 evaluable patients who received the former regimen, six achieved a complete remission and none achieved a partial remission. Among the 42 patients who received the latter regimen, three patients achieved a complete remission and two achieved a partial remission. The median durations of response were nine months and 5.5 months, respectively. Myelosuppression was more frequent in patients who received streptozotocin plus cyclophosphamide. It is clear from the results of these studies that major improvements will only be obtained through the discovery of more effective antitumor agents. Additional combination studies with currently available agents are not likely to lead to substantial improvements.

Occasional patients develop pancreatic tumors of islet cell origin. These tumors may be functional or nonfunctional. Islet cell tumors originating from the α cell may produce glucagon and cause hyperglycemia and dermatitis. Tumors of β cell origin may secrete insulin and cause hypoglycemic attacks. Occasional tumors may secrete gastrin which causes gastric hypersecretion, ulceration, diarrhea, and steatorrhea. A syndrome of flushing, watery diarrhea, hypokalemic acidosis, gastric hypochlorhydria, and hypercalcemia has been described with islet cell tumors. Rarely, islet cell tumors may secrete ACTH, serotonin, or parathormone. Islet cell tumors may metastasize to the liver, lung, bone, or brain. Generally, they follow an indolent course with a median survival of more than five years. Functioning tumors may cause debilitating symptoms that are difficult to control. Only a few patients have been treated with antitumor agents, and most investigators have limited experience with these tumors.

Broder and Carter (1973) reported 52 patients with pancreatic islet cell tumors who were treated with streptozotocin. Twelve patients had received prior 5-FU and three had responded. The majority of patients received streptozotocin on a weekly schedule to total doses of 8–10 mg/m². Thirty-nine patients could be evaluated for a biochemical response and 30 patients had measurable disease. Ten patients had return of insulin and glucose concentrations to normal, 11 patients had a 50% reduction in the abnormal values, and four patients had a 25% reduction, all lasting for more than one month. Five patients with measurable disease achieved a complete remission, and six achieved a partial remission. Among patients with measurable disease, the response rate was 36% for patients with a functioning tumor and 38% for patients with a nonfunctional tumor. The duration of measurable response varied from 123 to 980+ days with a median of 398+ days. These data plus other reports in the literature clearly indicate the efficacy of streptozotocin in these tumors, with an overall response rate of 35% in 71 patients with measurable disease (Bedikian et al. 1981).

Several other drugs have been evaluated in pancreatic islet cell tumors, but only a few patients have been treated (Table 3). Alloxan, diazoxide, glucagon, chlorpromazine, L-asparaginase, adrenal corticosteroids, and ACTH have been used to temporarily ameliorate symptoms but none of these agents have

Table 3. *Chemotherapy of Islet Cell Carcinoma*

Agent	Patients	Responses	References
Streptozotocin	71	25	Bedikian et al. 1981
			Broder and Carter 1973
Adriamycin	10	2	Bedikian et al. 1981
Tubercidin	8	5	Bedikian et al. 1981
5-Fluorouracil	12	3	Bedikian et al. 1981
Methyl CCNU	5	1	Bedikian et al. 1981
5-FU + Streptozotocin	60	37	Bedikian et al. 1981
			Moertel et al. 1980
5-FU + Streptozotocin +			
Tubercidin	10	10	Irish et al. 1979
			Kraybill et al. 1976

produced lasting tumor regressions. Tubercidin is an antibiotic that causes islet cell necrosis in animals. Only a few patients have been treated with this drug, but partial remissions have been obtained in five of eight patients (Bedikian et al. 1981).

Moertel and his colleagues have reported a prospective randomized trial of streptozotocin alone compared to streptozotocin plus 5-FU in patients with pancreatic islet cell carcinoma (Moertel et al. 1980). Fourteen (34%) of 41 patients treated with streptozotocin responded whereas 25 (63%) of 40 patients who received the combination responded (p = .01). The complete response rates were 12% and 33% (p < .05). Responses were observed in patients with both functional and nonfunctional tumors. The median duration of response was 17+ months for patients achieving a response and 24+ months for patients achieving a complete remission. Hence, 5-FU appears to add to the efficacy of streptozotocin in the management of these tumors. The combination of 5-FU, tubercidin, and streptozotocin has been administered to about 10 patients. All of these patients showed at least some objective response; hence, this regimen deserves further evaluation.

Primary hepatic tumors are uncommon in the United States although they are the most common visceral carcinoma of males in many areas of Africa and the Orient. Ninety percent of these tumors are hepatomas, 5% to 10% are cholangiocarcinomas, and the remainder are mixed tumors (Moertel 1974b). Rare types include hemangioendotheliomas, Kupffer cell sarcomas, hepatoblastomas (almost exclusively in children), and miscellaneous sarcomas. Less than 30% of patients are eligible for surgical resection, and of these only 16% survive five years. Radiation is an ineffective therapeutic modality for hepatic carcinomas.

During a 20-year period, 137 patients with hepatic carcinomas were referred to Memorial Hospital (El-Domeiri et al. 1971). Hepatocellular carcinoma was diagnosed in 97 patients, intrahepatic bile duct carcinoma in 21 patients, and miscellaneous tumors in the remaining patients. Tumor was localized to the liver in 57%, involved the abdomen in 10%, and metastasized in 31%, primarily to lung, bone, and brain. All 44 patients who received supportive care only died within six months. Of the 31 patients who received radiotherapy, 70% died within six months and all died within one year. All 13 patients who received systemic chemotherapy died within six months. The most effective therapy was partial hepatectomy which could be performed on 32 patients; five of them survived for at least five years. McBride (1976) reviewed the experience at our institution and found similar results. During a 30-year period, 173 patients were seen, of whom 68% had hepatocellular carcinoma and 26% had cholangiocarcinoma. Only 9% of these patients survived more than two years. Only 14% of the patients were candidates for partial hepatectomy and their median survival was only 20 months. Those patients treated with systemic chemotherapy (usually 5-FU) had a median survival of only eight months.

Geddes reported on results of therapy in a series of Bantu patients (Geddes et al. 1970). The average survival was only four months, and 80% were dead at six months. A small number of patients (four to eight in each treatment group) received single-agent chemotherapy with cyclophosphamide, hydroxyurea, mitomycin C, or actinomycin D. Their average survival was only 34 to 88 days from onset of therapy compared to 64 days for untreated patients.

Appropriate interpretation of therapeutic interventions depends upon adequate staging criteria, especially when the disease is being studied in such diverse populations as is the case with hepatoma. Primack et al. (1975) have identified important prognostic factors in 153 Ugandan patients with hepatoma. Statistically significant variables included duration of symptoms to diagnosis, development of abdominal collateral circulation, presence of ascites, weight loss, and impending liver failure. Biochemical and other laboratory parameters influencing survival included bilirubin, alkaline phosphatase, SGOT, α-fetoprotein, proline hydroxylase, and degree of cellular diferentiation. Extent of disease and presence of cirrhosis were not important prognostic factors. Using this information, these investigators devised a staging schema: Stage 1 patients had a median survival of about four months, Stage 2 patients, about two months, and Stage 3, less than one month.

Only a few chemotherapeutic agents have been evaluated adequately in the management of hepatic carcinomas (Table 4). Olweny and co-workers administered Adriamycin (75 mg/m^2 every three weeks) to 14 patients and achieved three complete remissions and eight partial remissions (Olweny et al. 1975). The only failures were those patients who died before receiving an adequate trial. The median survival was eight months, but those patients who achieved a complete remission did not experience improved survival. Subsequently, other investigators have attempted to duplicate these remarkable results with less success. Johnson et al. (1978) treated 44 patients, 36 of whom had a poor prognosis, with Adriamycin 60 mg/m^2 every three weeks. Fourteen patients (32%) showed objective response with loss of pain, decrease in hepatomegaly, and weight gain, including 11 patients with poor prognosis. The median

Table 4. *Single-Agent Chemotherapy of Hepatoma*

Agent	Patients	% Response	References
Adriamycin	154	27	Bedikian et al. 1981
5-Fluorouracil	94	10	Bedikian et al. 1981
Neocarzinostatin	52	20	McKelvey, Personal Communication
Mitomycin C	28	25	Bedikian et al. 1981 Frank and Osterberg 1960 Moertel 1974a
Dichloromethotrexate	16	0	Vogel et al. 1972

survival was only 14 weeks, but five patients who achieved a clinical complete remission remained in remission for 12 to 24 months. Vogel et al. (1977) treated 41 patients and only seven responded including four of 16 good-risk patients and three of 25 poor-risk patients. A problem with Adriamycin is the necessity of reducing the dose in the presence of liver impairment because the serum half-life is greatly prolonged.

5-FU has been used by several investigators and has shown only modest activity. Mitomycin C has produced a 25% response rate overall, but only a few patients have been treated in any series. Neocarzinostatin is a polypeptide antibiotic isolated from *Streptomyces carzinostaticus* which inhibits thymidine incorporation into DNA. In initial Japanese trials, five of eight patients with hepatoma were considered to have responded to this antitumor agent. A few patients responded in phase I trials in this country. Falkson et al. (1980) treated 30 evaluable patients, most of whom were black South Africans. Seven patients achieved a partial remission and the disease stabilized in nine patients. The median survival of all patients was six weeks, whereas the median survival for those patients who achieved a partial remission was 17 weeks.

Several combination regimens have been evaluated, but most studies included only a small number of patients (Table 5). In general, response rates have not been superior to those for single-agent regimens. The combination of 5-FU plus BCNU produced seven responses in 19 patients (Moertel 1975) and three patients survived for at least three years. Falkson and associates conducted a randomized trial in which they compared oral 5-FU, oral 5-FU plus streptozotocin, oral 5-FU plus methyl CCNU or Adriamycin (Falkson et al. 1978). Patients failing to respond to 5-FU regimens subsequently received Adriamycin. None of the 44 patients given 5-FU alone responded. Only four (12%) of 33 patients who received 5-FU plus streptozotocin and two (5%) of 44 patients who received 5-FU plus methyl CCNU responded. Three (10%) of the 31 patients given Adriamycin initially responded as did six (23%) of 26 who received it as secondary therapy. Hence, none of these regimens produced a major impact on the natural history of hepatic tumors.

Table 5. *Combination Chemotherapy of Hepatoma*

Regimen	Patients	% Response	References
5-FU + Methyl CCNU	44	5	Falkson et al. 1978
5-FU + Adriamycin	38	13	Baker et al. 1977
5-FU + BCNU	19	37	Moertel 1975
5-FU + Streptozotocin	33	12	Falkson et al. 1978
Adriamycin + Streptozotocin	13	15	Ihde et al. 1979
Adriamycin + Bleomycin	13	31	Ravry and Hester 1979
5-FU + Mitomycin C	6	33	Buroker et al. 1978

Chemotherapy administered via the hepatic artery appears to be the most effective treatment for unresectable hepatic cancer. El-Domeiri reported the best survival among patients who received intra-arterial chemotherapy (El-Domeiri et al. 1971). Six patients who received methotrexate or 5-FU by this route survived four months to three years. Likewise, Geddes reported an average survival of 291 days in five patients who received intra-arterial methotrexate (Geddes et al. 1970). However, four patients who received intra-arterial 5-FU survived an average of only 87 days. Matsumoto and co-workers treated patients with mitomycin C given weekly into the hepatic artery or every two to four months into the celiac artery (Matsumoto et al. 1976). The median survival was 130 days for eight patients receiving the weekly regimen and 178 days for 13 patients receiving the two to four monthly regimen, whereas eight patients who received combination chemotherapy intravenously survived a median of only 45 days. Al-Sarraf reported objective responses in nine of 16 patients who received intra-arterial 5-FU (Al-Sarraf et al. 1974). The median survival was 54 weeks for responders compared to only four weeks for nonresponders. Three of four patients who received intra-arterial 5-FU plus mitomycin C responded; one of these patients had been refractory to the same therapy administered intravenously. In our institution, Patt and his co-workers (unpublished) have treated eight evaluable patients with 5-FU, Adriamycin, and mitomycin C via the hepatic artery. One patient died at three months of unrelated causes and had no evidence of tumor at autopsy examination. Five patients who achieved partial remissions have survived for six months to 19+ months. Two patients who failed to respond died at three and six months. It is difficult to compare patients who received intra-arterial chemotherapy to patients who received intravenous chemotherapy because of differences in selection criteria; nevertheless, intra-arterial chemotherapy does appear to produce superior results.

Carcinomas of the gallbladder and bile ducts are uncommon in the United States, although gallbladder carcinoma appears to be a special problem among American Indians due to the prevalence of cholecystitis. Only 0.08% of referrals to our institution are for carcinoma of the gallbladder (Perpetuo et al. 1978). Since most patients have pre-existent cholecystitis and the two diseases cause similar symptoms, the interval between onset of symptoms and diagnosis of carcinoma may be prolonged. In our series of 75 patients, curative resection was possible in only 5%. The median survival of all patients was 5.2 months, although a few patients survived for more than three years. Only 47 patients with carcinoma of the extrahepatic bile ducts have been referred to this institution over a 30-year period (Bedikian et al. 1980). In more than half of these patients, the tumor had either invaded the liver or metastasized to other organs. Only five patients were eligible for curative resection of their tumor. The median survival of all patients was only eight months; 15% survived more than two years.

Experience with chemotherapy in managing these malignant tumors has been extremely limited. In the series from our institution, none of 36 patients with gallbladder carcinoma responded to chemotherapeutic agents, including 5-FU, Adriamycin, and nitrosoureas. However, their median survival was 5.8 months compared to four months for patients who received no chemotherapy (p = .05). Twenty-one patients with bile duct carcinoma were treated with chemotherapy at our institution. Six patients achieved partial remissions lasting two to five months. Responses were obtained with 5-FU (three), neocarzinostatin (one), and combination regimens (two). Responding patients survived significantly longer than nonresponding patients (8.5 months vs. two months, p = .005). A few patients have been included in studies of various single-agent and combination regimens used for gastrointestinal carcinomas. No conclusions can be drawn due to the inadequate numbers of patients. Of 29 patients with gallbladder carcinoma treated with fluoropyrimidines, 50% were alive at four months and four patients survived more than one year (Davis et al. 1974). The median survival for 12 patients with bile duct carcinomas was five months and three patients survived more than one year. In another series of 33 patients with gallbladder carcinoma, 13 received chemotherapy and had a median survival of 20 weeks whereas the remaining patients had a median survival of only eight weeks (p < .01) (Oswalt and Cruz 1977). It should be emphasized that occasional patients have achieved disease-free survival for prolonged periods, in rare patients for as long as five years. Hepatic artery infusions of chemotherapy may be superior to intravenous infusions. Misra et al. (1977) observed nine responders of 13 patients who received intra-arterial 5-FU and mitomycin C for gallbladder carcinoma. One patient had been refractory to previous therapy administered intravenously.

At the present, therapy is unsatisfactory for most patients with carcinomas of the pancreas, liver, gallbladder, and bile ducts. The most encouraging results have been obtained with streptozotocin in the management of islet cell carcinomas. The systematic investigation of therapeutic regimens in managing pancreatic carcinoma, which has only been attempted in recent years, is likely to identify effective new agents and combinations. Intra-arterial infusion therapy appears promising for hepatic tumors and new agents and combinations need to be investigated via this route.

ACKNOWLEDGMENTS

This investigation was supported in part by Contract # N01-CM-57042 and Grant # CA 05831, awarded by the National Cancer Institute, Department of Health and Human Services.

REFERENCES

Abderhalden, R. T., R. M. Bukowski, C. W. Groppe, J. S. Hewlett, and J. K. Weick. 1977. Streptozotocin (STZ) and 5-fluorouracil (5-FU) with and without mitomycin C (MITO) in the treatment of pancreatic adenocarcinoma (Abstract). Proc. ASCO 18:301.

Alberto, P., D. Gangji, Y. Kenis, A. Brugarolas, A. Clarysse, and R. Sylvester. 1977. Phase II study of anhydro-Ara-5-fluorocytidine (AAFC) (Abstract). Proc. AACR 18:231.

Alberto, P., M. Rozencweig, D. Gangji, A. Brugarolas, F. Cavalli, P. Siegenthaler, H. H. Hansen, and R. Sylvester. 1978. Phase II study of anhydro-Ara-5-fluorocytidine in adenocarcinoma of gastrointestinal tract, epidermoid carcinoma of lung, head and neck, breast carcinoma and small cell anaplastic carcinoma of lung. A study report of the E.O.R.T.C. early clinical trial cooperative group. Eu. J. Cancer 14:195–201.

Al-Sarraf, M., T. S. Go, K. Kithier, and V. K. Vaitkevicius. 1974. Primary liver cancer. A review of the clinical features, blood groups, serum enzymes, therapy, and survival of 65 cases. Cancer 33:574–582.

Awrich, A., W. S. Fletcher, J. H. Klotz, J. P. Minton, G. J. Hill, J. B. Aust. T. B. Grage, and P. M. Multhauf. 1979. 5-FU versus combination therapy with tubercidin, streptozotocin, and 5-FU in the treatment of pancreatic carcinomas: COG protocol 7230. J. Surg. Oncol. 12:267–273.

Baker, L. H., J. H. Saiki, S. E. Jones, J. S. Hewlett, R. W. Brownlee, R. L. Stephens, and V. K. Vaitkevicius. 1977. Adriamycin and 5-fluorouracil in the treatment of advanced hepatoma: A southwest oncology group study. Cancer Treat. Rep. 61:1595–1597.

Bedikian, A. Y., M. Valdivieso, and G. P. Bodey. 1981. Systemic chemotherapy for advanced gastrointestinal cancer: A general review. South. Med. J. (in press).

Bedikian, A. Y., M. Valdivieso, A. DeLaCruz, R. Martin, M. Luna, V. F. Guinee, and G. P. Bodey. 1980. Cancer of the extrahepatic bile ducts. Med. Pediat. Oncol. 8:53–61.

Bitran, J. D., R. K. Desser, M. F. Kozloff, A. A. Billings, and C. M. Shapiro. 1979. Treatment of metastatic pancreatic and gastric adenocarcinomas with 5-fluorouracil, Adriamycin, and mitomycin C (FAM). Cancer Treat. Rep. 63:2049–2051.

Broder, L. E., and S. K. Carter. 1973. Pancreatic islet cell carcinoma. II. Results of therapy with streptozotocin in 52 patients. Ann. Intern. Med. 79:108–118.

Buroker, T. R., P. N. Kim, L. H. Baker, V. Ratanatharathorn, B. Wojtaszak, and V. K. Vaitkevicius. 1978. Mitomycin-C alone and in combination with infused 5-fluorouracil in the treatment of disseminated gastrointestinal carcinomas. Med. Pediat. Oncol. 4:35–42.

Buroker, T. R., P. N. Kim, C. Groppe, J. McCracken, R. O'Bryan, F. Panettiere, J. Costanzi, R. Bottomley, G. W. King, J. Bonnet, T. Thigpen, J. Whitecar, C. Haas, V. K. Vaitkevicius, B. Hoogstraten, and L. Heilbrun. 1979. 5-FU infusion with mitomycin-C vs. 5-FU infusion with methyl-CCNU in the treatment of advanced upper gastrointestinal cancer. A southwest oncology group study. Cancer 44:1215–1221.

Carter, S. K., and R. L. Comis. 1975. The integration of chemotherapy into a combined modality approach for cancer treatment. VI. Pancreatic adenocarcinoma. Cancer Treat. Rev. 2:193–214.

Davis, H. L., G. Ramirez, and F. J. Ansfield. 1974. Adenocarcinomas of stomach, pancreas, liver, and biliary tracts. Survival of 328 patients treated with fluoropyrimidine therapy. Cancer 33:193–197.

De Jager, R. L., G. B. Magill, R. B. Golbey, and I. H. Krakoff. 1976. Combination chemotherapy with mitomycin C, 5-fluorouracil, and cytosine arabinoside in gastrointestinal cancer. Cancer Treat. Rep. 60:1373–1375.

El-Domeiri, A. A., A. G. Huvos, H. S. Goldsmith, and F. W. Foote, Jr. 1971. Primary malignant tumors of the liver. Cancer 27:7–11.

Engstrom, P. F., R. B. Catalano, and R. H. Creech. 1976. Phase II study of methyl-CCNU (NSC-9544) in advanced gastrointestinal cancer. Cancer Treat. Rep. 60:285–287.

Falkson, G., C. G. Moertel, P. Lavin, F. J. Pretorius, and P. P. Carbone. 1978. Chemotherapy studies in primary liver cancer. A prospective randomized clinical trial. Cancer 42:2149–2156.

Falkson, G., D. Von Hoff, D. Klaassen, H. Du Plessis, C. F. Van Der Merwe, A. M. Van Der Merwe, and P. P. Carbone. 1980. A phase II study of neocarzinostatin (NSC-157365) in malignant hepatoma. An eastern cooperative oncology group pilot study. Cancer Chemother. Pharmacol. 4:33–36.

Frank, W., and A. E. Osterberg. 1960. Mitomycin C (NSC-26980)—An evaluation of the Japanese Reports. Cancer Chemother. Rep. 9:114–119.

Gastrointestinal Tumor Study Group. 1979. Comparative therapeutic trial of radiation with or without chemotherapy in pancreatic carcinoma. Int. J. Radiat. Oncol. Biol. Phys. 5:1643–1647.

Geddes, E. W., and G. Falkson. 1970. Malignant hepatoma in the Bantu. Cancer 25:1271–1278.

Hall, S. W., R. S. Benjamin, W. K. Murphy, M. Valdivieso, and G. P. Bodey. 1979. Adriamycin, BCNU, ftorafur chemotherapy of pancreatic and biliary tract cancer. Cancer 44:2008–2013.

Ihde, D. C., P. A. Bunn, M. H. Cohen, and J. D. Minna. 1979. Combination chemotherapy of hepatocellular carcinoma with Adriamycin (ADM) and streptozotocin (STZ) (Abstract). Proc. ASCO 20:410.

Irish, C. E., A. Awrich, D. Moseson, C. Davenport, H. S. Moseley, and W. S. Fletcher. 1979. 5-Fluorouracil, tubercidin, streptozotocin and Adriamycin: Effective agents in the management of functioning and advanced islet cell tumors of the pancreas (Abstract). Proc. AACR 20:361.

Johnson, P. J., R. Williams, H. Thomas, S. Sherlock, and I. M. Murray-Lyon. 1978. Induction of remission in hepatocellular carcinoma with doxorubicin. Lancet 1:1006–1009.

Kaplan, R. S. 1978. Phase II trial of ICRF-159, β-2-deoxythioguanosine (β-2-TGdR), and galactitol (GAL) in advanced measurable pancreatic carcinoma. A study of the gastrointestinal tumor study group (GITSG) (Abstract). Proc. ASCO 19:335.

Kovach, J. S., C. G. Moertel, A. J. Schutt, R. G. Hahn, and R. J. Reitemeier. 1974. A controlled study of combined 1,3-bis-(2-chloroethyl)-1-nitrosourea and 5-fluorouracil therapy for advanced gastric and pancreatic cancer. Cancer 33:563–567.

Krauss, S., T. Sonoda, and A. Solomon. 1979. Treatment of advanced gastrointestinal cancer with 5-fluorouracil and mitomycin C. Cancer 43:1598–1603.

Kraybill, W. G., Jr., D. D. Anderson, T. D. Lindell, and W. S. Fletcher. 1976. Islet cell carcinoma of the pancreas: Effective therapy with 5-fluorouracil, streptozotocin, and tubercidin. Am. Surg. 42:467–470.

Matsumoto, Y., T. Suzuki, H. Ono, A. Nakase, and I. Honjo. 1976. Evaluation of hepatoma chemotherapy by α-fetoprotein determination. Am. J. Surg. 132:325–328.

McBride, C. M. 1976. Primary carcinoma of the liver. Surgery 80:322–327.

McCracken, J. D., P. Ray, L. K. Heilbrun, V. K. Vaitkevicius, J. H. Saiki, S. E. Rivkin, A. H. Rossof, and T. N. Moore. 1980. 5-Fluorouracil, methyl-CCNU, and radiotherapy with or without testolactone for localized adenocarcinoma of the exocrine pancreas. A southwest oncology group study. Cancer 46:1518–1522.

Misra, N. C., M. S. D. Jaiswal, R. V. Singh, and B. Das. 1977. Intrahepatic arterial infusion of combination of mitomycin-C and 5-fluorouracil in treatment of primary and metastatic liver carcinoma. Cancer 39:1425–1429.

Moertel, C. G. 1974a. Exocrine pancreas, *in* Cancer Medicine, J. F. Holland and E. Frei, III, eds. Lea & Febiger, Philadelphia, pp. 1559–1570.

Moertel, C. G. 1974b. The liver, *in* Cancer Medicine, J. F. Holland and E. Frei, III, eds. Lea & Febiger, Philadelphia, pp. 1541–1547.

Moertel, C. G. 1975. Clinical management of advanced gastrointestinal cancer. Cancer 36:675–682.

Moertel, C. G., D. S. Childs, Jr., R. J. Reitemeier, M. Y. Colby, Jr., and M. A. Holbrook. 1969. Combined 5-fluorouracil and supervoltage radiation therapy of locally unresectable gastrointestinal cancer. Lancet 2:865–867.

Moertel, C. G., H. O. Douglas, J. Hanley, and P. P. Carbone. 1976. Phase II study of methyl-CCNU in the treatment of advanced pancreatic carcinoma. Cancer Treat. Rep. 60:1659–1661.

Moertel, C. G., H. O. Douglas, Jr., J. Hanley, and P. P. Carbone. 1977. Treatment of advanced adenocarcinoma of the pancreas with combinations of streptozotocin plus 5-fluorouracil and streptozotocin plus cyclophosphamide. Cancer 40:605–608.

Moertel, C. G., P. Engstrom, P. T. Lavin, R. D. Gelber, and P. P Carbone. 1979. Chemotherapy of gastric and pancreatic carcinoma. Surgery 85:509–513.

Moertel, C. G., J. A. Hanley, and L. A. Johnson. 1980. A randomized comparison of strep-tozotocin (STZ) alone vs. STZ plus 5-fluorouracil (5-FU) in the treatment of metastatic islet cell carcinoma (Abstract). Proc. AACR 21:415.

Moertel, C. G., A. J. Schutt, R. J. Reitemeier, and R. G. Hahn. 1976. Therapy for gastrointestinal cancer with the nitrosoureas alone and in drug combination. Cancer Treat. Rep. 60:729–732.

Olweny, C. L. M., T. Toya, E. Katongole-Mbidde, J. Mugerwa, S. K. Kyalwazi, and H. Cohen. 1975. Treatment of hepatocellular carcinoma with Adriamycin. Preliminary communication. Cancer 36:1250–1257.

Oswalt, C. E., and A. B. Cruz, Jr. 1977. Effectiveness of chemotherapy in addition to surgery in treating carcinoma of the gallbladder. Rev. Surg., 436–438.

Perpetuo, M. D. C. M. O., M. Valdivieso, L. K. Heilbrun, R. S. Nelson, T. Connor, and G. P. Bodey. 1978. Natural history study of gallbladder cancer. A review of 36 years experience at M. D. Anderson Hospital and Tumor Institute. Cancer 42:330–335.

Primack, A., C. L. Vogel, S. K. Kyalwazi, J. L. Ziegler, R. Simon, and P. P. Anthony. 1975. A staging system for hepatocellular carcinoma: Prognostic factors in Ugandan patients. Cancer 35:1357–1364.

Ravry, M. J. R., and M. Hester. 1979. Phase II study of Adriamycin (ADR) plus bleomycin (Bleo) for the treatment of hepatocellular and biliary tract carcinoma (Abstract). Proc. ASCO 20:415.

Schacter, L., R. M. Bukowski, J. S. Hewlett, C. Groppe, J. Weick, and R. Reimer. 1979. Combination chemotherapy with 5-fluorouracil (5-FU), Adriamycin (AD), mitomycin C (MITO C), and streptozotocin (STZ) of pancreatic adenocarcinoma (Abstract). Proc. AACR 20:420.

Schein, P. S., P. T. Lavin, C. G. Moertel, S. Frytak, R. G. Hahn, M. J. O'Connell, R. J. Reitemeier, J. Rubin, A. J. Schutt, L. H. Weiland, M. Kalser, J. Barkin, H. Lessner, R. Mann-Kaplan, D. Redlhammer, M. Silverman, M. Troner, H. O. Douglass, Jr., S. Milliron, J. Lokich, J. Brooks, J. Chaffe, A. Like, N. Zamcheck, K. Ramming, J. Bateman, H. Spiro, E. Livstone, and A. Knowlton. 1978. Randomized phase II clinical trial of Adriamycin, methotrexate, and actinomycin-D in advanced measurable pancreatic carcinoma. A gas-trointestinal tumor study group report. Cancer 42:19–22.

Smith, F. P., J. S. Macdonald, P. V. Woolley, D. F. Hoth, T. A. Smythe, L. Lichtenfeld, B. Levin, and P. S. Schein. 1979. Phase II evaluation of FAM, 5-fluorouracil (F), Adriamycin (A) and mitomycin-C (M), in advanced pancreatic cancer (PC) (Abstract). Proc. AACR 20:415. 1979.

Smith, F. P., and P. S. Schein. 1979. Chemotherapy of pancreatic cancer. Sem. Oncol. 6:368–377.

Stephens, R. L., B. Hoogstraten, C. Haas, and G. Clark. 1978. Pancreatic cancer treated with carmustin, fluorouracil, and spironolactone. Arch. Intern. Med. 138:115–117.

Stolinsky, D. C., R. P. Pugh, and J. R. Bateman. 1975. 5-Fluorouracil (NSC-19893) therapy for pancreatic carcinoma: Comparison of oral and intravenous routes. Cancer Chemother. Rep. 59:1031–1033.

Vaitkevicius, V. K., L. H. Baker, T. R. Buroker, P. N. Kim, and M. L. Reed. 1974. Chemotherapy of gastrointestinal adenocarcinoma, in Cancer Chemotherapy (The University of Texas System Cancer Center M. D. Anderson Hospital and Tumor Institute Annual Clinical Conference on Cancer, 1974). Year Book Medical Publishers, Chicago, pp. 263–278.

Vogel, C. L., R. H. Adamson, V. T. DeVita, D. G. Johns, and S. K. Kyalwazi. 1972. Preliminary clinical trials of dichloromethotrexate (NSC-29630) in hepatocellular carcinoma. Cancer Chemother. Rep. 56:249–258.

Vogel, C. L., A. C. Bayley, R. J. Brooker, P. P. Anthony, and J. L. Ziegler. 1977. A phase II study of Adriamycin (NSC-123127) in patients with hepatocellular carcinoma from Zambia and the United States. Cancer 39:1923–1929.

Waddell, W. R. 1973. Chemotherapy for carcinoma of the pancreas. Surgery 74:420–429.

Wiggans, R. G., P. V. Woolley, III, J. S. Macdonald, T. Smythe, W. Ueno, and P. S. Schein. 1978. Phase II trial of streptozotocin, mitomycin-C and 5-fluorouracil (SMF) in the treatment of advanced pancreatic cancer. Cancer 41:387–391.

Gastrointestinal Cancer, edited by
John R. Stroehlein and
Marvin M. Romsdahl.
Raven Press, New York © 1981.

Large Bowel Cancer—Introduction

Murray M. Copeland, M.D.

National Large Bowel Cancer Project;
The University of Texas System Cancer Center, Houston, Texas

The multifaceted approach to identifying the causes, early diagnosis, and improved treatment regimens of colorectal cancer are characterized by the activities of the National Large Bowel Cancer Project in applying new knowledge to the solution of this important health problem (National Cancer Institute 1977).

The following eight broad program areas have been developed:

1. The identification of large bowel cancer causes and their inhibitors.
2. The identification and clarification of biochemical and molecular controls.
3. The identification of individuals at high risk for developing large bowel cancer.
4. The early diagnosis and prevention of the disease.
5. The application of modern pharmacologic methods in the development of new chemotherapeutic treatments.
6. The application of modern tumor immunobiological methods in developing methods of managing and preventing large bowel cancer.
7. Research treatment.
8. The promotion of interdisciplinary communications and collaborative research programs.

Currently in the United States, except for easily detectable and curable skin cancer, large bowel cancer ranks second in incidence of neoplastic diseases in both men and women, probably affecting 114,000 persons in 1980 (American Cancer Society 1980). It is believed to be an environmental, "man-made" disease. This is deduced from the incidence and mortality patterns around the world (Doll, Muir and Waterhouse 1970). Japan, parts of Central and South America, and Africa exhibit a low incidence of colonic cancer, and the Anglo-Saxon countries and parts of Western Europe, a high incidence. Within Scandinavia, Denmark has a high incidence of colonic cancer but Finland has a low incidence (Weisburger et al. 1977, Reddy et al. 1978).

The difference in incidence of colonic cancer between a high-risk country like the United States and a low-risk country like Japan is 5.4 to 1, but for rectal cancer this difference is merely of the order of 1.3 to 1 (Segi and

Kurihara 1972); this suggests that cancer of the rectum may be caused by factors different from those that cause colonic cancer. Rectal cancer does not vary as much in incidence between high- and low-risk regions, and it exhibits a more pronounced sex-linked effect, with a male/female ratio of 1.4 to 1 for rectal cancer but near unity for colonic cancer. Furthermore, the incidence of rectal cancer has shown a decreasing trend, while that of colon cancer is constant or showing a slight increase. These compared statistics indicate that a distinction needs to be made between rectal and colon cancer.

Fetal antigens that initially appeared specific for colorectal cancer have recently been found in a variety of neoplastic and non-neoplastic diseases. These have aroused new interest and activity in the development of improved means of early diagnosis of colorectal cancer and other primary malignant neoplasms. These efforts have also led to better understanding of certain aspects of pathogenesis in the development of cell culture systems of neoplastic tissues from the colon and other parts of the gastrointestinal tract.

A critical issue is whether or not to screen for colorectal cancer. Among the considerations are: the expected benefits and risks, sensitivity and specificity of available screening and diagnostic tests, cost effectiveness, and patient compliance. Screening programs in progress strongly suggest a survival benefit to those patients with a positive screening test, but a much longer follow-up period is necessary. Screening efforts directed toward high-risk groups are more productive than screening of the standard risk population. Therefore, for now, it appears realistic to practice secondary prevention on identification and eradication of precursor lesions, thus altering the potential incidence of evolving cancer.

Granted the existence of ongoing clinical trials and the study of treatment models for enhancing increased survival, the practicing physician and surgeon must have adequate knowledge concerning the currently acceptable guidelines for the care of the colorectal cancer patient.

The potpourri of presentations this afternoon will reflect the current status of factors bearing upon early diagnosis and the management of colorectal cancer by surgery and/or radiation therapy. (Tomorrow morning's session will place emphasis on chemotherapy, immunotherapy, and regional approaches to the management of colorectal cancer.)

REFERENCES

American Cancer Society. 1980. Cancer Facts and Figures, American Cancer Society, New York, p. 9.

Doll, R., C. S. Muir, and J. Waterhouse. 1970. Cancer Incidence in Five Continents (UICC). Springer-Verlag, Berlin.

National Cancer Institute. 1977. Program Description: The National Organ Site Programs Division of Cancer Research Resources and Centers. Published by the National Organ Site Programs Branch, DCRRC, NCI, April.

Reddy, B. S., A. Hedges, K. A. Laakso, and E. L. Wynder. 1978. Fecal constituents of a high-risk North American and a low-risk Finnish population for the development of large bowel cancer. Cancer Lett. 4:217–222.

Segi, M., and M. Kurihara. 1972. Cancer Mortality for Selected Sites in 24 Countries: No. 6, 1966–67, Japan Cancer Society.

Weisburger, J. H., B. S. Reddy, and E. L. Wynder. 1977. Colon cancer: Its epidemiology and experimental production. Cancer 40:2414–2420.

Gastrointestinal Cancer, edited by
John R. Stroehlein and
Marvin M. Romsdahl.
Raven Press, New York © 1981.

Precursor Conditions and Monitoring of High-Risk Colon Cancer Patients

Henry T. Lynch, M.D.,* William A. Albano, M.D.,†
B. Shannon Danes, M.D., Ph.D.,‡ Jane Lynch, R.N.,*
and Patrick M. Lynch, J.D.

*Departments of *Preventive Medicine/Public Health and †Surgery and
Preventive Medicine, Creighton University School of Medicine, Omaha, Nebraska,
and ‡Department of Medicine, Laboratory for Cell Biology,
Cornell University Medical College, New York, New York*

INTRODUCTION

Colon cancer "precursors" have customarily been considered to include only those lesions or states (i.e., adenomatous polyps, long-standing ulcerative colitis with dysplasia) which, if untreated, progress invariably or with a high probability to invasive cancer. However, several of the hereditary colon cancer predisposing syndromes that we shall discuss lack such premonitory signs. For this reason, we shall operationally use the term "precursor" in a broader sense so as to also include those in vitro markers of aberrant enzymatic activity, cellular kinetics, cytogenetics, or immunity that may be potentially linked pathogenetically to colon cancer. Ongoing research into such markers will be reviewed and one system, namely endoreduplication in long-term fibroblast cultures, will be highlighted as a model system.

Unfortunately, as we shall see, these in vitro systems are still very much in an experimental stage. Consequently, in the second half of our discussion, we shall stress the role of family history per se in defining that group of patients most likely to harbor colon cancer and its physical precursors. We shall conclude with a brief overview of currently recommended diagnostic and therapeutic measures for patients from families having either of the two classes of syndromes under consideration, namely those with and those without adenomatous polyposis of the colon.

Familial Polyposis Coli (FPC)

Adenomatous polyps as colon cancer precursors pose a dilemma when only one or a few are present in a given patient. The size of individual polyps, their number and location in the colon or upper gastrointestinal tract, and the age of the patient in question must all be considered in the decision logic relevant to any patient's colon cancer risk. The problems of such modest polyp expression in patients lacking other clinical signs, family histories of FPC, or other hereditary colon cancer syndromes are beyond the scope of this discussion.

There is a consensus that patients manifesting multiple adenomatous polyposis but lacking a family history of this trait must represent a germinal mutation of the FPC gene. Yet it is possible that an affected patient with a negative family history (even if showing a florid polyposis phenotype) may be an example of autosomal recessively inherited disease. These may include Turcot's syndrome or other, as yet to be determined, disorders in which a "negative" family history may not preclude primary genetic etiology. In other cases, key relatives may have been insufficiently ascertained, died of other causes prior to manifesting the trait, shown reduced penetrance of the deleterious gene, or been the product of undisclosed false paternity. In all such cases, unequivocal identification of a gene locus, or product thereof, would be of inestimable value, both in terms of clarifying genetic models and, more importantly, in establishing a more valid diagnosis.

Supposing that a positive family history is clearly shown, there remains the issue of the minimum number of polyps required to establish the diagnosis in a given patient. Many clinicians (Dukes 1930, Dukes 1951, Lockhart-Mummery 1925) have long adhered to the requirement of 100 to 200+ polyps as a minimum diagnostic criterion for FPC. However, it has been observed (Lynch et al. 1979a) that within families showing FPC, individuals with florid manifestations of this disease (including malignant transformation) have had a parent, sibling, or progeny with only isolated colonic polyps, but characteristically early onset of colonic cancer (Figure 1). Many variations upon this theme have been reported to us by other investigators and many other such cases may simply have been considered trivial in prior family studies. Given these circumstances, how is one to evaluate a young patient who is known to be genotypically at risk for the FPC gene, but who presents with only a single adenomatous polyp? It becomes quite clear that in this context, expression of an isolated polyp may be of only limited diagnostic assistance to the clinician. As stated previously, more definitive laboratory signs of FPC genotypes are necessary. Their utility can only be established through longitudinal study of families according to ongoing protocols described below.

Nonpolyposis Coli Syndromes

The two disorders to be discussed in this section are the cancer family syndrome (CFS) (Figure 2) and hereditary site-specific colon cancer (HSCC) (Figure 3), neither of which involve the phenotype of multiple adenomatous polyps of the colon and rectum. Criteria for the CFS include: (1) an increased frequency of adenocarcinoma of the colon, endometrium, and ovary (Lynch and Lynch 1979b) and, to a lesser extent, carcinoma of the breast (Lynch et al.

C-205

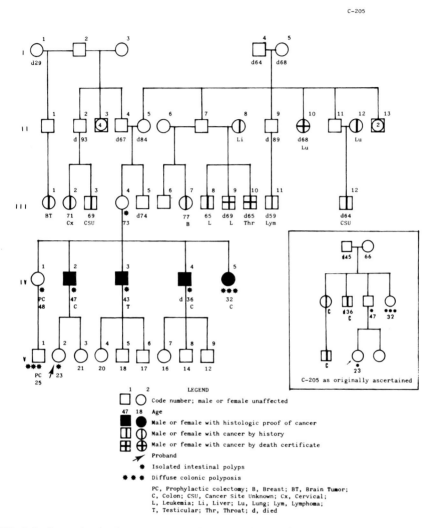

FIG. 1. Pedigree showing heterogeneous polyp expression in a family with familial polyposis coli (FPC). (Reproduced from Lynch et al. 1979, with permission of Journal of Medical Genetics.)

1973a), stomach (Lynch et al. 1979c), and perhaps other histologic varieties (Law et al. 1977); (2) in the case of colon cancer, a significant excess of proximal colon involvement (Lynch et al. 1977a) (Table 1); (3) significantly early age of onset (mean of approximately 45 years) (Lynch et al. 1979c) when compared to sporadically occurring counterparts in the general population (mean onset approximately 65 years); (4) an excess of multiple primary cancer in affected patients (Lynch et al. 1977b); (5) pedigree expression consistent with an autosomal dominant mode of genetic transmission (Lynch et al.

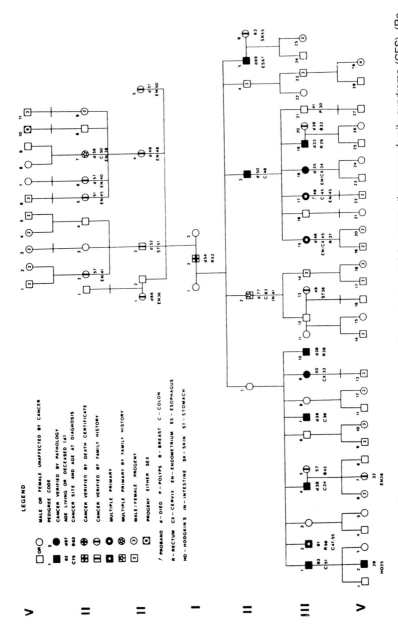

FIG. 2. Pedigree of a family showing vertical transmission of colon/endometrial cancer—the cancer family syndrome (CFS). (Reproduced from Lynch et al. 1977, with permission of Annals of Surgery.)

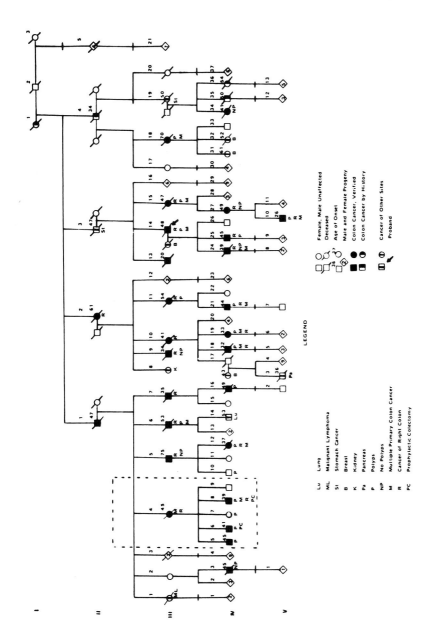

FIG. 3. Pedigree of a family with hereditary site-specific colon cancer (HSCC). (Reproduced from Lynch et al. 1977, with permission of Archives of Surgery.)

Table 1. *Proximal Colonic Cancer Frequencies Among 19 Families*

Family #	Total Colon Cancer Occurrence* (Initial Diagnosis Only)	First Occurrence at Proximal Colon	Percent
1	7	7	100
33	27	11	41
51	6	3	50
120	7	5	71
196	11	4	36
200	7	6	86
30	4	4	100
35	3	2	67
115	7	6	86
113	5	4	80
164	6	4	67
199	4	4	100
250	6	2	33
007	2	2	100
198	26	21	81
069	4	4	100
194	3	1	33
010	2	1	50
203	2	1	50
	139	92	66

*Only tumors which have been verified as to subsite have been included; all families include additional cases in which colon cancers could not be verified or could not be verified as to subsite.

1979c); (6) occasional occurrence of sebaceous adenoma, epitheliomas, and carcinomas in patients with visceral cancer (referred to as Torre's syndrome when occurring in individual patients) (Bitran and Pellettiere 1974, Rulon and Helwig 1973, Lynch et al. 1981); and (7) an increased frequency of prolonged survival in patients with syndrome cancers (Lynch et al. 1978a).

Hereditary site-specific colon cancer (HSCC) differs only in that it lacks the spectrum of extracolonic tumors which characterizes the CFS. Because of this, it is certainly at least arguable that HSCC may simply represent one point on the continuum of CFS tumor expression.

In these disorders, the identification of precursor lesions would obviously be of even greater clinical value than in the FPC syndromes (see subsequent discussion of marker systems under investigation.

As noted, cutaneous signs previously considered to be manifestations of Torre's syndrome (sebaceous adenoma, sebaceous epithelioma, sebaceous carcinoma, and possibly keratoacanthoma) have been observed in several patients from CFS kindreds (Lynch et al. in press). Because of their relative infrequency in patients affected with the CFS, the occurrence of these lesions would appear to be of greater use in retrospectively identifying an affected family than as a guide to cancer risk in an individual at-risk patient.

Precursor Conditions and/or Biomarkers

Tetraploidy: A Model for In Vitro Markers

In vitro research in heritable cancer syndromes has been based on the hypothesis that a cell, such as those derived from a skin biopsy, considered normal by all criteria, when grown in culture, would demonstrate such mutant cancer-prone genotypes irrespective of its cancer expression in vivo.

The occurrence of an in vitro cellular abnormality in consecutive generations, that is, vertical transmission from the clinically affected to his offspring, would be considered evidence of an in vitro expression of a cancer-prone mutation. Thus, an opportunity would be given to identify in vitro increased risk for colonic cancer prior to clinical expression.

In vitro studies done in several laboratories (Pfeffer et al. 1976, Kopelovich et al. 1979, Danes 1975 and 1976a, Danes and Alm 1979, Danes 1980, Danes et al. 1980b) have demonstrated that skin cells from affecteds and some at-risk family members from families with heritable colon cancer syndromes show cellular abnormalities presumably due to the in vitro expression of a germinal mutation. One of these abnormalities was increased in vitro tetraploidy.

Methodology

Skin biopsies were obtained from each family member studied. A coded number was assigned to each biopsy, which was the only identification used until the studies on in vitro tetraploidy had been completed. Skin cultures were established from these split thickness biopsies by standard culture methods (Danes and Alm 1979) (Figure 4).

In standardization of an assay for occurrence of in vitro tetraploidy, the following relevant observations were made. Increased tetraploidy appeared to be an in vitro rather than an in vivo phenomenon because the occurrence of tetraploidy was constant in some cultures from the first subculture, but in

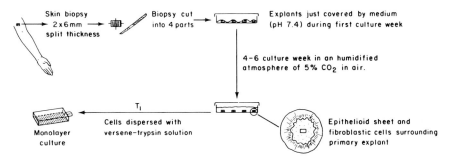

FIG. 4. Methodology used in the establishment of monolayer (mixed fibroblast and epithelioid) cultures from human skin biopsies.

others its occurrence increased during the first 15 culture weeks after initiation of the explant culture (Danes et al. 1980a). The occurrence of tetraploidy in all subcultures derived from a single explant culture was similar (Danes 1975 and 1976a, Danes and Alm 1979). False-negative results could have been recorded if the occurrence of in vitro tetraploidy was determined only before the fifteenth culture week. Therefore, chromosome preparations (Danes 1975) were made during three culture periods (4–9, 9–15, and 15–29 weeks in culture). As ingredients of the culture medium, such as serum from different species, have been known to influence stability of chromosomes (Parshad and Sanford 1968), only one serum source (fetal calf) was used in both primary explant and monolayer cultures.

Only explant cultures containing epithelium prior to the first subculture were included, as it has previously been determined that increased tetraploidy was observed only in cultures containing epithelium (Danes 1978). It was appreciated that until cultures of known cell type (i.e., cultures containing either epidermal cells or fibroblasts solely) are available, the occurrence of tetraploidy in each cell type could not be determined.

Occurrence of In Vitro Tetraploidy in Skin Cultures Derived from Members of Families with Heritable Colon Cancer Syndromes

Normals (Family Members-by-Marriage)—The occurrence of tetraploidy in dermal cultures established from 90 (ages 9–73 years) of the 97 normals (ages 9–73 years) was 0–7% (Figure 5). The percentage of cells showing tetraploidy was approximately the same in all the subcultures established

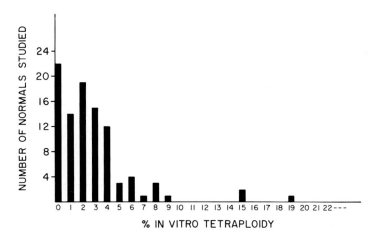

FIG. 5. Percentage of dividing cells showing tetraploidy in cultures from skin biopsies from 97 normals (family members-by-marriage without a family history of colon cancer). (Reproduced from Danes, B. S. 1981, with permission of *Cancer*.)

from a single biopsy from all of these normals and stayed within this range throughout 29 culture weeks. Cultures from the other seven (ages 16–53 years) showed increased tetraploidy (8%–19%). Cultures established from a second biopsy from each of the seven showed approximately the same percentage of tetraploidy. None of these seven had a family history of colonic cancer, but four had a family history of other solid tumors (breast, skin, ovary, and urogenital tract).

The association of increased in vitro tetraploidy and a family history of solid tumors other than colonic suggested that one of the in vitro expressions of other cancer-prone genes may be the increased occurrence of in vitro tetraploidy. Since 7% of an unrelated group (7 of 97) of normals (defined as individuals without a family history of colonic cancer) showed increased in vitro tetraploidy, such studies on larger groups with and without family histories of cancer should be undertaken to determine the occurrence and relevance to clinical cancer of increased in vitro tetraploidy in such groups.

Familial Polyposis Coli (FPC)—Cultures established from 28 FPC affecteds from 16 of the 19 FPC families studied (Figure 6A) showed no increased tetraploidy (0–7%). Of the 14 family members at increased risk from eight of these FPC families, none showed increased tetraploidy (0–7%) (Figure 6B). Cultures established from five affecteds from three families with FPC, clinically indistinguishable from the other FPC affecteds studied, showed increased tetraploidy (8%–14%). Of the six members at increased risk from two of these FPC families, three had increased in vitro tetraploidy (10%, 11%, 18%) and three did not (1%, 3%, 7%) (Figure 6B).

Increased in vitro tetraploidy was therefore found not to be useful in detecting the polyposis gene in the majority of FPC families. However, in those three FPC families in which increased tetraploidy was found in all affecteds studied (Figure 6A, Tables 2, 3), this cellular abnormality would be informative.

All 19 families studied were considered to have FPC on the basis of adenomatosis of the colon without any extracolonic disease. The finding that three showed increased in vitro tetraploidy and 16 did not suggested that the clinical phenotype, colonic polypsis, was not the result of the same mutation—this genetic difference not being detected in vivo but rather in vitro.

Familial Colon Cancer in Association with Discrete Polyps (DP)—In the three families studied (Tables 2, 3), the cultures from the three affecteds showed increased tetraploidy (9%–13%). Of the four at-risk family members studied, one showed increased in vitro tetraploidy (11%) and three did not (0–4%).

The finding of increased in vitro tetraploidy in all affecteds studied in three unrelated families added credence to this clinically defined syndrome (based on relative number of colonic polyps) (Woolf et al. 1955). If further family studies substantiate these observations, this cellular abnormality should be of clinical value.

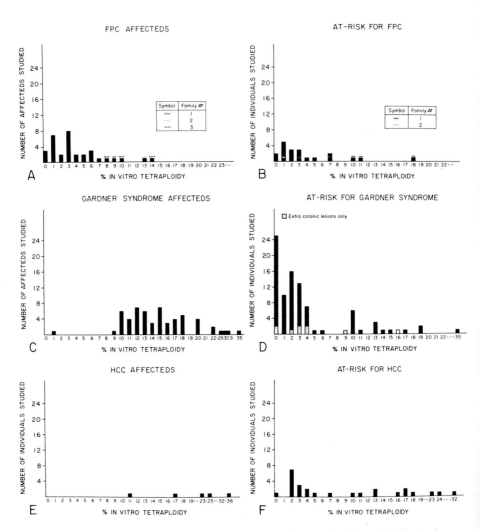

FIG. 6. Percentage of dividing cells showing tetraploidy in cultures derived from skin biopsies from: **A.** 33 clinically affected FPC and **B.** 20 at risk members from 19 FPC families, **C.** 57 clinically affected GS and **D.** 91 at risk members from 16 GS families, **E.** 5 clinically affected HCC and **F.** 26 at risk members from four HCC families. (Reproduced from Danes, B. S. 1981, with permission of *Cancer*.)

Gardner Syndrome (GS)—In the 16 GS families studied (Figures 6C, D, Tables 2, 3), increased in vitro tetraploidy (9%–35%) was observed in cultures from 56 of the 57 GS affecteds studied. One affected (male, age 40 years, with clinical stigmata of GS—fibromas, epidermoid cysts, lipomas, and adenomatosis of the colon for which a colectomy had been performed—and whose family history was unknown because he was an orphan) did not have increased in vitro tetraploidy (1%). Cultures derived from a second biopsy obtained two years later showed a similar percentage of tetraploid mitoses. Of

Table 2. *Occurrence of In Vitro Tetraploidy in Families with Heritable Colon Cancer*

| Syndrome | Number of Families Studied | Occurrence of In Vitro Tetraploidy of all Clinically Affected Members Studied within Each Family (no. of families) | | Potential Application of Increased In Vitro Tetra- ploidy to Families* | |
		Normal	Increased	Identification of At-Risk Status	Detection of Heterogeneity
FPC	19	16	3	No	Yes
DP	3		3	Yes	No
GS	16	1	15	Yes	Yes
OS	3		3	Yes	No
TS	2	2		No	No
HCC	4		4	Yes	No

Abbreviations (references): FPC—Familial polyposis coli (Dukes, 1952); DP—familial colon cancer in association with discrete polyps (Woolf et al., 1955); GS—Gardner syndrome (Gardner, 1972); OS—Oldfield syndrome, familial polyposis coli with sebaceous cysts (Oldfield, 1954); TS—Turcot syndrome (Turcot et al., 1959); HCC—heritable colon cancer without polyposis coli (Kluge, 1964, Peltokallio & Peltokallio, 1966).

*Based on the occurrence of in vitro tetraploidy in skin cultures reported in text.

the 91 family members at risk from 15 unrelated GS families (Figure 6D), 18 showed increased in vitro tetraploidy (9%–35%) and 73 did not (0–6%). The ranges of in vitro tetraploidy within each of the 15 GS families with increased in vitro tetraploidy were similar.

Such consistency supported the concept that one of the in vitro cellular expressions of the germinal mutation for the Gardner Syndrome was an increase in the occurrence of tetraploidy. Such a cell marker has potential value for three kinds of family members (those with full, partial, or no expression of the Gardner gene).

Table 3. *Identification of Family Members with Cancer-Prone Genotypes Based on Increased In Vitro Tetraploidy*

| Syndrome* | Number Of Families Studied | Total Number Members Studied | Increased In Vitro Tetraploidy | | | | |
| | | | All Affecteds (+) | Family Members At Risk | | Observed (+/Total) | Expected (+/Total) |
				+	−		
GS	15	147	56	2** 16	7** 66	74/147	74/147
HCC	4	31	5	11	15	16/31	16/31
DP	3	7	3	1	3		
FPC	3	11	5	3	3		
OS	3	13	10	1	2	11/13	7/13

*Abbreviations: GS—Gardner syndrome; HCC—heritable colon cancer without polyposis coli; DP—familial colon cancer in association with discrete polyps; FPC—familial polyposis coli; OS—Oldfield syndrome, familial polyposis coli with sebaceous cysts.

**With extracolonic lesions.

Table 4. Clinical and Cell Culture Phenotypes of Six Clinically Affected Members in Two Generations from a Family with the Gardner Syndrome

Generation#: # within Generation	Sex	Age at Dx	G.I. Pathology				Age at	Extra Colonic Tissue Growths					In Vitro Studies	
			Polyposis	Minute Polyps	Gastric Adenomatosis	Colectomy		Fibromas	Epidermoid (Cysts)	Sebaceous (Cysts)	Osteomas	Desmoid Tumors	Age at Biopsy	Tetraploidy
III:2	♂	38	+				39	+	−	+	−	−	48, 50	+
IV:1	♂	13	+		+		14	−	−	−	−	−	23	+
IV:2	♂	21	+	+			21	−	−	−	−	−	19	+
IV:4	♂	18	+				18	−	−	+	+	−	28	+
IV:6	♂	14	+					−	−	+	−	−	14, 15	+
IV:7	♀	13	+				18	−	−	−	−	−	18	+

+ = present; − = not present

In the first group (with full expression), the diagnoses had been made on the basis of the clinical phenotype. Variation in extracolonic growths in this group did not influence the in vitro observations (Table 4). The finding that the skin cultures established from 56 of the 57 GS affecteds studied showed increased tetraploidy only substantiated the clinically established diagnosis.

In GS, the extracolonic connective tissue growths usually appear in the first decade of life and the colonic adenomatosis by the end of the second decade. However, this time course is not invariably observed in every GS affected. Although infrequently encountered, in the second group (with only partial expression—extracolonic lesions with normal colons) seven members from two GS families have been studied (Table 5), three (ages 41, 45, 90 years) well beyond the expected age for colonic disease, and showed no increased tetraploidy (Table 5). The absence of increased tetraploidy in skin cultures from the four youngest investigated with only extracolonic lesions might have been due to any one of three possibilities: (1) The occurrence of tetraploidy in cultured skin cells might be age-dependent, as the occurrence of in vivo polyps is known to be (Gardner 1972, Pierce 1972). However, increased in vitro tetraploidy has been reported in skin cultures derived from clinically asymptomatic members at risk as early as five years of age (Danes and Krush 1977). Age of the donor of the skin biopsy from normals (not at risk) and clinically GS affecteds has been shown not to influence the occurrence of in vitro tetraploidy. (2) The possibility that epithelioid cells from the epidermis had not been included in the cell population studied from these three must be considered. Until pure epidermal cultures can be established, variation in the proportion of epidermal cells to fibroblast cells (shown not to have increased tetraploidy) (Danes 1976b) could produce an erroneously low incidence of

Table 5. *Clinical and Cell Culture Phenotypes of Seven Members with only Extracolonic Lesions in Two Families with the Gardner Syndrome*

Family #	Member Studied #	Colonic Polyposis	Cysts	Fibromas	Osteomas	Dentition Abnormalities	Age at Biopsy (Yrs.)	% Tetraploidy*
1	1	−	+				90	4
2	1	−	+				45	3
	2	−	+	+			41	2
	3	−				+	25	0
	4	−	+	+		+	14	4
	5	−	+	+	+	+	2	0
	6	−	+		+		4	3

All Clinically affecteds in both families showed full expression including colonic polyposis and extracolonic connective tissue growths.

*Based on number of metaphases showing tetraploidy divided by total number of metaphases scored blind on slides having at least 100 divisions per slide.

+ = present; − = not present.

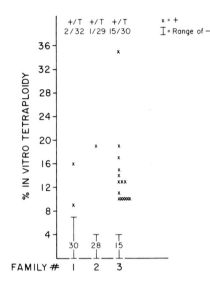

FIG. 7. The occurrence of in vitro tetraploidy in skin cultures derived from members at risk of three Gardner syndrome families studied: member at risk with (X) and without (given as a range with the number of members in each family) increased in vitro tetraploidy.

tetraploidy. (3) Increased tetraploidy may be expressed in skin cultures derived only from those individuals with the Gardner gene who will ultimately develop colonic polyps and, if not treated, cancer.

In the third group (without any clinical expression of GS) the at-risk members could be divided into two groups on the basis of in vitro tetraploidy (Figures 6D, 7, Table 3). All 18 at-risk members studied who showed increased in vitro tetraploidy would be expected to ultimately show such colonic disease, and the 73 at-risk members without increased in vitro tetraploidy would not, since they had not inherited the GS gene (Figure 6D, Table 3).

The need to identify, through cell culture studies, family members who have inherited a cancer-prone gene depended on the age at which the clinical signs were recognized within such families. Of the 57 affecteds studied, 12 were between the ages of 8 and 18 years. As a consequence, only 18 of the 91 members at risk had increased in vitro tetraploidy, since the majority of those family members having the GS gene had been identified through their extracolonic lesions in the first decade of life. When the total GS clinically affecteds with increased tetraploidy (56) were added to those detected in vitro (18), 74 of the total 147 GS family members (affecteds and at-risk) studied had increased in vitro tetraploidy, which was the 50% expected to have inherited the GS gene in this autosomal dominant disorder (Table 3).

Oldfield Syndrome (OS)—In the three families with OS (Table 2, 3), all 10 affecteds showed increased in vitro tetraploidy (8%–17%). Of the three at-risk members from two of these OS families studied, one showed increased tetraploidy (20%) and two did not (1, 4%). On the basis of only three OS families studied, these biomarkers appeared to be an in vitro expression of the OS mutant genotype.

Turcot Syndrome (TS)—Two TS affecteds studied did not show increased in vitro tetraploidy (0, 1%) (Table 2). This cellular abnormality did not distinguish the TS cultured skin cell from that of normals.

Heritable Colon Cancer Syndrome without Polyposis (HCC)—In the four HCC families studied (Figures 6E, F, 8, Tables 2, 3), five affecteds showed increased in vitro tetraploidy. Of the 26 members at risk from four HCC families studied, the cultures from 11 showed increased tetraploidy (10%–32%) and 15 did not (0–7%) (Danes et al. 1980b).

In HCC, there were no clinical signs to identify those family members who had inherited an increased risk for colonic cancer. Identification of members in such families through cell culture studies prior to its clinical expression as a colonic adenocarcinoma producing colonic symptoms would have clinical value. Although only four families have been studied (Figures 6E, F, Table 3), all five affecteds and 42% (11/26 studied) of at-risk family members studied have shown increased in vitro tetraploidy (Figure 8).

Interpretation and Conclusions on Increased In Vitro Tetraploidy

The occurrence of in vitro tetraploidy was not specific for any of the genotypes studied but appeared to be an in vitro expression, probably one of many so far unrecognized, of cultured skin cells from several of the autosomal

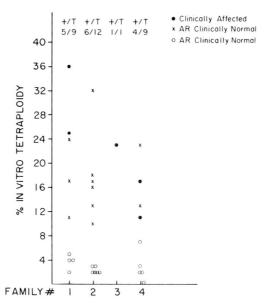

FIG. 8. The occurrence of in vitro tetraploidy in skin cultures derived from four HCC families: clinically affected (•), family members at risk for HCC with (X) and without (○) increased tetraploidy. (Reproduced from Danes, B. S. 1981, with permission of *Cancer*.)

dominant heritable colon cancer syndromes studied (majority of the Gardner syndrome, familial colon cancer syndromes in association with discrete polyps, familial polyposis with sebaceous cysts, and heritable colon cancer without polyposis coli) and not for cells with other such germinal mutations (familial polyposis coli and the Turcot syndrome).

On the basis of the occurrence of in vitro tetraploidy, both familial polyposis coli and the Gardner syndrome could be further divided into two subgroups. Familial polyposis with and without sebaceous cysts could be separated according to the occurrence of in vitro tetraploidy. Such differences between and within syndromes of this colon cancer group supported the concept, long assumed on the basis of clinical differences, that they are not all due to the same mutation but represent distinct genetic entities, these genetic differences not being detected in vivo but rather in vitro (Danes and Alm 1979, Danes 1980).

From this in vitro research, it was concluded that increased in vitro tetraploidy should be used to detect increased risk for colonic cancer only if family studies are done to determine that all clinically affecteds show this in vitro abnormality and vertical transmission can be documented. Until this method of identification of increased risk for colon cancer has been proven to be 100% accurate, all family members at risk, irrespective of their cell culture status, should receive close clinical observation. The significance of increased in vitro tetraploidy in a clinically asymptomatic family member should be that the attending physician be informed so that this member will receive appropriate cancer surveillance.

HL-A

HL-A typing was performed on 115 members of CFS-Family N (Lynch et al. 1975). In cancer-prone branches of the family, 20 of 21 members with cancer had one HL-A haplotype, namely HL-A-2/HL-A-12 (relative odds equal 6.30), including some deceased family members who had haplotypes assigned. Eleven of 12 family members with cancer in the branches prone to this disease, who were actually typed, had HL-A-2/HL-A-12 (relative odds equal 6.06). Although many more CFS kindreds will have to be studied in order to establish linkage of a cancer susceptibility gene to the HL-A locus, the rather extraordinary association of HL-A-2/HL-A-12 to cancer within this large family is suggestive of such linkage ($p < 0.025$). This nonparametric test of association is conservatively biased in that most members of the sixth generation were young and, while at risk, were less likely to clinically manifest cancer. The pervasiveness of the HL-A 2-12 haplotype and the high frequency of cancer in those with HL-A2-12, particularly in the maternal line of the proband (overall relative odds of 6.30), are strongly suggestive.

CEA

In 1973(b), Lynch and Guirgis presented preliminary data revealing a cluster of increased levels of plasma carcinoembryonic antigen (CEA) in a kindred manifesting the CFS. Guirgis et al. (1978) later reported these observations in four families manifesting the syndrome. Finally, Guirgis, Lynch, and others (1978) analyzed CEA in six extended kindreds manifesting the CFS and found that cancer patients and relatives at high genetic risk had a significantly higher mean value of $\sqrt{CEA}$ than relatives at low genetic risk. However, an unexpected finding was that unrelated *spouses* (used as controls) had mean levels of $\sqrt{CEA}$ which were strikingly similar to those of their direct line mates, suggesting the existence of a connubial effect on $\sqrt{CEA}$ levels. Subsequently, Lynch et al. (1978b) described a pattern of five immunochemical markers (including CEA) among several members of a pedigree manifesting familial malignant melanoma and other associated malignant neoplasms. In addition, these investigators offered a model for the putative connubial CEA phenomenon in the CFS (Figure 9). In this model, the high risk relative is taken to be a carrier of the putative cancer gene which causes derepression of an ubiquitous oncogene. This process may then directly trigger the host's immune response, or it may accomplish the same result through influencing the premonitory target organs (colon and endometrium), resulting in subsequent CEA elevation. Secondary effects of this process, either through the de-

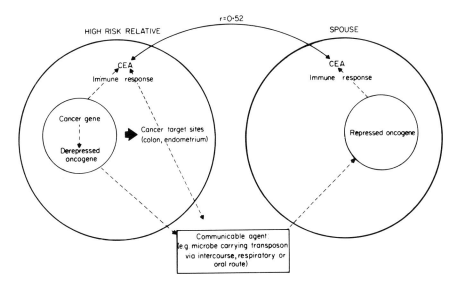

FIG. 9. Schematic diagram which provides a speculative, integrative model as a partial explanation for the putative connubial CEA phenomenon in the cancer family syndrome. (Reproduced from Lynch et al. 1978, with permission of Scandinavian Journal of Immunology.)

repressed oncogene or the premonitory cancer target organ tissue, may induce a communicable factor capable of eliciting specific (presumably genetic) information such as CEA production in the spouses. Conceivably, the derepressed oncogene could release transposons (Nevers and Saedler 1977) which are then incorporated into microbes and subsequently exchanged through husband and wife via intercourse or respiratory/oral passages. Such microbe-carrying transposons, acting in concert with the genome, could secondarily influence the immune response and/or CEA precursor, leading to differential CEA elevation. While speculative, this model is intended to provoke further study of the connubial phenomenon.

Plasma CEA determinations in all of these investigations were performed at Hoffman-LaRoche laboratories using the methods of Hansen et al. (1974).

Elevated CEA values have since been found to cluster in families prone to retinoblastoma (Felberg et al. 1976), in patients with medullary thyroid carcinoma (Isaacson and Judd 1976), ataxia telangiectasia (Sugimoto et al. 1978), epidermolysis bullosa (Rochman et al. 1979), and possibly Gardner's syndrome (Krush, personal communication).

An increasing body of evidence linking a possible infectious component in the etiology of cancer has been seen recently in the case of such lesions as Burkitt's lymphoma, nasopharyngeal carcinoma, Hodgkin's disease, osteogenic sarcoma, uterine cervical cancer, prostatic cancer, and hepatoma.

Cytoskeletal Actin in Cultured Skin Fibroblasts

Kopelovich et al. (1980) studied cytoskeletal architecture by immunofluorescence in cultured skin fibroblasts from individuals with FPC, and from high risk patients from CFS kindreds. This investigation confirmed previous findings of altered distribution of actin-containing cables in skin fibroblasts from patients with FPC. However, patients at risk from CFS kindreds and normal controls showed no disturbance of cytoskeletal patterns. As such, this phenotypic marker may be useful in identifying FPC gene carriers, but it does not appear to provide a marker capability in the CFS. It is also consistent with our assumption of the existence of separate genotypes for CFS and FPC.

SV40 T-Antigen

SV40 T-antigen has been observed rarely in members of high risk families. It has been postulated that multiple genetic factors may regulate this phenomenon (Blattner et al. 1978).

Lubiniecki et al. (1980) observed T-antigen expression in 24 of 31 skin fibroblast cell lines from members of CFS Family G of Warthin and found these to be significantly elevated when compared to healthy controls. It was of interest, however, that the pattern of elevation did not correspond to the patient's cancer risk. The T-antigen values were also independent of the age and sex, as well as the branch, of family and generation of the cell donor. Of further biological interest was the fact that cell lines from CFS-G tended to divide more frequently than cell lines from controls. Furthermore, this tendency was inversely related to T-antigen elevation in Family G cell lines. No such correlation was observed in the control cell lines.

In conclusion, SV40 T-antigen assay does not fit the criterion for a marker of cancer risk in CFS-G so far as a dominantly inherited cancer risk is concerned. This conclusion is drawn by the fact that individuals with normal values in certain branches of the family had offspring with elevated SV40 T-antigen values. The inverse association between cell division and SV40 T-antigen expression is seemingly unique to Family G. The explanation of this phenomenon remains elusive, although it may reflect the genetic makeup of Family G or possibly the fact that the range and variance of T-antigen expression values for this kindred were larger than for any other group. Finally, while elevated T-antigen is not clearly associated with cancer risk, it is possible that such elevated expression of SV40 T-antigen may be indicative of increased cancer risk at the group or family levels but not at the individual level, and that multiple genetic factors regulate T-antigen expression (Lubiniecki et al. 1980).

We have presented these SV40 T-antigen observations in CFS-G in order to provoke further inquiry into this at present elusive phenomenon. While the results clearly do not qualify as a "precursor" as we have defined the term, they do suggest a cancer risk at the "group level" in a manner not unlike some of the implications we have advanced for the communicable CEA model in the CFS.

Proliferative Lesions of Colonic Epithelial Cells

Human colonic epithelial cells may develop characteristics of malignant cells and still appear normal by conventional morphological evaluation. These epithelial cells, during their evolution to malignant cells, may pass through phases in which they demonstrate increasingly abnormal proliferative characteristics (Figure 10). Lipkin (1974) has defined this process as follows: (1) in Phase 1, a proliferative lesion develops and the colonic epithelial cells fail to repress DNA synthesis during their maturation. They develop an enhanced ability to proliferate and, in turn, develop a net retention (or accumulation) of cells in the mucosa; (2) in the case of a Phase 2 proliferative lesion, cells begin to develop properties that enable them to be retained in the colonic mucosa in increasing numbers. The morphologic changes may be accompanied by differentiation-specific molecular errors which result in the abnormal persistence of metabolic pathways leading to enhanced DNA synthesis. These proliferative cellular lesions have been demonstrated by Lipkin to occur in familial multiple adenomatous polyposis coli (FPC). They have

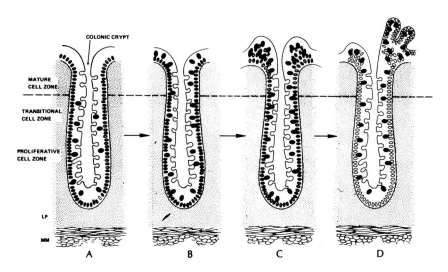

FIG. 10. One sequence of events to account for the location of abnormally proliferating colonic epithelial cells before and during the formation of polypoid neoplasms in man and rodent. **A** shows location of proliferating and differentiating epithelial cells in normal colonic crypt. Dark cells illustrate thymidine labeling in cells that are synthesizing DNA and preparing to undergo cell division. As cells pass from proliferative zone through the transitional zone, DNA synthesis and mitosis are repressed, and migrating epithelial cells leave the proliferative cell cycle to undergo normal maturation before they reach the surface of the mucosa. **B** shows the development of a Phase 1 proliferative lesion in colonic epithelial cells as they fail to repress the incorporation of thymidine ^{3}H into DNA and begin to develop an enhanced ability to proliferate. The mucosa is flat and the number of new cells born equals the number extruded without excess cell accumulation in the mucosa. **C** shows the development of a Phase 2 proliferative lesion in colonic epithelial cells. The cells incorporate thymidine ^{3}H into DNA and also have developed additional properties that enable them to accumulate in the mucosa in increasing numbers. **D** shows further differentiation of abnormally retained proliferating epithelial cells into pathologically defined neoplastic lesions including adenomatous polyps and villous papillomas. (Reproduced from Lipkin 1977, with permission of *Cancer*.)

also been observed in individuals in the general population who develop isolated colon cancer and in rodents after a chemical carcinogen is given.

Of pertinence to the CFS, Lipkin et al. (1980) have identified strikingly similar Phase 2 proliferative lesions of the distal colonic crypts in patients affected and at high risk for the CFS. While based on limited numbers, this study is being expanded to include a larger number of patients at high cancer risk.

Recognitive Immunity

The mixed leukocyte culture (MLC) has provided an in vitro measurement of cellular immunity. Lymphocyte reactivity in MLC represents a response to foreign histocompatibility antigens which are only subtly different from those of the responding cells. As such, it represents the recognition phase of the in vivo allograft response and becomes an in vitro measurement relevant to the malignant situation (Bach 1974). The MLC requires the interaction of both lymphocytes and macrophages and, therefore, the MLC can be adapted to examine both lymphocyte and macrophage function during the response to foreign histocompatibility antigens (Twomey and Sharkey 1972). Berlinger et al. (1977) have reported pilot data suggestive of a decreased response to in vitro stimulation on the part of affected and high risk members from families prone to colon cancer and lacking polyposis. Of 18 offspring of patients with hereditary colon cancer, eight demonstrated deficient cellular immunities measured by significantly decreased MLC responses. Interestingly, patients from polyposis families failed to show such a response in MLC. It is possible that the subclinical immune defect is genetically transmitted and contributes in some unknown way to the genesis of colon cancer. The second possibility is that the immune defect is an epigenetic phenomenon which could be secondary to an environmental carcinogen or an oncogenic virus, both potential immunosuppressive agents. Further work is ongoing in an effort to identify more fully the significance of recognitive immunity in the CFS.

Clinical/Management Aspects

Overview

Clinical/management considerations are based upon the known pathogenesis of the hereditary colon cancer syndromes in question, but require as a precondition the selection of family members most likely to express the cancer phenotype.

Age, diet, and geography (Goligher et al. 1975) are statistically associated with colorectal cancer and can suggest mass *screening* in certain circumstances (despite its poor sensitivity and specificity), but only when it can be done very inexpensively, as with occult fecal blood testing.

However, more aggressive measures can only be encouraged when the risk ascribable to an individual patient is several orders of magnitude greater than that predicated upon the above factors. A point is reached at which patient compliance and cost benefit ratios require the separation of hereditary cancer syndromes from chance aggregations. Limitations in the present state of the biomarker art are such that the most clinically informative "precursor" is an adequate interpretation of a suitably detailed pedigree and, when present, a polyposis phenotype.

Prognosis

Survival differences between hereditary colon cancer syndromes portend innate biological characteristics within the respective cancer-prone genotype subsets. They also harbor implications for monitoring.

Clinical decisions in the management of hereditary colon cancer are presently modified by an increasing knowledge of the natural history of this entity

Table 6. *Five-Year Survival Colon Cancer Site-Specific*

	Non-Polyposis Genetic	Total Colon Population
Ascending Colon	56.8%*	34.6%*
Transverse Colon	50.0%	33.5%
Descending Colon	33.3%	46.3%
Recto-sigmoid Colon	33.3%	34.7%
Multiple Sites	50.0%	29.6%
All Locations	52.8%*	35.3%*

*Statistically significant

and the widespread clinical application of sophisticated diagnostic techniques. In an attempt to assess prognosis in hereditary colon cancer, the presenting clinical stage and survival of 117 cancer patients from 18 unrelated, nonpolyposis hereditary colon cancer-prone families were studied. This population was then compared to findings from the American College of Surgeons (ACS), long-term colon cancer audit. The presenting clinical stage was similar in both series (Table 6).

However, the five-year survival differed significantly between the two samples. The overall five-year survival in the ACS study was 35%, as compared to a survival of 53% in the hereditary colon cancer group (p < .05). Improved survival was noted in the hereditary colon cancer population for each clinical stage, but primarily in lesions confined to the muscular wall and without nodal involvement (Albano et al. unpublished data).

Screening and Diagnostic Techniques

Barium studies of the lower gastrointestinal tract have achieved a high degree of sophistication and are universally available. The use of double air contrast barium studies has allowed for the diagnosis of increasingly small mucosal lesions, 1–2 cm (Miller 1975). Endoscopy has advanced rapidly with the flexible colonoscope which now permits visualization of the entire colon (Penfold et al. 1977). Reports from ongoing cancer screening projects have demonstrated a significant reduction in rectal cancer mortality and incidence among patients screened with routine proctosigmoidoscopy with removal of all polyps (Hertz et al. 1960). Colonoscopy, while an ideal diagnostic tool, is obviously not cost effective for screening the general population. However, its use in detecting cancer in asymptomatic high risk family members (those at 50% risk for colonic cancer) may be practical under certain circumstances.

Decision Logic and Precursor Signs

Adenomatous polyps are invaluable precursor signs. Multiple polyps may gain even greater power as a cancer predictor in those cancer syndromes with extracolonic phenotypic presentations, e.g., Gardner's syndrome. Familial polyposis coli syndromes (FPC), though uncommon, are usually much more familiar to the clinician than the more commonly occurring nonpolyposis coli cancer syndromes, such as the CFS. Cancer secondary to FPC is the only hereditary colon cancer with well-established, clinically proven, and virtually universally accepted management implications. Unfortunately, even this classic precursor marker is occasionally associated with confusing clinical presentations, as already discussed (Figure 1).

On the horizon, however, though far from universally available, are the several markers with a potential as premalignant precursor signs for hereditary colon cancer. Ideally, nonaffected high risk family members may, in time, be able to be screened through the use of these precursor signs in order to establish a susceptibility index which will allow for a more accurate and definitive management plan. These precursor markers include subtle histologic changes within polyps or in colon mucosae, such as the degree of pseudostratification of the glandular epithelium and the amount of glandular branching (Kozuka 1975a, Kozuka et al. 1975), skin fibroblast tetraploidy (Danes 1978), colonic mucosal cell proliferation index (Lipkin 1974), immunologic factors (Goldrosen et al. 1977, Neilan 1980), cytoskeletal actin changes in cultured skin fibroblasts (Kopelovich et al. in press), and tumor markers including CEA (Arnaud et al. 1980). The clinical use of such research tools, though extremely challenging and thought-provoking, has unfortunately not been sufficiently studied to enable clinical/management decisions.

Management of nonaffected high risk family members can be separated into those within multiple polyposis families versus those within hereditary nonpolyposis coli syndromes. The screening of patients with unexpressed familial polyposis phenotypes is presently associated with a more flexible approach due to its heterogeneity and advances in diagnostic techniques.

FPC Syndromes

Screening for polyps should begin early in life with biannual occult fecal blood determinations beginning at the age of 10. The polyp phenotype is usually expressed in the rectum and sigmoid colon which makes proctosigmoidoscopy the most important screening tool. Due to technical difficulties as well as problems in compliance, endoscopic screening should not begin until the age of 15, unless the patient has become symptomatic. Proctoscopic studies should be continued annually until the age of 45, and then performed at two-year intervals for life. In asymptomatic patients, a baseline double contrast barium study should be performed at age 20.

The treatment of FPC when the precursor phenotype of polyps is manifested is based upon the number, histology, and location of polyps. In individuals manifesting more than 100 polyps, total proctocolectomy is recommended, although the use of a continent ileostomy or a sphincter-saving operation may be considered. In patients with 10 to 100 polyps, when the rectum is not extensively involved (less than 6 to 8 polyps), total abdominal colectomy with ileorectal anastomosis is favored. In these cases, biannual endoscopic examination with fulguration of polyps must be performed. It should be remembered that females, younger patients, and individuals with multiple/recurrent rectal polyps have an increased proclivity to develop rectal cancer. The difficulty of retroperitoneal fibrosis in Gardner's syndrome may make subsequent proctectomy quite difficult or impossible. If the rectum is preserved in patients with rectal polyps, a 59% incidence of rectal cancer occurs within 23 years postcolectomy. In these cases, careful consideration of elective proctectomy should be made 10 years following initial colon resection. In patients with less than 10 polyps, when the rectum is not extensively involved, biannual colonoscopic evaluation with subsequent polypectomy is recommended. Colectomy should be considered if polyps continue to recur or if cellular atypia is noted on removed polyps.

Nonpolyposis Coli Syndromes

FPC syndromes, although dramatic in phenotypic presentation, account for only a fraction of hereditary colon cancer disorders. Nonpolyposis hereditary colon cancer syndromes, when identified on the basis of family history and pedigree analysis, demand close and careful surveillance as their primary clinical management. The favorable natural history, especially in early lesions, and improved diagnostic techniques, coupled with timing of prophylactic colectomy, make this approach feasible.

As previously described, most forms of nonpolyposis hereditary colon cancer syndromes involve a predilection for the right side of the colon (Table 1), occur at an early age, and show an excess of multiple primary cancers. Recommended screening of asymptomatic high risk relatives should therefore be instituted by age 20 and should stress biannual occult fecal blood determinations. This approach would appear superior to the traditional rectal exam and proctosigmoidoscopy since lesions are predominantly right-sided. Full colon endoscopy or proctoscopic evaluation with double air contrast barium studies are indicated on a two-year basis. As hereditary colon cancer is in general a disease of younger individuals, the most critical screening interval is between ages 30 and 55. Hereditary nonpolyposis colon cancer syndromes frequently are associated with neoplasia of other organs. If these syndrome tumor associations are found in the subject family, screening specific to the high risk organs should be promptly initiated (Lynch et al. 1977c), since they also occur earlier in life than their sporadic counterparts.

Treatment of the predicted tumor presents its own challenge to the clinician. Assuming the tumor is of low clinical stage (as it should be if the early detection program has been conscientiously followed), total abdominal colectomy with ileorectal anastomosis is recommended because of the predisposition to multiple colon primaries. This allows the attending physician to continue surveillance of the remaining colon and rectum with office proctosigmoidoscopy.

Other specific organs, especially endometrium and ovary in women from CFS kindreds, should be evaluated preoperatively. If associated malignant disease is found, appropriate treatment should be instituted. If indicated on the basis of definitive hereditary cancer syndrome identification, high risk organs (i.e., uterus, ovaries) should be considered for prophylactic removal at the time of primary colon surgery.

As often happens, hereditary colon cancer syndrome delineation may be made subsequent to primary surgical therapy. In these cases, the remaining colon should be evaluated with colonoscopy or proctosigmoidoscopy with double air contrast barium enema. Such studies should be repeated annually, due to the high incidence of second primaries. Postoperative occult fecal blood determinations should be performed routinely on all patients having manifested colon cancer, from such kindreds, on a four-month basis. Should subsequent malignant neoplastic lesions be found, total abdominal colectomy should be considered. Other organs at high risk must undergo intensive surveillance for life. It must be noted that as with all cancer patients, treatment must be individualized; certainly intensive multi-organ screening or prophylactic procedures are not indicated for the patient with advanced colon cancer.

Chronic Ulcerative Colitis (CUC)

Retrospective studies have demonstrated an association between dysplasia throughout the colon mucosae in excised CUC specimens removed for cancer. It is now believed that epithelial dysplasia is a distinct precursor to the development of colon cancer Since dysplasia may be difficult to determine, a second opinion may be warranted. Recommendations for management include total colonoscopy beginning approximately five years after the onset of the disease. Biopsies (from multiple areas throughout the colon) are performed when the disease is quiescent. If colonoscopy is not available, proctosigmoidoscopy with double air contrast barium enema may be acceptable in that when dysplasia is found, it is most frequently in the rectum. Patients with epithelial dysplasia should be considered for proctectomy.

COMMENT

The diagnostician's talents may be most effectively utilized when the signs of hereditary colon cancer have both a high sensitivity and specificity. We have discussed the matter of broadly defined precursors in relation to their potential efficacy in monitoring high risk patients. Because of the experimental nature of the in vitro studies emphasized in this discussion, it is obvious that clinical management must now rely heavily upon the more traditional physical signs (as in polyposis syndromes) or the criteria derived from family history and pedigree evaluation, as in nonpolyposis syndromes.

While the laboratory work described offers an immediate potential as clues to carcinogenesis, we hope to have offered a rationale for their eventual inclusion in the clinician's armamentarium, given anticipated improvement in their sensitivity and specificity. Hence, we see ways in which precursor signs can be utilized for the generation and ultimate testing of hypotheses relevant to both etiology and carcinogenesis in addition to their role in monitoring high risk patients. Since increased proliferation of colonic mucosa at the distal colonic crypts appears to be common to both FPC and the hereditary non-polyposis coli syndromes, one might speculate that this particular phenomenon provides an integral link to carcinogenesis in the hereditary colon cancer syndromes; along the same line, increased in vitro tetraploidy occurs in both Gardner's syndrome and in nonpolyposis coli patients. Certain questions immediately arise, namely "Are these phenomena peculiar only to those thus far studied genetically predisposing colon cancer disorders, and, in turn, is there a separate mechanism which might be linked to malignant transformation of colonic mucosa in sporadic varieties of colonic cancer? Are we dealing with the requirement for greater environmental carcinogenic insult in sporadic varieties of cancer so that in the presence of a significant lesser degree of proliferation at the distal colonic mucosa, for example, malignant transformation may be promoted?" It becomes readily apparent that any single precursor sign—in this case, mucosal cell proliferation or increased in vitro tetraploidy—assumes major importance in the spheres of genetics, environmental carcinogenesis, and, in turn, in monitoring strategy.

As we see today's research tools evolve into tomorrow's clinically applicable precursor markers, specific management protocols will be developed which, it is hoped, will significantly reduce the mortality from this disease.

ACKNOWLEDGMENTS

This study was partially supported by the National Cancer Institute, Grant No. CA 27831-01.

The in vitro studies were made possible through a grant from the National Large Bowel Cancer Project of the National Cancer Institute Division of Cancer Research (CA 15973) and supported in part by the Danes Medical Research Fund, Cornell University Medical College.

REFERENCES

Arnaud, J. P., C. Koehl, and M. Adloff. 1980. Carcinoembryonic antigen in diagnosis of colorectal carcinoma. Dis. Colon. Rectum 23:141–144.

Bach, F. H. 1974. Normal histocompatibility antigens as a model for tumors. Am. J. Clin. Pathol. 62:173–183.

Berlinger, N. T., C. Lopez, M. Lipkin, J. E. Vogel, and R. A. Good. 1977. Defective recognitive immunity in family aggregates of colon carcinoma. J. Clin. Invest. 59:761–769.

Bitran, J., and E. V. Pellettiere. 1974. Multiple sebaceous gland tumors and internal carcinoma: Torre's syndrome. Cancer 33:835–836.

Blattner, W. A., A. S. Lubiniecki, J. J. Mulvihill, P. Lalley, and J. F. Fraumeni. 1978. Genetics of SV40 T-antigen expression: studies of twins, genetic syndromes, and cancer families. Int. J. Cancer 22:231–238.

Danes, B. S. 1975. The Gardner syndrome: a study in cell culture. Cancer 36:2327–2333.

Danes, B. S. 1976a. The Gardner syndrome: increased tetraploidy in cultured skin fibroblast. J. Med. Genet. 13:52–56.

Danes, B. S. 1976b. Increased tetraploidy: cell-specific for the Gardner gene in the cultured cell. Cancer 38:1983–1988.

Danes, B. S. 1978. Increased in vitro tetraploidy: tissue specific within the heritable colorectal syndromes with polyposis coli. Cancer 41:233.

Danes, B. S. 1981. Occurrence of in vitro tetraploidy in the heritable colon cancer syndromes. Cancer (in press).

Danes, B. S., and T. Alm. 1980. In vitro evidence of genetic heterogeneity within the heritable colon cancer syndromes with polyposis coli. (In preparation).

Danes, B. S., and T. Alm. 1979. In vitro studies on adenomatosis of the colon and rectum. J. Med. Genet. 16:417–422.

Danes, B. S., T. Alm, and A. M. O. Veale. 1980a. Modifying alleles in the heritable colorectal cancer syndromes with polyps, in Colorectal Cancer, Prevention, Epidemiology, and Screening, S. Winawer, D. Schottenfeld, and P. Sherlock, eds. Raven Press, New York, pp. 73–81.

Danes, B. S., S. Bulow, and L. B. Svendsen. 1980b. Hereditary colon cancer syndromes: an in vitro study. Clin. Genet. 18 (in press).

Danes, B. S., and A. J. Krush. 1977. The Gardner syndrome: a family study in cell culture. J. Natl. Cancer Inst. 58:771–775.

Dukes, C. E. 1930. The hereditary factors in polyposis intestini or multiple adenomata. Cancer Rev. 5:241–256.

Dukes, C. E. 1951. Familial intestinal polyposis. Ann. Eugen. 17:1–50.

Felberg, N. T., J. B. Michelson, and J. A. Shields. 1976. CEA family syndrome: abnormal carcinoembryonic antigen (CEA) levels in asymptomatic retinoblastoma family members. Cancer 37:1397–1402.

Freedman, V. H., and S. I. Shin. 1974. Cellular tumorigenicity in nude mice: correlation with cell growth in semi-solid medium. Cell 3:355–359.

Gardner, E. J. 1972. Discovery of the Gardner syndrome. Birth Defects Orig. Art. Ser. 8:48–51.

Goldrosen, M. H., D. Rohrdanz, B. Sabatino, G. P. Burns, and E. D. Holyoke. 1977. Age-related impairment of tumor-associated lymphocytotoxicity in patients with colonic adenocarcinoma. Dis. Colon Rectum 20:561–565.

Goligher, J. C., H. L. Duthie, and H. H. Nixon. 1975. Surgery of the Anus, Rectum, and Colon. Macmillan Pub. Co., New York, 1164 pp.

Guirgis, H. A., H. T. Lynch, R. E. Harris, and J. P. Vandevoorde. 1978. Carcinoembryonic antigen (CEA) in the cancer family syndrome. Cancer 40:1574–1578.

Guirgis, H. A., H. T. Lynch, R. E. Harris, and J. P. Vandevoorde. 1978. Genetic and communicable effects on carcinoembryonic antigen expressivity in the Cancer Family Syndrome. Cancer Res. 38:2523–2528.

Hansen, H. J., J. J. Snyder, E. Miller, J. P. Vandevoorde, O. N. Miller, C. R. Hones, and J. J. Burns. 1974. Carcinoembryonic antigen (CEA) assay. Hum. Pathol. 5:139.

Hertz, R. E. L., M. R. Deddish, and E. Day. 1960. Value of periodic examinations in detecting cancer of the rectum and colon. Postgrad. Med. 27:290–294.

Isaacson, P., and M. A. Judd. 1976. Carcinoembryonic antigen in medullary carcinoma of the thyroid. Lancet 2:1016–1017.

Klug, T. 1964. Familial cancer of the colon. Acta chir. scand. 127:292–398.

Kopelovich, L., M. Lipkin, W. A. Blattner, J. F. Fraumeni, H. T. Lynch, and R. E. Pollack. 1980. Organization of cytoskeletal actin in cultured skin fibroblasts from individuals at high risk of colon cancer. Int. J. Epidemiol. (in press).

Kopelovich, L., L. M. Pfeffer, and N. Bias. 1979. Growth characteristics of human skin fibroblasts in vitro. A simple experimental approach for the identification of hereditary adenomatosis of the colon and rectum. Cancer 43:218–223.

Kozuka, S. 1975. Premalignancy of the mucosal polyp in the large intestine. I. Histologic gradation of the polyp on the basis of epithelial pseudostratification and glandular branching. Dis. Colon Rectum 18:483–493.

Kozuka, S., M. Nogaki, T. Ozeki, and S. Masumori. 1975. Premalignancy of the mucosal polyp in the large intestine. II. Estimation of the periods required for malignant transformation of mucosal polyps. Dis. Colon Rectum 18:494–500.

Law, I. P., R. B. Herberman, R. K. Oldham, J. Bouzoukis, S. M. Hanson, and M. C. Rhode. 1977. Familial occurrence of colon and uterine carcinoma and of lymphoproliferative malignancies. Cancer 39:1224–1228.

Lipkin, M. 1974. Phase 1 and phase 2 proliferative lesions of colonic epithelial cells in diseases leading to colonic cancer. Cancer 34:878–888.

Lipkin, M., E. Deschner, W. Blattner, J. F. Fraumeni, and H. T. Lynch. 1980. Tritiated thymidine incorporation into colonic epithelial cells of subjects in colon cancer prone families. Abstract 752. Proceedings of AACR/ASCO Annual Meeting.

Lockhart-Mummery, J. P. 1925. Cancer and heredity. Lancet 1:427–429.

Lubiniecki, A. S., H. T. Lynch, W. A. Blattner, and H. A. Guirgis. 1980. Increased expression of SV40 T-antigen and cell division in skin fibroblast cell lines derived from a family at high risk of carcinoma (Family G of Warthin). (in press).

Lynch, H. T., W. A. Bardawil, R. E. Harris, P. M. Lynch, H. A. Guirgis, and J. F. Lynch. 1978a. Multiple primary cancer and prolonged survival. Dis. Colon Rectum 21(3):165–168.

Lynch, H. T., and H. A. Guirgis. 1973b. Carcinoembryonic antigen in families. JAMA 224:1042.

Lynch, H. T., H. A. Guirgis, R. E. Harris, B. C. Frichot, J. F. Lynch, and J. P. Vandevoorde. 1978b. Familial clustering of plasma carcinoembryonic antigens (CEA) in the Cancer Family Syndrome. Scand. J. Immunol. 8 (Suppl. 8):465–470.

Lynch, H. T., H. A. Guirgis, R. E. Harris, P. M. Lynch, J. F. Lynch, R. C. Elston, R. C. P. Go, and E. Kaplan. 1979c. Clinical, genetic, and biostatistical progress in the Cancer Family Syndrome. Front. Gastroenterol. 4:142–150.

Lynch, H. T., R. E. Harris, P. M. Lynch, H. A. Guirgis, J. F. Lynch, and W. A. Bardawil. 1977b. Role of heredity in multiple primary cancer. Cancer 30:1849–1854.

Lynch, H. T., R. E. Harris, C. H. Organ, H. A. Guirgis, P. M. Lynch, J. F. Lynch, and E. J. Nelson. 1977c. The surgeon, genetics, and cancer control: the Cancer Family Syndrome. Ann Surg. 16:434–440.

Lynch, H. T., A. J. Krush, and H. A. Guirgis. 1973a. Genetic factors in families with combined gastrointestinal and breast cancer. Am. J. Gastroenterol. 59(1):31–40.

Lynch, H. T., and P. M. Lynch. 1979b. Tumor variation in the Cancer Family Syndrome: ovarian cancer. Am. J. Surg. 138:439–442.

Lynch, H. T., P. M. Lynch, K. L. Follett, and R. E. Harris. 1979a. Familial polyposis coli: Heterogeneous polyp expression in 2 kindreds. J. Med. Genet. 16:1–7.

Lynch, H. T., P. M. Lynch, R. Fusaro, and J. Pester. The Cancer Family Syndrome: rare cutaneous phenotypic linkage of Torre's syndrome. Arch. Int. Med. 141:607–611.

Lynch, H. T., R. J. Thomas, P. I. Terasaki, A. Ting, H. A. Guirgis, A. R. Kaplan, J. F. Lynch, and C. Kraft. 1975. HLA in cancer family "N." Cancer 36:1315–1320.

Lynch, P. M., H. T. Lynch, and R. E. Harris. 1977a. Hereditary proximal colonic cancer. Dis. Colon Rectum 20:661–668.

Miller, R. E. 1975. Examination of the colon. Current Problems in Radiology, Vol. V, Number 2, 40 pp.

Neilan, B. A. 1980. Lack of correlation of T and B lymphocytes with stage of colorectal carcinoma. Dis. Colon Rectum 23:65–67.

Nevers, P., and H. Saedler. 1977. Transposable genetic elements as agents of gene instability and chromosomal rearrangements. Nature 268:106.

Oldfield, M. C. 1954. The association of familial polyposis of the colon with multiple sebaceous cysts. Br. J. Surg. 41:534–541.

Parshad, R., and K. K. Sanford. 1968. Effect of horse serum, fetal calf serum, bovine serum, and fetuin on neoplastic conversion and chromosomes of mouse embryo cells in vitro. J. Natl. Cancer Inst. 41:767–779.

Peltokallio, P., and V. Peltokallio. 1966. Relationship of familial factors to carcinoma of the colon. Dis. Colon Rectum 9:367–370.

Penfold, J. L. B., T. M. Talbott, A. W. M. Marino, Jr., R. J. Spencer, and C. E. Culp. 1977. Early detection of colonic cancer by colonoscopy. Dis. Colon Rectum 20:85–88.

Pfeffer, L., M. Lipkin, O. Stutman, and L. Kopelovich. 1976. Growth abnormalities of cultured skin fibroblasts derived from individuals with hereditary adenomatosis of the colon and rectum. J. Cell Physiol. 89:29–37.

Pierce, E. R. 1972. Pleiotropism and heterogeneity in hereditary intestinal polyposis. Birth Defects Orig. Art. Ser. 8:52-62.

Rochman, H., M. Cooper, N. B. Esterly, and E. A. Bauer. 1979. Carcinoembryonic antigen: increased plasma levels in recessive epidermolysis bullosa. J. Invest. Dermatol. 72:262-263.

Rulon, D. G., and E. G. Helwig. 1973. Multiple sebaceous neoplasms of the skin: an association with multiple visceral carcinomas, especially of the colon. Am. J. Clin. Pathol. 60:745-752.

Sugimoto, T., T. Sawada, M. Tozawa, T. Kodowaki, T. Kusunoki, and N. Yamaguchi. 1978. Plasma levels of carcinoembryonic antigen in patients with ataxia telangiectasia. J. Pediatr. 92:436-439.

Turcot, J., J. P. Depres, and F. St. Pierre. 1959. Malignant tumors of the central nervous system associated with familial polyposis of the colon: report of two cases. Dis. Colon Rectum 2:464-468.

Twomey, J. J., and O. Sharkey. 1972. An adaptation of the mixed lymphocyte culture test for use in evaluating lymphocyte and macrophage function. J. Immunol. 108:984-990.

Woolf, C. M., R. C. Richards, and E. J. Gardner. 1955. Occasional discrete polyps of the colon and rectum showing an inherited tendency in a kindred. Cancer 8:403-408.

Gastrointestinal Cancer, edited by
John R. Stroehlein and
Marvin M. Romsdahl.
Raven Press, New York © 1981.

The Radiologic Diagnosis of Carcinoma
of the Colon

Gerald D. Dodd, M.D.

*Department of Diagnostic Radiology, The University of Texas System Cancer Center
M. D. Anderson Hospital and Tumor Institute, Houston, Texas*

At present, cancers of the large bowel are detected mainly by rectosig-moidoscopic and radiologic examinations. In the United States, rectosig-moidoscopy discovers about 45,000 cases of cancer per year while radiologic examination detects an additional 30,000. The overall survival rate for colo-rectal carcinoma is about 50%, but it has been estimated that three of every four affected individuals might be cured if the lesion were detected early. In fact, few rectosigmoid cancers escape the proctologist, and wider application of proctosigmoidoscopy should result in earlier diagnosis in at least three fifths of all patients. Conversely, approximately 3.4 million roentgenographic examinations of the colon are performed annually in the United States and every radiologist is, or should be, aware that 15% to 18% (Cooley et al. 1960, Vynalek 1947, British Cancer Survey 1952, Ramsey 1956, Allcock 1958, Brown and Colvert 1947, Clark and Jones 1970) of all cancers are missed on the first examination only to be obvious on a second study done within months or a year or two.

Why are such cancers overlooked by competent radiologists? Among the reasons cited are redundancy of the bowel, the large diameter of the cecum and other parts of the colon, multiple lesions, and human interpretive or observational error. Added to these might be the improper use of barium sulphate preparations, failure to employ adequate technical methods, inade-quate instrumentation, and imprecise interpretive criteria. However, most of these are of secondary importance to proper cleansing of the bowel. The barium enema is a diagnostic tool intended to reveal mucosal abnormalities, the morphology of which have a definite diagnostic significance. When prop-erly performed it is a precise procedure capable of not only demonstrating but also categorizing the type of disease present. This precision can be achieved only if the mucous membrane is accessible to the contrast material. It is the failure to understand this necessity that is responsible for the poorly per-formed studies, the misdiagnoses, and the low esteem in which the procedure is often held.

The diagnostic potential of the barium enema has been demonstrated by Welin (1967). Employing a special modification of the double contrast method, he has shown that the majority of colon neoplasms, both benign and malignant, can be diagnosed by the technique. Lesions between 0.5 and 1 cm can be detected routinely, and the sensitivity of the examination will include many neoplasms 2 to 3 mm in diameter. Needless to say, accuracy of this magnitude depends upon the proper performance of the examination from all aspects. It is the purpose of this discussion to present, briefly, the basic requirements of an acceptable study and the results that may be anticipated when these are met.

PREPARATION

The problem of cleansing of the colon is a complex one from both the physiologic and the pharmacologic standpoint. Although a variety of preparatory regimes has been described, the majority of radiologists and clinicians are dissatisfied with their present method. For the most part, recommendations for colon cleansing are based upon testimonials or upon comparison of preparation A vs. preparation B. Many studies suffer from lack of controls and other faults in experimental design. The few satisfactory comparisons available differ widely in the criteria employed. Nevertheless, while it is obvious that properly randomized studies are needed, adequate preparation can usually be obtained if a few basic principles are followed. Unquestionably, it is of value to maintain the patient on a low residue or liquid diet for at least 18 to 24 hours prior to examination. Hydration is also essential since it prevents absorption of moisture from the stool and permits a more satisfactory response to the laxative.

The laxative or laxatives chosen should be reasonably potent. While castor oil is most frequently employed, it is unpleasant to the taste, and combinations of other laxatives may be equally effective. At The University of Texas M. D. Anderson Hospital and Tumor Institute we have, for some years, employed the preparation developed by Garland Brown (1968). While there is no clear evidence that this regime is superior to all others, it has been quite satisfactory in the majority of adults. The preparatory sequence begins with a low residue diet starting at noon the day prior to examination. Hydration with orally administered liquids begins concurrently and is continued until the time of the examination. A combination of laxatives is employed, including an initial saline cathartic for bulk evacuation (magnesium citrate) followed by a contact irritant (Bisacodyl). A 2,000 cc tap water enema is given in the Department of Diagnostic Radiology at least one hour prior to the contrast study. No medication is added to the water enema; the 2,000 cc volume is sufficient to stimulate evacuation. Usually 30 to 45 minutes are sufficient to assure complete explusion of the cleansing enema. In our experience this sequence will adequately prepare the colon for single or double contrast examination in at least 90% of adult patients.

CHOICE OF PROCEDURE

The debate between advocates of the single column–high kilovoltage technique and those who prefer the double contrast examination continues. The comparative statistics of Figiel (1969) and Welin (1967) are of interest in this respect. As a strong advocate of high kilovoltage–single column techniques, Figiel has reported finding polyps in 7.5% of patients in the course of routine examinations. By comparison, Welin, in a series of 36,000 consecutive air contrast studies, found polyps in 12.5%. This latter rate equaled the frequency of polyps found at routine autopsies at the same institution. The 40% difference between the two techniques would appear significant and favors the use of the double contrast examination for the majority of patients.* It is our impression that a properly performed double contrast study is superior to the single column variety and will result in a consistently higher information yield. While changes in contour or filling defects can be demonstrated by the single column–high kilovoltage method, minor alterations of the mucous membrane pattern are best appreciated when visualization of the mucosal surface is possible. This is readily apparent in the early stages of Crohn's disease. Aphthoid or linear ulcerations are readily recognizable by double contrast techniques but, since they do not alter the bowel contours, cannot be appreciated by standard single contrast examination (Figure 1A). The same is true for the small irregularities that characterize adult lymphoid hyperplasia (Figure 1B), and the pseudopolyps of ulcerative colitis (Figure 1C).

It should also be noted that many of the reasons given for missed diagnoses on conventional barium enemas are negated by the double contrast approach, i.e., redundancy and overlap of the flexures, a large diameter of the cecum and other parts of the colon, etc. The major complaints leveled against the double contrast method are an excessive number of false-positive lesions due to retained fecal material, obscuration of the sigmoid by barium-filled ileal loops, added discomfort to the patient, and the extra time and effort required for performance and interpretation. By and large these are manifestations of improper technique and inexperience; as such they are subject to control and correction. For practical purposes the double contrast enema is now the procedure of choice at The University of Texas M. D. Anderson Hospital.

RADIOGRAPHIC TECHNIQUE

In the performance of adequate double contrast studies, it is essential that thorough radiographic coverage of the mucous membrane be obtained. This can only be done by multiple films in multiple projections. Rosengren (1977) has found that a minimum of ten films per examination is necessary to provide total coverage of the colon in rats with artificially induced cancers. Although

---

*The incidence of polyps in Scandinavia and the United States is essentially the same.

A

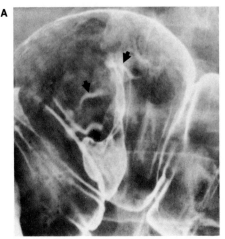

B

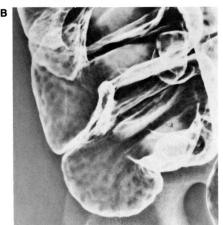

FIG. 1. Minor abnormalities affecting the mucous membrane of the colon. **A.** Linear ulcers of the hepatic flexure in a patient with proven Crohn's disease. The ulcerations are limited to the mucous membrane and cannot be seen in profile. **B.** Lymphoid hyperplasia of the cecum. Note that the margins of the bowel show little hint of the submucosal nodules. **C.** Inflammatory polyps of the colon in a patient with quiescent nonspecific ulcerative colitis.

C

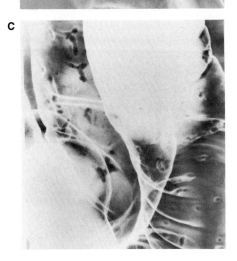

there are differences in anatomy, a comparable number of films are needed in the human being. The redundancy and circular nature of the bowel requires a sufficient number of projections to assure that the entire circumference of the lumen is visualized in profile. If this is not done, the presence of small lesions cannot be excluded and, indeed, very large lesions may be overlooked due to puddling of the barium (Figure 2).

Minimum film coverage requires 14 × 17 films of the abdomen in the prone, supine, erect, and lateral decubitus projections. Of these, the supine, lateral decubitus, and erect projections are probably the most important (Figure 3). Oblique films may be useful on occasion, but they are not a requisite and should be omitted in younger individuals to minimize radiation dosage.

Also of great importance are the lateral and angled projections of the rectum and sigmoid. The latter are made with the patient in both the supine and prone position with the tube angled 30° cephalad and caudad, respectively. These projections provide excellent coverage of the rectosigmoid and place it well within the province of the radiologist (Figure 4).

The double contrast method does not negate the need for spot filming under fluoroscopic control. Oblique films of all flexures and redundancies are essen-

A   B

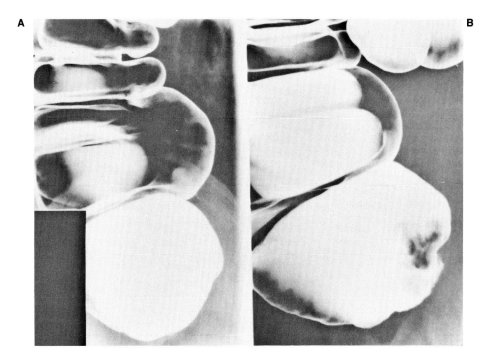

FIG. 2. Effect of position on the visualization of intraluminal lesions. **A.** In the anteroposterior projection, there is no apparent abnormality of the cecum. **B.** In the left anterior oblique projection, redistribution of the barium and air permits visualization of a carcinoma of the cecal tip.

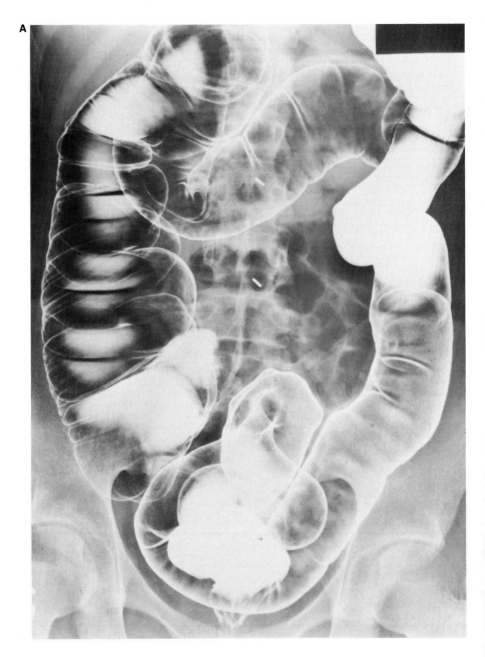

FIG. 3. Standard radiographic projections. **A.** Supine projection. (*contd*)

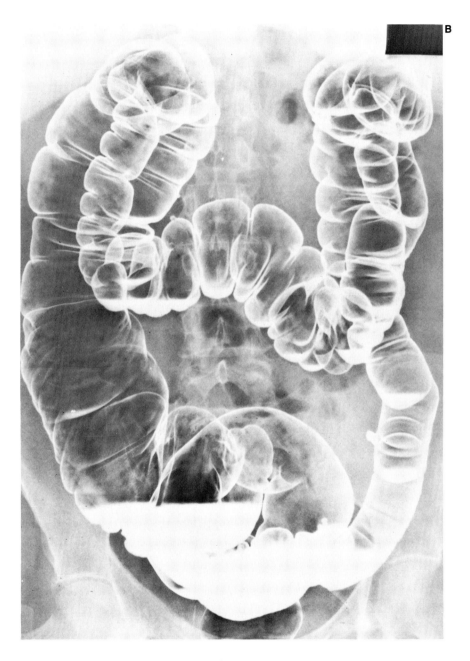

FIG. 3 (*contd*). **B.** Erect posteroanterior projection. (*contd*)

C

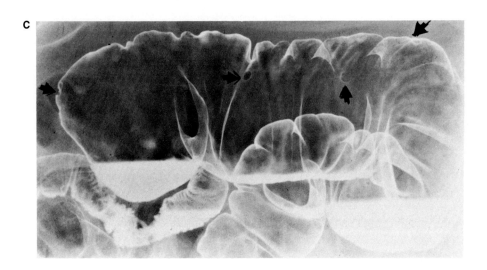

FIG. 3 (*contd*). **C.** Right lateral decubitus projection. There are a number of small polyps in the cecum and ascending colon (arrows). In the prone and supine views, excess barium gravitates to the dependent portion of the bowel and may obscure significant disease. In the erect and decubitus projections, the distribution of the excess barium can be recognized and a true view of the mucosal pattern obtained.

tial and should be made with the patient in both the erect and the supine position. The manipulation of the patient under fluoroscopic control often serves to displace intraluminal artifacts and to provide step-by-step coverage of the mucosal surface (Figure 5).

CONTRAST MEDIA

There is considerable difference between the barium mixture required for single column studies and that utilized for double contrast enemas. In the former, a relatively dilute solution is necessary to permit penetration by the x-ray beam. High voltage techniques, when coupled with compression, permit the examiner to "see through" the barium column. However, in larger-than-average patients, areas not susceptible to compression may not be sufficiently penetrated to permit the visualization of intraluminal defects. In Miller's experience (1975), a 15% weight-volume mixture is optimal for this technique.

In double contrast enemas, the primary requirement is uniform coating of the bowel wall without attendant flocculation or fragmentation. The barium suspension must be considerably more concentrated than that used for single column studies, preferably on the order of an 85% weight-volume mixture. Because of the increased viscosity, a relatively large bore tip and tubing is needed; usually a minimum internal diameter of 3/8th inch is necessary.

A

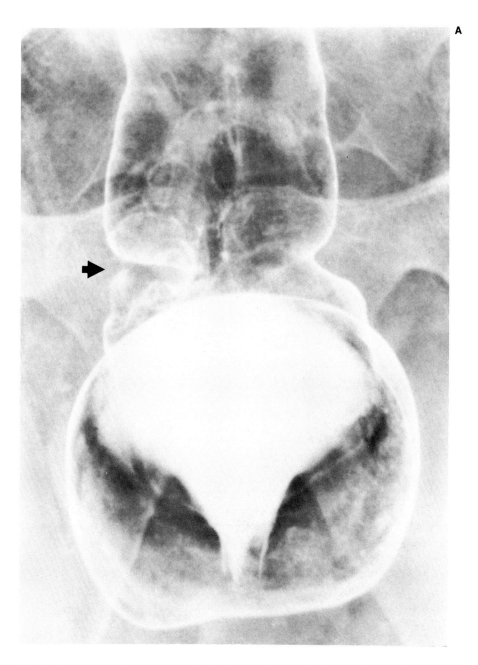

FIG. 4. Visualization of the rectosigmoid. **A.** 30° angled view with the patient prone. There is a recurrent carcinoma at the suture line following a low anterior resection (arrow). (*contd*)

B

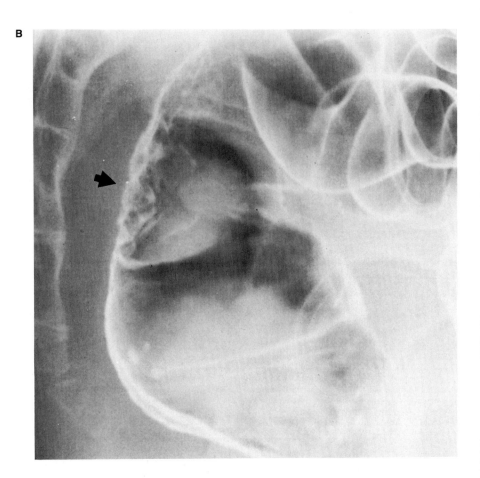

FIG. 4 (*contd*). **B.** Lateral rectum. There is a plaque-like villous adenoma of the posterior rectal wall (arrow).

The quantity of air required will vary with the individual examination, but for practical purposes, a total of 2,500 cc or more is required for the average adult. Although the discomfort of the insufflation has been prominently listed as one of the drawbacks of the double contrast study, the administration of 2 mg of glucagon intramuscularly (1 mg intravenously) usually minimizes the problem. For those patients who are apprehensive, Valium may also be used (Miller 1975). Additionally, according to Ferrucci and Benedict (1971), an

FIG. 5. Spot films of the colonic flexures. **A.** Posteroanterior view of the splenic flexure (erect). **B.** Anteroposterior film of the hepatic flexure (erect). There is a villous adenoma of the proximal transverse colon and a carcinoma of the lateral wall of the ascending colon (arrows). All superimposed segments of the bowel should be uncoiled under fluoroscopic control and spot films made of each.

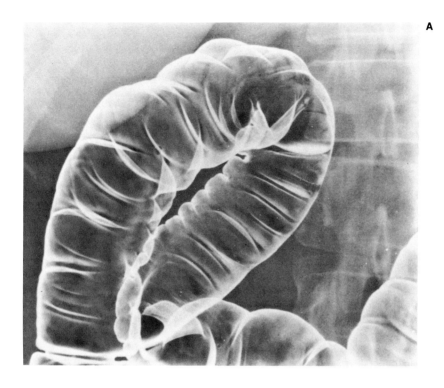

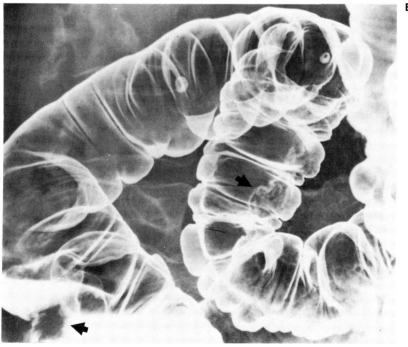

antispasmodic is useful for reducing spasm, defining localized narrowings, or combating functional inability to retain the enema.

DIAGNOSTIC CRITERIA

The basic roentgen signs of a well-developed carcinoma of the colon are those of mass and mucosal destruction. These are well known and require no further elaboration. Such cancers may be overlooked due to faulty preparation or technical error, but are readily diagnosed with a properly performed study. The more important problem lies in the demonstration and classification of small polypoid tumors. If benign, no treatment other than observation or colonoscopic removal may be necessary. Conversely, the malignant variety afford the best opportunity for cure, and reliable diagnostic criteria are of the utmost importance. Youker et al. (1968, 1973) have listed the following as pertinent:

1. Size
   The probability of malignancy increases with size. In their experience, less than 5% of polypoid tumors under 1 cm in diameter are malignant, whereas approximately one third of those between 1 and 2 cm, and two thirds of those greater than 2 cm are of the malignant variety (Figure 6B).
2. Pedicle Formation
   In polyps with a well-defined pedicle, the chances for malignancy are small (Figure 6A).
3. Base Configuration
   With those tumors showing a well-defined base, the probability of malignancy is on the order of 3%. If, however, the base is oblong or if, in profile, the width of the polypoid mass exceeds its height, the probability of malignancy is greatly increased (Figure 6C).
4. Indented Base
   Notching of the base implies invasion of the wall of the bowel and is applicable only to broad-based polypoid masses; pedunculated polyps may show an indentation related to traction which is of no significance. Although inflammatory changes may produce similar findings, the indented base is so commonly associated with malignancy that this should be the diagnosis until proven otherwise (Figure 6D).
5. Rough Surface
   An irregular surface of a polypoid tumor is far more common in malignant than benign masses (Figure 6B).
6. Doubling Time
   The probability of malignancy in polyps that require 1,200 or more days to double in size is on the order of 13%. With doubling times of 1,200 days or less, the probability rises to 87%.

The significance of these findings, when considered in the aggregate, is illustrated by a statistical analysis of the criteria. The chances of a polyp being

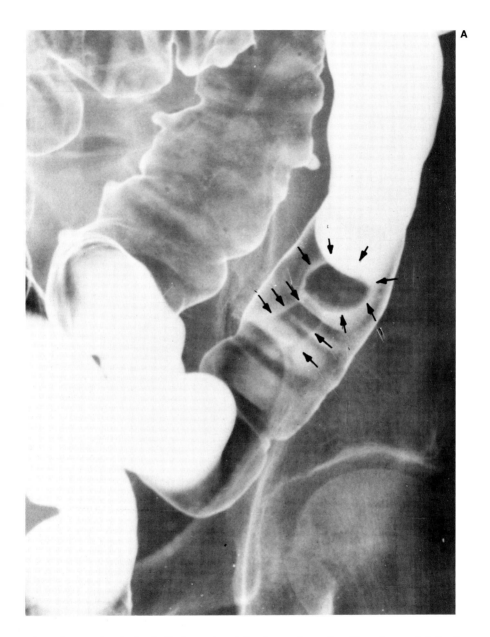

FIG. 6. Diagnostic criteria. **A.** Benign polyp of the descending colon. There is a well-defined pedicle. (*contd*)

malignant are but 1 in 92 if the tumor is less than 1 cm in diameter, has a smooth surface, and shows no indentation at its base. By contrast, if the tumor exceeds 2 cm in diameter, has a roughened surface, and shows an indented base, the chances of malignancy increase to 23 in 27.

B

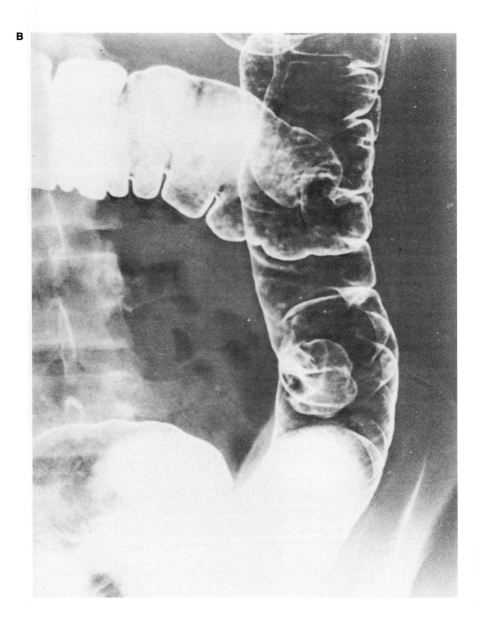

FIG. 6 (*contd*). **B.** Malignant polyp of the descending colon. The greatest diameter exceeds 1 cm and the margins are irregular. (*contd*)

These observations have recently been confirmed by Rosengren (1977) in an animal model. Following the induction of benign and malignant tumors to the colons of rats, double contrast techniques were used to locate, classify, and follow the neoplasms. Ninety-three percent of all histologically proven malig-

C

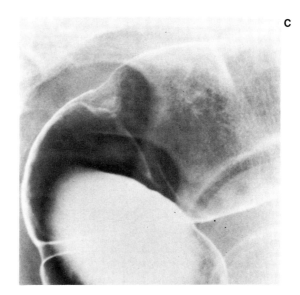

FIG. 6 (*contd*). **C.** Polypoid carcinoma of the posterior rectal
wall. The width of the base of
the tumor exceeds its height. **D.**
Polypoid carcinoma of the
transverse colon. There is
notching of the bowel wall at
the base of the polyp, which is
indicative of invasion.

D

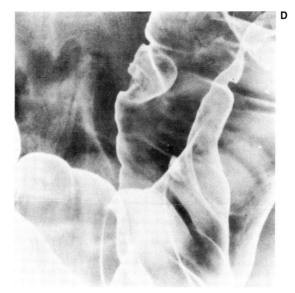

nant tumors were identified, and a correct distinction between benign and
malignant tumors was made in 92% of instances (171 of 185 tumors).

DISCUSSION

Although the barium enema is the most frequently requested examination
for the diagnosis of carcinoma of the colorectum, the fact that one in five
cancers is overlooked is unacceptable. It has been estimated by Eyler (1969)

that 75% of all cancers missed are due to the radiologist mistaking the tumor for retained fecal material or reporting "no gross disease" without insisting upon repetition of the examination. The results of delay in diagnosis are particularly unfortunate when the natural history of these tumors is considered. Eklund et al. (1974) observed a mean linear growth rate of 0.61 mm per month in 30 patients with proven colorectal cancer. The average time required for the tumors to increase from 1 to 5 cm in diameter was 5.4 years. This slow rate of growth offers an opportunity for cure that is not reflected in other tumors of the gastrointestinal tract.

The potential for early diagnosis by barium enema is underscored by the work of Welin (1967, 1976). On the basis of roentgen findings, 1,062 patients were subjected to surgery. In 204 cases, polyps were definitely malignant, and an additional 855 showed some degree of cellular atypia. Follow-up examination showed distal metastases in only two of the patients.

It is ironic that the means of implementing earlier diagnosis and treatment have been at hand for many years; what has been lacking has been a refinement of the techniques, an effort to define high-risk populations, and an attempt to make available to these populations the existing diagnostic modalities. Although sigmoidoscopy and the barium enema are the two most reliable tools now readily available, fiberoptic colonoscopes have made rapid technical strides and are being introduced into clinical practice at an ever-increasing rate. However, there are definite limitations on the facility with which colonoscopy can be performed on every patient. Significant problems may be encountered with redundancy of the sigmoid, spasm, fixation of the bowel, partially obstructing lesions, or the instrumentation time required when the examination includes the ascending colon and cecum. It is therefore reasonable, at this time, to regard the barium enema as the most readily available method for examining the proximal colon. The average cost per examination is relatively high ($100–$150), but is acceptable when compared with colonoscopy charges which are from two to six times greater. Much of the double contrast examination is performed by trained nonmedical personnel; with proper support facilities, a high volume of patients can be achieved. Since the methods can be developed in virtually every hospital, the examination is within reach of the average patient and can also be used to screen high-risk populations.

It is a mistake to place colonoscopy and the barium enema in a competitive position; the two methods ideally complement one another. Detection by the enema should be followed by colonoscopic verification and biopsy. The two procedures, when used in tandem, should considerably reduce the number of laparotomies performed for the confirmation or exclusion of early colonic cancer. The complementary use of the two modalities has been described by Williams et al. (1974), who routinely use some form of barium enema, preferably the double contrast type, before colonoscopy. It has been their experience that properly performed radiologic examinations identify 98% of colonoscopically diagnosed polyps greater than 1 cm in diameter and up to 95% of polyps over 0.5 cm in diameter. It must be emphasized that such accuracy can only be achieved by meticulous attention to detail on the part of the radiologist. He must assume a responsibility not only for the technical and interpretive aspects of the examination, but also for the education of his colleagues from other services and the preparation of the patient. When he does so, a high degree of accuracy may be anticipated and the number of asymptomatic and potentially curable cancers will increase proportionately.

SUMMARY

The barium enema is a highly accurate and readily available procedure which is capable of diagnosing benign and malignant tumors of the colon at a very early stage. This level of accuracy is dependent upon the radiologist assuming complete responsibility for the preparation of the patient and the examination of the entire colon; he cannot excuse mistakes on the grounds of incomplete preparation nor can he assume that certain portions of the large bowel are not within his province. While reasonable results may be obtained with the high kilovoltage—single contrast method, it is our opinion that the double contrast examination is a more sensitive technique and therefore should be the method of choice.

REFERENCES

Allcock, J. M. 1958. An assessment of the accuracy of the clinical and radiological diagnosis of carcinoma of the colon. Br. J. Radiol. 31:272–277.
British Empire Cancer Campaign, Survey of Cancer in London. 1952. (As quoted by Allcock, 1958).
Brown, C. H., and J. R. Colvert. 1947. Analysis of roentgen ray diagnosis in carcinoma of cecum and ascending colon. Ann. Intern. Med. 27:936–943.
Brown, G. 1968. The Direct Air Contrast Colon Examination: A Monograph. Garland R. Brown, Ft. Wayne, Indiana.
Clark, A. M., and I. S. C. Jones. 1970. Diagnostic accuracy and diagnostic delay in carcinoma of the large bowel. NZ Med. J. 71:341–347.
Cooley, R. N., C. H. Agnew, and G. Rios. 1960. Diagnostic accuracy of the barium enema study in carcinoma of the colon and rectum. Am. J. Roentgenol. 84:316–331.
Eklund, G., C. Lindstrom, and J. E. Rosengren. 1974. Appearance and growth of early carcinomas of the colon—rectum. Acta Radiol. 15:670–679.
Eyler, W., Moderator. 1969. Panel on patient preparation for colon examinations, *in* Proceedings of First Standardization Conference—1969, Detection of Colon Lesions, American College of Radiology ad hoc Committee on Detection of Cancer of the Colon, p. 108.
Ferrucci, J. T., and K. T. Benedict. 1971. Anticholinergic-aided study of the gastrointestinal tract. Radiol. Clin. North Am. 9:23–39.
Figiel, S. J. 1969. Colon examination technique, *in* Proceedings of First Standardization Conference—1969, Detection of Colon Lesions, American College of Radiology ad hoc Committee on Detection of Cancer of the Colon, pp. 132–143.
Miller, R. 1975. Examination of the colon. Curr. Probl. Radiol. 5:2.
Ramsey, G. S. 1956. Negative x-ray report in cancer of the colon. Br. J. Surg. 43:576–579.
Rosengren, J. E. 1977. Radiographic investigation of experimentally induced colonic tumors in the rat. Malmo General Hospital.

Vynalek, W. J., L. L. Saylor, and R. Schrek. 1947. Carcinoma of the colon: A statistical analysis. Surg. Gynecol. Obstet. 84:669–677.

Welin, S. 1967. Results of the Malmo technique of the colon examination. JAMA 199:369–371.

Welin, S., and G. Welin. 1976. The Double Contrast Examination of the Colon Experience with the Welin Modification. Geor Thieme Verlag, Germany. 111 pp.

Williams, C. B., R. H. Hunt, H. Loose, R. H. Riddell, Y. Sakai, and F. T. Swarbrick. 1974. Colonoscopy in the management of colon polyps. Br. J. Surg. 61:673–682.

Youker, J. E., S. Welin, and G. Main. 1968. Computer analysis in the differentiation of benign and malignant polypoid lesions of the colon. Radiology 90:794–797.

Youker, J. E., W. J. Dodds, and S. Welin. 1973. Colonic polyps, *in* Alimentary Tract Roentgenology. Vol. 2, A. R. Margulis and H. J. Burhenne, eds. C. V. Mosby, St. Louis, pp. 1037–1067.

Gastrointestinal Cancer, edited by
John R. Stroehlein and
Marvin M. Romsdahl.
Raven Press, New York © 1981.

Surgical Management of Colorectal Neoplasms

Oliver H. Beahrs, M.D.

Mayo Medical School, Rochester, Minnesota

Surgical resection of cancer of the colon, rectum, and anus remains the primary treatment for cancer of the large bowel. In many respects it should be considered local treatment, in that the surgical procedure removes the segment of bowel in which the tumor is located and those regional tissues that can be safely sacrificed. Unfortunately, it has no effect on tumors that have spread distantly or where infiltration has occurred into tissues at the margin of the resection.

Although there are several recommendations regarding staging of cancer of the colon, the one originally proposed by Dukes for cancer of the rectum remains the most acceptable. Its use has been extended to the colon and it has undergone several modifications. That recommended by Astler is the modification of the Dukes' classification that we use in evaluating our cases (Astler and Coller 1954). A Dukes' A lesion is one that is localized to the mucosa and in which the regional nodes contain no metastasis. B_1 is a tumor that is infiltrating into the muscularis but has not penetrated it. A B_2 lesion is one in which tumor extends through the muscularis into the immediately adjacent tissues, but in which the regional nodes are negative. A C_1 tumor is one in which the tumor penetrates the bowel wall, and the immediately adjacent nodes contain metastasis. A C_2 lesion is one in which the primary lesion has penetrated the full thickness of the bowel wall, and lymph nodes beyond the immediate regional area are also positive. If one wished to identify the entire spectrum of the extent of a cancer, a Dukes' O might be considered an in-situ lesion, while a Dukes' D would be any lesion with distant metastasis.

Unfortunately, on a clinical-diagnostic basis it is not always possible to be accurate in staging a cancer, and for this reason if all patients are to benefit from surgical treatment, some patients have to be overtreated to prevent other patients from being undertreated. Staging is more accurate when done after surgical resection and detailed study of the resected specimen. It is unfortunate if a resection more extensive than necessary to remove the cancer is carried out (especially if it entails removal of the anus); but a greater error is to have been conservative in the extent of the resection only to jeopardize the future well-being of the patient.

A philosophical statement as to the best cancer operation is expressed by Miles:

> "There are, I hold, two main principles to be observed in the surgical treatment of cancer of the rectum, and indeed of all cancers wherever they are found: first, the operation should be based on a knowledge of the demonstrable facts of pathology, and, second, the most extensive operation possible in conformity with that knowledge should be performed on all patients no matter how small or early the local manifestation of the disease may seem to be." (Miles 1926.)

While a few decades ago the risk of surgery of the colon and rectum was significantly high, today it is reasonably safe. In the late 1930's, the risk of operation on the colon and rectum generally carried a 20% mortality rate. With the advent of chemotherapeutic agents in the early 1940's and antibiotics later, the hospital mortality dropped to about 5%. Today with the availability of a wide spectrum of antibiotics, improved anesthesia, blood transfusions, and other supportive aides (cardiac and pulmonary support), mortality rates are reported in the 1% to 2% range, with death being caused by complications other than those associated with the operative procedure.

Many effective preoperative bowel preparations are used today. Most important is a good mechanical cleansing of the bowel together with antibiotics as proposed by Washington and Judd in their double blind study (Washington et al. 1974). Their method has been most effective for us, and is as follows:

BOWEL PREPARATION

Two Days Before Surgery
    Diet: Minimal residue.
    Mechanical preparation: At 12 noon, 15 ml of Phosphosoda. In p.m. before 6:00, two tap-water enemas (1,000 ml with patient in knee-chest position).
    Antibiotics: Neomycin 1 gm (9 a.m.; 1, 5, 9 p.m.). Tetracycline 250 mg (9 a.m.; 1, 5, 9 p.m.)

One Day Before Surgery
    Diet: Minimal residue. NPO after midnight.
    Mechanical preparation: At 8 a.m., 15 ml of Phosphosoda. At 9 a.m. and 6 p.m., three tap-water enemas (1,000 ml with patient in knee-chest position). If not clear, two more enemas. If still not clear, notify service.
    Antibiotics: Neomycin 1.5 gm (9 a.m.; 1, 5, 9 p.m.). Tetracycline 250 mg (9 a.m.; 1, 5, 9 p.m.)

Day of Surgery
    Diet: NPO
    Mechanical preparation: Rectal aspirations at 6 a.m. and every two hours until surgery.

There is little controversy over the surgical management of cancers of the abdominal colon, since they can be removed by segmental, partial, or total colectomy without altering the external anatomy or bowel function through the anal canal. The extent of the colonic resection is important, but it rests with the judgement of the surgeon. It should be as extensive as indicated to offer the patient the best chance of cure of the cancer and any other co-existing disease.

Controversy does exist when the cancer is in the rectosigmoid, rectum, or anus. If the philosophy as expressed by Miles is to be followed, then a combined abdominoperineal resection would have to be carried out in almost all cases. Although the mortality rate of this procedure is very low, it does leave the patient with altered anatomy—a colostomy—and with it altered function. As previously stated, it is unfortunate if a colostomy has been done but the prognosis is not altered for the patient; however, it is also unfortunate if the surgical approach has been compromised to avoid a colostomy only to jeopardize the future well-being of the patient.

However, by using all available data as to history, physical findings, and pathology to arrive at surgical judgement, lesser procedures than the combined abdominal resection are justified in well-selected cases. If the surgeon is conservative in arriving at his surgical judgement, few patients will be undertreated.

The anterior resection and low anterior resection offer a reasonable compromise for most lesions of the lower colon and upper rectum, in that an adequate resection proximally, laterally, and distally for a distance of close to 5 cm below the lesion is possible. Intestinal continuity can be re-established by an anastomosis, using one of several techniques, with a very low mortality and morbidity rate.

In evaluating 902 cases of anterior resection (556 anterior resections where the anastomosis was made between the bowel segments proximally with peritoneal cover and also distally with peritoneal cover, and 346 cases of low anterior resection where the bowel distally had no peritoneal cover), it was found that the prognosis was directly related to the anatomic extent of the tumor on pathologic examination. It was significantly altered, according to the symptoms, to the level of the tumor above the anus, the size of the tumor, or the degree of differentiation (Wilson and Beahrs 1976). For lesions that were localized, the five-year survival rate was 79%. When one node was metastatic, it was 64%, but when four or more nodes were positive for cancer it dropped to 30%. The mortality rate for the series was 2%, and the cause of death was unrelated to the surgical procedure in all cases. There was a 6% incidence of leakage of the anastomosis but in no incidence did this lead to mortality and in only seven cases was a temporary proximal colostomy necessary. These survival figures compare very favorably with those for combined abdominoperineal resection done in a series of 1,766 cases, in which survival rates were 68% for localized lesions, 41% when nodes were metastatic, and 55% for all cases (Mayo et al. 1959). The corresponding survival rates for anterior resection in the series were 64%, 37%, and 51%.

Since anterior resection can be accomplished for lesions of the lower sigmoid colon, rectosigmoid, and upper third of the rectum, it remains the most viable alternative; it can be done safely, it removes the primary tumor, regional tissues, and the segment of bowel in which the tumor is located, and it preserves normal external anatomy and bowel function.

The difficulty in decision-making arises for many cancers of the middle third of the rectum and all cancers of the lower third of the rectum. In these cases, a lower anterior resection is technically difficult when possible, or is not feasible at all. For such lesions, a combined abdominal resection is necessary as the best cancer operation. Since many of the lesions are small or localized (Dukes' A or B_1 or B_2) and since only approximately 50% or fewer will have regional spread, a lesser operation offers the patient a chance of cure without alteration in body function.

Jackman (1961), in the careful selection of 252 tumors which were small, pedunculated, and well differentiated, and of which half were in situ and often asymptomatic, treated the lesions by excision and fulguration. In this group of patients, 96% survived at five years. This illustrates that with expert selection of favorable cancers, local treatment can be successful.

Culp treated more advanced lesions in 80 patients with medical complications that increased the risk of major surgery, and 50% survived (Culp and Jackman 1974). This is largely based on the fact that overall about 50% of the cases would have been localized tumors without regional spread at the time of treatment. Madden (Madden and Kandalaft 1971), Turnbull, and Crile (Crile and Turnbull 1972) have had similar experiences in the treatment of both high- and low-risk patients. Fulguration under general anesthesia for destruction of cancer at times requires multiple operations, hospitalization, and high cost, and it is associated with some morbidity. The secret of success when approaching the treatment of cancer in this manner is the conservative and proper selection of patients. It has been recognized that about 25% of patients with only nodal spread survive at least five years when treated by the Miles procedure. Most of these patients would have been lost to disease if managed conservatively.

In addition to excision, fulguration, and fractional electrodesiccation, cryosurgery might also be used for the local destruction of tumor. Likewise, Papillon (1975), Sischy (Sischy et al. 1980), and others have suggested intracavitary radiation in high doses with low penetration as a preferred local treatment for highly selected lesions. Again this proves successful if, in fact, the lesions are localized. Unfortunately, Dukes' A lesions are associated with a 10% incidence of regional nodal metastasis and Dukes' B tumors with an incidence of 12%. Therefore, local treatment would fail in these cases.

For lesions of the mid rectum and lower rectum where it is desirable that a segmental resection of the bowel be carried out and yet it is thought unlikely that an anastomosis from above can be accomplished, the surgeon might consider a combined endorectal pull-through operation or other pull-through operations. Or he might use the transsacral approach to accomplish the anastomosis; however, these operations are not supported by many.

Ninety-five percent of cancers of the colon and rectum are adenocarcinomas. Lesions of the anal canal and anus, which comprise only 1% to 2% of cancers of the large bowel, are most frequently squamous cell epithelioma followed by basaloid carcinoma (cloacogenic carcinoma). In addition, infrequently seen lesions are Paget's disease, basal cell epithelioma, melanoma, and adenocarcinoma. When these lesions are invasive there is no alternative except to do an abdominoperineal resection. Originally, it was thought that the basaloid lesion had a worse prognosis than the squamous cell tumor, but in a review of 64 of the former and 113 of the latter, the prognosis was approximately the same (63 vs. 59 at five years and 48 vs. 44 at 10 years) (Beahrs and Wilson 1976). Again, the major factor in determining the prognosis was the extent of the disease at the time of treatment.

The place of inguinal node dissection in the management of anal cancer is uncertain since clinically evident metastasis or nodal metastasis found at the time of elective groin dissection indicates an extremely poor prognosis.

Perianal and squamous cell cancer (that within 5 cm of the anal verge) is often identified early and for this reason might be treated by excision, radiation, or other conservative measures with excellent results. However, if local treatment requires destruction of the external anal sphincter, then radical treatment is best done.

Finally, the stage of the disease at the time of treatment is the most important single factor in the prognosis of colorectal-anal cancer. Therefore, the treatment of known precancerous lesions and the proper selection of treatment based on the best assessment of extent of the cancer will offer most patients a chance of cure.

REFERENCES

Astler, V. B., and F. A. Coller. 1954. The prognostic significance of direct extension of carcinoma of the colon and rectum. Ann. Surg. 159:846.

Beahrs, O. H., and S. M. Wilson. 1976. Carcinoma of the anus. Ann. Surg. 184:422–427.

Crile, G., Jr., and R. B. Turnbull, Jr. 1972. The role of electrocoagulation in the treatment of carcinoma of the rectum. Surg. Gynecol. Obstet. 135:391–396.

Culp, C. E., and R. J. Jackman. 1974. Reappraisal of conservative management of certain selected cancers of the rectum, *in* Surgery of the Gastrointestinal Tract, J. S. Najarian and J. P. Delaney, eds. Intercontinental Medical Book Corp., New York, pp. 511–520.

Jackman, R. J. 1961. Conservative management of selected patients with carcinoma of the rectum. Dis. Colon Rectum. 4:429–434.

Madden, J. L., and S. Kandalaft. 1971. Electrocoagulation in the treatment of cancer of the rectum, a continuing study. Ann. Surg. 174:530–538.

Mayo, C. W., J. M. Waugh, E. S. Judd, B. M. Black, G. A. Hallenbeck, O. H. Beahrs, and A. H. Bulbulian. 1959. Surgical management of carcinoma of the rectum and rectosigmoid. Postgrad. Med. 26:375–385.

Miles, W. E. 1926. Cancer of the Rectum. Harrison. London.

Papillon, J. 1975. Resectable rectal cancers. Treatment by curative endocavitary irradiation. JAMA 231:1385–1387.

Sischy, B., J. H. Remington, S. H. Sobel, and E. D. Savlov. 1980. Treatment of carcinoma of the rectum and squamous carcinoma of the anus by combination chemotherapy, radiotherapy and operation. Surg. Gynecol. Obstet. 151:369–371.

Washington, J. A., W. H. Dearing, E. S. Judd, and L. R. Elveback. 1974. Effect of preoperative antibiotic regimen on the development of infection after intestinal surgery: Prospective, randomized, double-blind study. Ann. Surg. 180:567.

Wilson, S. M., and O. H. Beahrs. 1976. The curative treatment of carcinoma of the sigmoid, rectosigmoid and rectum. Ann. Surg. 183:556–565.

Gastrointestinal Cancer, edited by
John R. Stroehlein and
Marvin M. Romsdahl.
Raven Press, New York © 1981.

Elective Radiation Therapy in the Curative Treatment of Cancer of the Rectum and Rectosigmoid Colon

H. Rodney Withers, M.D., Ph.D.,* L. Cuasay, M.P.H.,†
K. A. Mason, M.A.,* M. M. Romsdahl, M.D., Ph.D.,‡
and J. Saxton, M.D.

*Department of Radiotherapy, †Department of Epidemiology, and
‡Department of Surgery, The University of Texas System Cancer Center
M. D. Anderson Hospital and Tumor Institute, Houston, Texas*

The success of surgery in controlling local disease in patients with adenocarcinoma of the rectum and rectosigmoid is limited by the pathobiology of the disease. Subclinical extension of disease along lymphatics or nerves, or directly through tissues, commonly leads to local recurrence in the pelvis. While the technical expertise of the surgeon may be a factor in reducing local recurrence rates, it is the nature of the disease process and the anatomy of the pelvis that ultimately preclude improved local control by surgery alone.

The reported local recurrence rates after surgery for adenocarcinoma of the rectum vary from less than 10% to greater than 70% (Gilchrist and David 1948, Dukes and Bussey 1958, Gilbertsen 1960, Deddish and Stearns 1961, Taylor 1962, Morson et al. 1963, Floyd et al. 1965, Glenn and McSherry 1966, Morson and Bussey 1967, Copeland et al. 1968, Griffen et al. 1969, Bacon 1971, Cohn 1971, Polk and Spratt 1971, Gunderson and Sosin 1974, Shindo 1974, Roswit et al. 1975, Moossa et al. 1975, Cass et al. 1976, Stevens et al. 1976, Walz et al. 1977, Withers and Romsdahl 1977, Gilbert 1978). This variation may be related to differences in the distribution of stages of disease in the various studies, or to the methods employed for diagnosis of local recurrence (e.g., clinical, second-look surgery, autopsy).

Clinical experience and radiobiological principles indicate that radiotherapy can increase local control rates if given in the pre- or postoperative period. The role of radiotherapy in this combined approach is the elimination of subclinical disease extending beyond the margins of surgical resection or implanted there during surgery. Since the number of tumor cells to be ster-

---

*Present Address: Department of Radiation Oncology, University of California Los Angeles, Los Angeles, California.

ilized in patients undergoing "curative" surgery is relatively small, the dose of radiation may be considerably less than that which would be necessary if the surgeon did not remove the macroscopically detectable disease or if therapy was delayed until local recurrence became detectable. The purpose of this paper is to compare the results of treating a group of patients by surgery and elective postoperative radiotherapy with the historical results of surgery alone at M. D. Anderson Hospital.

SELECTION OF PATIENTS FOR ANALYSIS

Patients were included in the analysis if the following criteria were met:

1. The tumor was primary (as distinct from recurrent) adenocarcinoma staged 2A–4B.
2. Surgical excision was considered "complete."
3. No distant metastases were detectable at the time of surgery (including metastasis to ovaries).

Patients dying in the immediate postoperative period were excluded. Records of patients were identified through files in the Departments of Epidemiology, Pathology, and Radiotherapy. Several hundred charts from throughout the period of analysis (1945–1979) are still to be reviewed. This report is, therefore, an interim one.

STAGING

Tumors were staged using the simplified nomenclature proposed by Withers and Romsdahl (1977) with the help of Peters (Table 1) to describe the pathological findings considered important in various modifications of Dukes' classification (Dukes 1932, Astler and Coller 1954, Gunderson and Sosin 1974).

Table 1. *Staging Nomenclature*

	Lymph Node Involvement	
Penetration of Bowel Wall	Negative	Positive
Confined to mucosa	1A	1B
Invading muscularis propria	2A	2B
Invading through full-thickness of muscularis propria (and through serosa if above peritoneal reflection)	3A	3B
Invading adjacent structures (histologically established)	4A	4B

RESULTS OF SURGERY ONLY

Results of surgical treatment as a single modality in 509 patients with Stages 2A to 4B cancer are shown in Figures 1-3. Several points are apparent from the data in Figures 1-3.

1. Prognosis correlated well with staging.

2. Lymph nodal metastasis was more significant than depth of bowel wall invasion in determining the probability of either local recurrence or distant metastasis.

3. Death from cancer occurred in about 30% of the total group. Failure of treatment was apparent as: (a) local recurrence only, (b) distant metastases only, or (c) coexistent local and metastatic disease.

Each of these three possibilities contributed approximately equally to the total 30% failure rate. Thus, local recurrence was a factor in approximately two thirds of all treatment failures.

4. Stages 2A, 3A, and 3B accounted for 91% of the cases fitting the criteria for inclusion in this analysis. Approximate death rates for these stages were 12.5%, 25%, and 50%, respectively. In Stage 2A patients, local recurrence was present in slightly less than half of those dying from cancer. In Stages 3A and 3B, however, the approximately equal three-way distribution of modes of treatment failure was evident.

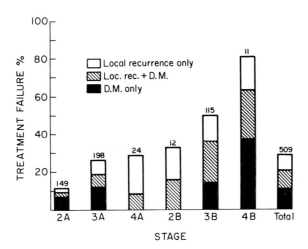

FIG. 1. The nature of treatment failure in 509 patients treated by surgery only as a function of tumor stage for Stages 2A through 4B cancer of the rectum and rectosigmoid. The pattern for the total group is shown in the histogram on the right. The numbers on each histogram represent the number of patients who had that stage disease. Failure was directly correlated with tumor stage. In the most common stages (2A, 3A, 3B), and overall, failure was fairly evenly distributed between three general categories—local recurrence alone, metastases alone, or coexistent local and metastatic recurrence.

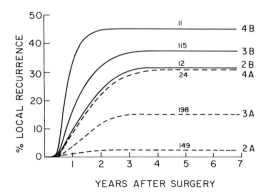

FIG. 2. Actuarial plots of the *total* incidence of local recurrence in Stages 2A through 4B cancer of rectum and rectosigmoid. Most recurrences are evident within three years, and on retrospective analysis most have suggestive symptoms within twelve months of surgery. The numbers on the lines represent the total number of patients in each stage.

5. In view of the distribution of patterns of failure after surgery alone (Figure 1), effective radiotherapy could influence the probability of local recurrence, and thereby improve the quality of survival, in approximately 20% of patients with Stages 3 and 4 disease (Figure 2).

6. Radiotherapy could improve the cure rate by up to 10% in individuals with Stages 3 and 4 disease (Figure 3).

RESULTS OF SURGERY AND POSTOPERATIVE RADIOTHERAPY

Postoperative radiotherapy was recommended if the tumor had penetrated the full thickness of the bowel wall, or if metastases were found in lymph nodes regardless of depth of bowel wall invasion. Occasionally, a patient with Stage 2A disease was treated, usually because of adherence of the tumor-

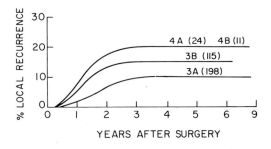

FIG. 3. Actuarial plots of local recurrence *in the absence of metastatic disease* in Stages 3A, 3B, 4A, and 4B cancer of the rectum. These curves indicate the potential increase in cure rate from effective elective radiotherapy given in conjunction with surgery.

bearing bowel to an adjacent structure. Not all patients irradiated postoperatively had had surgery at M. D. Anderson Hospital. However, analysis showed no difference between the intramural and extramural treatment groups, and therefore all patients having radiotherapy at M. D. Anderson Hospital were combined and compared with the surgery alone (control) group, all of whom had their surgery at M. D. Anderson Hospital. Staging was in all cases based on the report of M. D. Anderson Hospital staff pathologists. Most patients treated with the combination of surgery and radiotherapy had Stage 3 tumors (29 Stage 3A and 44 Stage 3B).

Actuarial plots of freedom from local recurrence as a function of time since surgery for patients with Stages 3A or 3B disease are presented in Figure 4. There is an improvement in local control in both stages as a result of the postoperative radiotherapy. Local recurrence has not occurred in patients with Stage 3A tumors. The incidence of local recurrence in patients with Stage 3B disease receiving combined treatment was the same as that for patients with Stage 3A disease treated by surgery alone. *All* local failures are included in the analysis, including one which developed in a patient who did not complete radiotherapy.

The patterns of failure in Stages 3A and 3B following treatment by surgery alone are compared in Figure 5 with those following the combined treatment. Since combined treatment reduced the incidence of local recurrence, the proportion of patients developing distant metastases as the only evidence of treatment failure was increased.

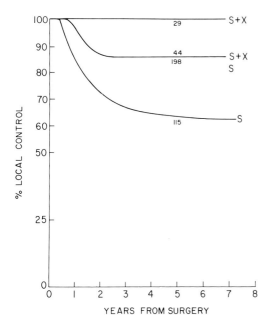

FIG. 4. Actuarial plots for local control of cancer of the rectum and rectosigmoid, Stages 3A and 3B, treated by surgery (S) or surgery plus elective radiotherapy (S+X). The numbers of the curves represent numbers of patients treated. All recurrences were included in the radiotherapy series even if, for example, the patient did not complete treatment.

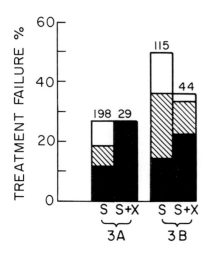

FIG. 5. Histograms comparing the distribution of modes of treatment failure for Stages 3A and 3B cancer of the rectum treated by surgery only (S) or surgery and elective radiotherapy (S+X). The histograms are as shown in Figure 1—i.e., solid = distant metastases alone, hatched = coexistent local and distant recurrence, and open = local recurrence alone. As local control is increased by radiotherapy the percentage of patients developing metastatic disease alone increases. The decrease in the incidence of local recurrences is significant.

COMPLICATIONS OF COMBINED THERAPY

The major complication from adjuvant postoperative radiotherapy is small-bowel obstruction. Surgical intervention for this complication was required in 17/97 patients treated with postoperative radiotherapy for the various stages of disease. Table 2 shows that this complication is three times more common than after surgery alone and is not dependent upon the type of surgery employed. This complication has decreased as the radiotherapy technique was modified to reduce the volume of small bowel exposed to high doses of radiation. Nevertheless, the present incidence is about 10%, with a median time to development of approximately six months from the initiation of postoperative radiotherapy.

An important difference between bowel obstruction developing after radiotherapy, compared with that after surgery alone, concerns its management. Irradiated bowel is often bound tightly in loops within the pelvis and is less elastic and more easily injured. The usual surgical management is to bypass

Table 2. *Incidence of Bowel Obstruction Requiring Surgery*

Surgery	A-P R	22/401	=	5.5%	⎰ 5.3%
	Ant. R	5/108	=	4.6%	⎱
Surgery + XRT	A-P R	8/52	=	15%	⎰ 17.5%
	Ant. R	9/45	=	20%	⎱

Incidence of bowel obstruction in 509 patients treated by surgery only and 97 patients treated by surgery and elective postoperative radiotherapy. A-PR refers to abdomino-perineal resections including exenterations while Ant. R refers to anterior resections including Hartmann's procedure. The incidence of obstruction after combined therapy has now been reduced to about 10% by modifying the treatment technique to reduce the volume of small bowel exposed to high doses.

the obstructed bowel, leaving it in situ. An approach more vigorous than gentle exploration, to determine whether adhesions causing the obstruction can be easily lysed, may lead to lacerations in irradiated bowel wall and to fecal peritonitis.

IMPROVING THE THERAPEUTIC RATIO

Surgery

The surgeon can improve the therapeutic ratio in a combined surgery-radiotherapy approach to cancer of the rectum and rectosigmoid by:

1. Marking areas of adherence or uncertainty of tumor excision using radiopaque metal clips (or other markers if clips are used for hemostasis). This will usually permit the radiotherapist to boost the dose to this area to improve the probability of local control. This is an important consideration since doses used in elective radiotherapy are chosen on the basis of an assumed small tumor load. The probability of sterilizing residual disease falls rapidly if the dose is not increased to account for an increase in tumor residuum.

2. Reconstructing a high pelvic floor to minimize the amount of small bowel remaining in the pelvis.

3. Primary closure of the perineal wound to reduce the interval between surgery and radiotherapy.

4. Bypassing irradiated small bowel if obstruction develops after radiotherapy.

Radiotherapy

The therapeutic ratio could be improved by increasing the rate of tumor control or decreasing the incidence of complications, or both.

Although doses and techniques have evolved over the eight year duration of our combined treatment program, the recent aim has been to give 4,500 rads midline dose through opposed antero-posterior fields using 25 MV photons, weighting the delivery 2:1 through the posterior portal, and supplementing this five-week treatment with about 600 rads mid-pelvis dose through a perineal or two lateral portals. Initially, treatment portals extended to cover para-aortic lymph nodes, but this is now considered ill-advised because of the high incidence of complications and the low probability of altering the prognosis of patients with disease which has extended this far from the primary site. Treatment fields should be the smallest thought likely to include residual disease, rarely extending above the sacral promontory.

In 44 Stage 3B patients the incidence of local recurrence was reduced two- to threefold from that in the surgery only controls. The therapeutic advantage could be increased by developing techniques to increase tumor dose without increasing the incidence of small-bowel complications. A worthwhile decrease in small-bowel injury could be achieved by limiting to about 4,000 rads the dose given to large volumes of small bowel through anterior and posterior portals. A similarly worthwhile improvement in local tumor control would be expected from increasing the tumor dose to 5,500–6,000 rads. This is not a straightforward problem; it depends on such factors as the energy of radiotherapy machines available, patient size, surgery and pathology findings, location and degree of small-bowel fixation postoperatively, and the clinician's best estimate regarding the size and location of the "target" volume. More of the tumor dose would be given through lateral and/or perineal fields, but this carries an attendant decrease in confidence that the potential tumor-bearing tissues are completely within an adequately dosed target volume.

Improved Selection of Patients

Only 15% to 40% of patients with Stages 3A through 4B disease develop local recurrence and therefore stand to benefit from elective radiotherapy (Figures 1, 2). An even smaller proportion may have their probability of cure improved (Figure 3). The risk-benefit ratio could be improved if the 15% to 40% of potential beneficiaries could be identified prospectively.

To determine whether certain groups of patients could be safely spared radiotherapy, several variables in the surgery control series were examined.

1. *Age and sex:* These were not significant variables.

2. *Operative procedure:* The local recurrence rates for different operative procedures performed for tumors located 10–25 cm from the anal margin were similar (Table 3).

3. *Number of lymph nodes containing metastases:* In 115 patients with Stage 3B tumors, the number of lymph nodes reported to be involved by metastatic tumor did not correlate well with local recurrence or survival (Table 4). This finding is similar to that of Copeland et al. (1968) for a large group of patients who also had "curative" resection, but contrary to that of earlier investigators (Dukes and Bussey 1958, Spratt and Spjut 1967) analyzing series that included patients having palliative as well as curative resections.

4. *Location of tumor:* Tumors close to the anal margin had a higher probability of local recurrence than did high rectal lesions (Table 5). Even Stage 2A tumors near the anus had an 8% probability of local recurrence. Earlier reports (Gilchrist and David 1948, Morson et al. 1963, 1967, Moossa et al. 1975) have also indicated a higher risk of local recurrence when the tumor is near the

Table 3. *Local Recurrence vs. Operation. 138 patients.*
*Tumor 10–25 cm**

Abdomino-perineal or exenteration	7/77	(9%)
Anterior resection (incl. Hartmann's)	7/61	(11%)

*Stages 2A to 4B

Table 4. *Prognostic Significance of Nodal Metastases—Stage 3*

Nodes Involved		Local Recurrence (%)		Metastases (%)		Death from Cancer (%)	
0	(3A)	31/198	(16)	37/198	(19)	56/198	(27)
1		12/35	(34)	9/35	(26)	14/35	(40)
2		6/21	(29)	8/21	(38)	11/21	(52)
3		7/14	(50)	6/14	(43)	9/14	(64)
4–5		8/17	(47)	6/17	(35)	8/17	(47)
>5		9/28	(32)	13/28	(46)	16/28	(57)

anus. However, distance from the anal margin did not provide any guide for *excluding* patients from adjuvant radiotherapy.

5. *Tumor adherence to adjacent structures:* Adherence of the tumor to an adjacent organ or the pelvic wall, or tumor-related difficulty of excision for other reasons (e.g., a large low lesion), was, of the variables studied, the best prognosticator for local recurrence (Figure 6). In Stage 3A tumors the rate of local recurrence in the adherent tumors was twice that for easily excised tumors, and in Stage 3B the difference was threefold. Morson et al. (1963) reported similiar observations.

These data suggest that the staging system may be improved by considering "adherence," as noted by the surgeon, to be as significant as invasion established histologically.

Although adherence or difficulty of excision has major prognostic implications, it is of limited usefulness in excluding patients from radiotherapy. Thus, the most favorable group, the easily excised nonadherent Stage 3A tumors, showed a local recurrence rate of 13% (19/146), with about one half of these patients (10/146) developing no evidence of distant metastases. Thus, local radiotherapy after the easy excision of nonadherent Stage 3A tumors could reduce local recurrence in up to 13% of patients and increase the cure rate by up to 7%. The need for postoperative radiotherapy in other subgroups of Stage 3 cancers of the rectum is more clear cut, since between 20% and 70% of patients may have an improved quality of survival (Figure 6), while the probability of survival may be increased 10% to 20% (Figure 3).

In summary, none of the variables studied proved to be reliable indices for excluding patients from postoperative radiotherapy. A similar conclusion was reached in a study reported by Moossa et al. (1975).

Table 5. *Percentage Probability of Local Recurrence*

Stage	No. Patients	Distance from Anal Margin (cm)				Overall
		1–4	5–8	9–12	≥13	
2A	149	8.2	3.5	4	0	4.7
3A	198	18	18	9	17	15.7
3B	115	50	29	25	29	36.5

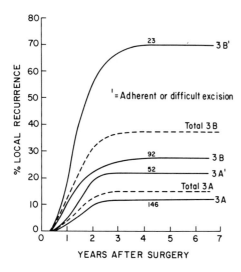

FIG. 6. Actuarial incidence of local recurrence (with or without coexistent distant metastases) in Stage 3 adenocarcinoma of the rectum as a function of adherence of tumor to adjacent structures or difficulty of excision for other tumor-related reasons. The dashed lines trace the overall local recurrence incidence for Stages 3A and 3B disease. Similar curves are shown for subgroups 3A and 3B in which excision was easy, and for subgroups 3A' and 3B' in which the tumor was excised with difficulty. Numbers on the lines represent the number of patients in the various groupings.

CONCLUSIONS

1. Radiotherapy given postoperatively reduces the incidence of local failure after "curative" resections for adenocarcinoma of the rectum and rectosigmoid (Gunderson 1976, Withers and Romsdahl 1977, Hoskins et al. 1980). Preoperative radiotherapy (Roswit et al. 1975, Stevens et al. 1976, Wassif et al. 1979), and probably also "sandwich" (pre- and postoperative) radiotherapy (Mohiuddin et al. 1980) can also accomplish this goal.

2. Radiotherapy is indicated when the tumor has extended to adjacent lymph nodes or when the primary tumor is adherent to or invading adjacent structures. We advise its use in easily excised Stage 3A tumors, but this may be debated since the local recurrence rate is only about 13%.

3. The major complication of radiotherapy is small-bowel obstruction. This should be treated by bypassing the irradiated bowel rather than by any attempt at lysis of adhesions or resection of irradiated loops of bowel bound down in the pelvis.

4. In principle, the ability of radiotherapy to eliminate subclinical disease may later encourage an evaluation of more conservative (sphincter-preserving) approaches for excising the macroscopically detectable tumor. It should be emphasized, however, that any surgical procedure that does not result in complete excision of macroscopically detectable cancer reduces the effectiveness of radiotherapy.

5. Selection of patients for postoperative radiotherapy has been based on the stage of the disease. Other parameters studied (e.g., location of tumor) did not discriminate adequately between patients at high and low risk of local recurrence.

ACKNOWLEDGMENTS

This work was supported in part by USPHS grant number CA 6294 awarded by the National Cancer Institute.

REFERENCES

Astler, V. A., and F. A. Coller. 1954. The prognostic significance of direct extension of carcinoma of the colon and rectum. Ann. Surg. 139:846–851.

Bacon, H. E. 1971. Present status of the pull-through sphincter-preserving procedure. Cancer 28:196–203.

Cass, A. W., R. R. Million, and W. W. Pfaff. 1976. Patterns of recurrence following surgery alone for adenocarcinoma of the colon and rectum. Cancer 37:2861–2865.

Cohn, I. J. 1971. Cause and prevention of recurrence following surgery for colon cancer. Cancer 28:183–189.

Copeland, E. M., L. D. Miller, and R. S. Jones. 1968. Prognostic factors in carcinoma of the colon and rectum. Am. J. Surg. 116:875–881.

Deddish, M. R., and M. W. Stearns. 1961. Anterior resection for carcinoma of the rectum and rectosigmoid area. Ann. Surg. 154:961–966.

Dukes, C. E. 1932. The classification of cancer of the rectum. J. Pathol. Bacteriol. 35:323–332.

Dukes, C. E., and H. J. R. Bussey. 1958. The spread of rectal cancer and its effect on prognosis. Br. J. Cancer 12:309–320.

Floyd, C. E., R. G. Cosley, and I. J. Cohn. 1965. Local recurrence of carcinoma of the colon and rectum. Am. J. Surg. 109:153–159.

Gilbert, S. G. 1978. Symptomatic local tumor failure following abdominoperineal resection. Int. J. Radiat. Oncol. Biol. Phys. 4:801–807.

Gilbertsen, V. A. 1960. Adenocarcinoma of the rectum—incidence and location of recurrent tumor following present-day operations performed for cure. Ann. Surg. 151:340–348.

Gilchrist, R. K., and V. C. David. 1948. Lymphatic spread of carcinoma of the rectum. Ann. Surg. 108:621–626.

Glenn, F., and C. K. McSherry. 1966. Carcinoma of the distal large bowel: 32 year review of 1026 cases. Ann. Surg. 163:838–849.

Griffen, W. O., L. J. Humphrey, and H. Sosin. 1969. The prognosis and management of recurrent abdominal malignancies. Curr. Probl. Surg. 3:3–41.

Gunderson, L. L. 1976. Radiation therapy: Results and future possibilities, *in* Clinics in Gastroenterology 5, P. Sherlock, and N. Zamcheck, eds. W. B. Saunders Ltd., East Sussex, U. K., pp. 773–776.

Gunderson, L. L., and H. Sosin. 1974. Areas of failure found at reoperation (second or symptomatic look) following 'curative surgery' for adenocarcinoma of the rectum. Cancer 34:1278–1292.

Hoskins, B., L. Gunderson, D. Dosoretz, and J. Galdabini. 1980. Adjuvant postoperative radiotherapy in carcinoma of the rectum and rectosigmoid. Int. J. Radiat. Oncol. 6:1379–1380.

Mohiuddin, M., R. R. Dobelbower, and S. Kramer. 1980. A new approach to adjuvant radiotherapy in rectal cancer. Int. J. Radiat. Oncol. Biol. Phys. 6:205–207.

Moossa, A. R., P. C. Ree, J. E. Marks, B. Levin, C. E. Pletz, and D. B. Skinner. 1975. Factors influencing local recurrence after abdominoperineal resection for cancer of the rectum and rectosigmoid. Br. J. Surg. 62:727–730.

Morson, B. C., and H. J. R. Bussey. 1967. Surgical pathology of rectal cancer in relation to adjuvant radiotherapy. Br. J. Radiol. 40:161–165.

Morson, B. C., E. G. Vaughn, and H. J. R. Bussey. 1963. Pelvic recurrence after excision of rectum for carcinoma. Br. Med. J. 2:13–18.

Polk, H. C., and J. S. Spratt. 1971. Recurrent colorectal carcinoma: Detection, treatment and other considerations. Surgery 69:9–23.

Roswit, B., G. A. Higgins, and R. J. Keehn. 1975. Preoperative irradiation for carcinoma of the rectum and rectosigmoid colon: Report of a national Veterans Administration randomized study. Cancer 35:1597–1602.

Shindo, K. 1974. Recurrence of carcinoma of large intestine. A statistical review. Am. J. Proctol. 25:80–90.

Spratt, J. S., Jr., and H. J. Spjut. 1967. Prevalence and prognosis of individual clinical and pathologic variables associated with colorectal carcinoma. Cancer 20:1976–1985.

Stevens, K. R., C. V. Allen, and W. S. Fletcher. 1976. Preoperative radiotherapy for adenocarcinoma of the rectosigmoid. Cancer 37:2866–2874.

Taylor, F. W. 1962. Cancer of the colon and rectum—a study of routes of metastases and death. Surgery 52:305–308.

Walz, B. J., E. R. Lindstrom, H. R. Butcher, and R. J. Baglan. 1977. Natural history of patients after abdomino-perineal resection. Implications for radiation therapy. Cancer 39:2437–2442.

Wassif, S. B., B. L. Langenhorst, and W. C. J. Hop. 1979. The contribution of preoperative radiotherapy in the management of borderline operability rectal cancer, *in* Adjuvant Therapy of Cancer II, S. E. Jones and S. E. Salmon, eds. Grune and Stratton, New York, pp. 613–620.

Withers, H. R., and M. Romsdahl. 1977. Postoperative radiotherapy for adenocarcinoma of rectum and rectosigmoid. Int. J. Radiat. Oncol. Biol. Phys. 2:1069–1074.

Directions for Future Research

Gastrointestinal Cancer, edited by
John R. Stroehlein and
Marvin M. Romsdahl.
Raven Press, New York © 1981.

Chemotherapeutic Management of Colorectal Cancer and Prospects for New Agents

Agop Y. Bedikian, M.D.,* Gerald P. Bodey, M.D.,*
Manuel Valdivieso, M.D.,* John R. Stroehlein, M.D.,†
David A. Karlin, M.D.,† Roland W. Bennetts, M.D.,†
Yehuda Z. Patt, M.D.,* and Michael A. Burgess, M.D.*

*Departments of *Developmental Therapeutics and †Medicine,
The University of Texas System Cancer Center
M. D. Anderson Hospital and Tumor Institute, Houston, Texas*

Cancer of the digestive system afflicts more patients throughout the world than cancer originating in any other organ system. Colorectal cancer is the most common malignant neoplasm arising from the gastrointestinal tract; it accounts for approximately 10% of all deaths from malignant neoplasms (Silverberg 1979). Over the past three decades, progress in the surgical treatment of colorectal cancer has been insignificant, affecting the patient's survival very little. More than half of patients with colorectal cancer die as a result of progression of their disease.

Chemotherapy for colorectal cancer has had increasingly widespread acceptance since it was demonstrated over two decades ago that 5-fluorinated pyrimidines, 5-fluorouracil (5-FU), and 5-fluoro-2-deoxyuridine (FUDR) were capable of producing reduction in tumor size in patients with metastatic cancer of the gastrointestinal tract. Subsequently, investigators have attempted to increase the therapeutic index of these agents by altering route, duration, or schedule of administration. Results of studies comparing the efficacy of 5-FU administered by different routes and schedules (Table 1) indicate that for 5-FU, the oral route is considerably inferior to the intravenous route, and that the weekly schedule is inferior to the loading dose. Administration of 5-FU by prolonged intravenous (IV) infusion has been shown to be less toxic, but had no significant superiority in response rate over simple administration by rapid IV injection using the five-day schedule. Overall, fluorinated pyrimidines produce objective responses in only 15% to 20% of treated patients. In this context, objective response is defined as a reduction of more than 50% in the sum of the product of the diameters of measurable lesions. These responses are usually only partial, lasting for a median time of four to five months.

Table 1. *Correlation of Dose Schedule and Response Rate in Controlled Trials with 5-FU in Colorectal Cancer*

Administration		Response			
Route	Schedule	Total No. Pts.	No. Pts.	%	References
Oral	Single dose, weekly	93	12	13	(Bateman et al. 1975)
Oral	5–6-day course	95	15	16	(Ansfield 1975, Hahn et al. 1975)
Intravenous	Single dose weekly	149	30	20	(Bateman et al. 1975, Ansfield 1975)
Intravenous	5-day course, rapid infusion	89	22	25	(Carroll et al. 1979, Seifert et al. 1975)
Intravenous	5-day course, slow infusion*	115	28	24	(Seifert et al. 1975, Reitemeier and Moertel 1969, Hartman et al. 1979)
Intravenous	Loading course	93	25	27	(Carroll et al. 1979, Hartman et al. 1979)

*Daily dose administered over 8 to 24 hours.

Before exerting its antitumor activity, 5-FU is converted to its nucleoside derivative, FUDR. Four studies comparing the antitumor activity of 5-FU and FUDR in colorectal cancer produced widely differing results. The response rates for FUDR varied from 4% to 42%. Overall, the response rate to 5-FU was 17% compared with 23% for FUDR (Table 2). Ftorafur, a fluorinated pyrimidine analog of 5-FU developed in the Soviet Union, has been shown to behave as a depot form of 5-FU. It has the advantage of being less myelotoxic than 5-FU. Administration of the drug intravenously has been found to be more toxic and less active than 5-FU. However, preliminary results with the oral formulation of ftorafur (Tegafur, by Mead Johnson) in our institution indicate better tolerance and antitumor activity. In this study patients with colorectal cancer with no prior chemotherapy are stratified by performance status and presence of liver metastasis and randomized to receive ftorafur 1 gm/m^2 po for 21 days or 5-FU 500 mg/m^2 daily × 4 followed by 250 mg/m^2 for 4 doses given on alternate days. Forty patients have been entered so far, 17 of whom are evaluable in each treatment group. The characteristics of the patients are similar. There were three partial remissions and five minor responses on the ftorafur treatment arm, compared with three partial remissions and two minor responses in the 5-FU-treated group. All six responding patients had good pretreatment performance status. Three patients who failed on 5-FU, subsequently, were treated with ftorafur and one had minor response. Objective tumor regressions in the liver were more common with ftorafur (50% vs. 33% respectively). No significant myelosuppression occurred with ftorafur while moderate neutropenia was dose-limiting with 5-FU. In contrast, gastrointestinal toxicity was dose-limiting in the ftorafur-treated group. Nausea, vomiting, and diarrhea were seen in a third to one half of treatment courses on either regimen. Mucositis was present during 32% of treatment courses of 5-FU, an incidence twice that seen with ftorafur. In contrast to intravenous formulation, neurologic symptoms occurred in 2% of courses of ftorafur and were mild. Ftorafur by the schedule used in this study appears as effective as 5-FU.

Methotrexate and Baker's antifol or triazinate are folate inhibitors. Unlike methotrexate, Baker's antifol has the advantage of being able to penetrate cells passively. Phase II trials of this drug in patients with colon cancer showed response rates of 10%–18%. However, because of the increased incidence of mucocutaneous and gastrointestinal toxicities associated with the administration of Baker's antifol to patients with abnormal liver functions, the drug is less commonly incorporated in multidrug chemotherapy regimens for colorectal cancer than one would expect based on its antitumor activity.

PALA (N-(phosphonacetyl)-L-aspartate) and AAFC (anhydro-ara-5-fluoro-cytidine) have shown minimal activity against colorectal cancer. PALA is a recently evaluated antimetabolite that inhibits de novo pyrimidine bio-synthesis by blocking the activity of aspartate carbamoyl transferase (ACTase). Phase II trial of PALA in colorectal cancer in our institution, comparing the single dose with 5-day dose schedules administered at 2-week intervals, resulted in no partial or complete responses in 27 evaluable patients (Valdivieso, personal communication). During a phase II trial at the Clinical Oncology Branch of the National Cancer Institute, PALA administered by the 5-day schedule every 3 weeks resulted in no partial or complete responses in

Table 2. *Efficacy of Antimetabolites in Colorectal Cancer*

| | Total No. Pts. | Response | | References |
		No. Pts.	%	
5-FU	321	55	17	(ECGSTC 1967, Ansfield and Cuerri 1963, Young et al. 1960, Moertel and Reitemeier 1969)
FUDR	226	51	23	(Ansfield and Cuerri 1963, Young et al. 1960, Moertel and Reitemeier 1969, Somal et al. 1978, Moertel 1978a)
Ftorafur	111	14	13	(Ansfield et al. 1980, Buroker et al. 1977b, 1979)
Methotrexate	95	13	14	(ECGSTC 1967, Moertel et al. 1970, Sullivan et al. 1967)
PALA	84	1	1	(Carroll et al. 1980, Van Echo et al. 1980)
Baker's antifol	54	8	15	(McCreary et al. 1977, Padilla et al. 1978)
AAFC*	54	2	4	(Kemeny et al. 1978, Alberto et al. 1978)

*AAFC = anhydro-ara-5-fluorocytidine

21 evaluable patients with large bowel cancer (Van Echo et al. 1980). Phase II trial at the Mayo Clinic using the 5-day q 6 weeks schedule resulted in one partial response in 17 evaluable patients with colorectal cancer (Eagan, personal communication). The observed antitumor activity of PALA alone seems to be inadequate to produce remissions in man. AAFC is an antimetabolite synthesized at the Memorial Sloan-Kettering Cancer Center. It has two possible mechanisms of action: as a DNA polymerase inhibitor like Ara-C, and as a thymidylate-synthetase inhibitor, like 5-FU. In a phase II study in patients with colorectal cancer, Kemeny and co-investigators observed only one minor response in 22 evaluable patients (Kemeny et al. 1978).

Table 3. *Efficacy of Other Antitumor Agents in Colorectal Cancer*

Treatment	Total No. Pts.	Response No. Pts.	%	References
Mitomycin C	257	50	19	(Crooke and Bradner 1976, Buroker et al. 1978a)
Methyl CCNU	244	27	11	(Douglass et al. 1976, 1978, Baker et al. 1976a, Moertel et al. 1976, Posey and Morgan 1977, Taylor et al. 1979)
Anguidine	161	6	4	(Murphy et al. 1978, Adler et al. 1979, Diggs et al. 1978, Bukowski et al. 1980)
VP-16-213	157	6	4	(Perry et al. 1976, Issell and Crooke 1979, Radice et al. 1979, Douglass et al. 1979b)
ICRF-159	120	8	7	(Moertel 1975a, Paul et al. 1979, Douglass et al. 1979a, Bellet et al. 1976)
BCNU	105	15	14	(Moertel et al. 1976)
CCNU	103	9	9	(Moertel et al. 1976)
AMSA	98	1	1	(Leichman et al. 1980, McNamee et al. 1980)
DTIC	84	7	8	(Slavik 1976)
Methyl GAG	73	4	5	(Knight et al. 1980, Killen et al. 1980)
Vindesine	71	6	8	(Bedikian et al. 1979a, Carroll et al. 1979, Rossof et al. 1979, Stambaugh 1980)
Chlorozotocin	59	2	3	(Hoth et al. 1978, Talley et al. 1979)
Dianhydrogalactitol	53	2	4	(Perry et al. 1976, De Jager et al. 1979)
Cis-platinum	51	0	0	(Kovach et al. 1973, Somal et al. 1978)

Many other chemotherapeutic agents have been evaluated for activity against colorectal cancer (Table 3); of these only carmustine (BCNU), methyl CCNU, and mitomycin have shown consistent activity and have been extensively used in combination with 5-FU. Lomustin (CCNU), DTIC, ICRF-159 (a nonpolar derivative of ethylenediaminotetraacetic acid) and vindesine (desacetyl vinblastine amide sulfate, a derivative of vinblastine) have shown only modest activity in patients refractory to 5-FU. Recently, several new antitumor agents were evaluated in patients with colorectal cancer refractory to 5-FU-containing regimens. Anguidine (protein synthesis inhibitor), VP-16-213 (a semi-synthetic product derived from podophyllotoxin), chlorozotocin, methyl GAG (polyamine synthesis inhibitor), and dianhydrogalactitol (a diepoxide) had minimal activity, while AMSA (a new acridine derivative) and cis-platinum had no activity against large bowel cancer. These results may not predict activity when the drugs are administered to patients with no prior exposure to chemotherapy. Several new antitumor agents have been inadequately evaluated in managing colorectal cancer (Table 4). A recently completed phase II trial with PCNU in our institution resulted in objective tumor regressions in 6 of 28 evaluable patients with colorectal cancer (Bedikian, unpublished data). Two patients achieved partial responses. Although the hematologic toxicity of PCNU was similar to that of other nitrosoureas, the gastrointestinal toxicities were remarkably milder. Metoprine is a lipid soluble inhibitor of dihydrofolate reductase. Phase II trial with metoprine in 24 patients with advanced colorectal cancer has resulted in two partial responses lasting 5+ and 6+ months (Lynch et al. 1980). Low response rates obtained with PCNU and metoprine should not be a deterrent to proceeding with further evaluation of these agents in untreated patients with advanced colorectal cancer.

None of the previously mentioned chemotherapeutic agents used alone consistently produces response rates above 30% or significantly prolongs

Table 4. *Efficacy of New Antitumor Agents in Colorectal Cancer*

Treatment	Total No. Pts.	Response No. Pts.	%	References
Diglycoaldehyde	35	1	3	(Douglass et al. 1979b)
PCNU*	33	4	12	(Friedman et al. 1980, Stewart et al. 1980)
Bruceantin	24	0	0	(Bedikian et al. 1979b)
Metoprine	24	2	8	(Lynch et al. 1980)
Maytansine	23	0	0	(Blum et al. 1978, Ravry et al. 1980)
9-HME†	16	0	0	(Clarysse et al. 1980)
Neocarzinostatin	8	0	0	(Issell et al. 1979)
VM-26	6	0	0	(Radice et al. 1979)

*PCNU = 1-(2-chloroethyl)-3-(2,6-dioxo-3-piperidyl)-1-nitrosourea
†9-HME = 9-hydroxy-methyl-ellipticinium

Table 5. *Reported Response Rates with 5-Fluorouracil-Methyl CCNU Combination in Colorectal Cancer*

References	Total No. Pts.	Response No. Pts.	%
(Baker et al. 1976b)	142	45	32
(Buroker et al. 1978b)	133	21	16
(Engstrom et al. 1980)	88	9	10
(Moertel 1978a)	61	10	16
(Lokich et al. 1977)	52	2	4
(Kane et al. 1978)	36	6	17
(Posey and Morgan 1977)	35	14	40
(Ravry 1977)	21	3	14
(Fischetti et al. 1978)	20	2	10
(Berman et al. 1978)	14	3	21
(Mario et al. 1979)	12	2	17

duration of survival of patients with colorectal carcinoma. Recent evidence indicates that even the available drug combinations produce only a modest increase in response rates without affecting the survival duration of patients with colorectal cancer. The most frequently used two-drug combination is 5-FU with methyl CCNU (Table 5). The response rate to this combination in 11 studies including 614 patients varied from 4% to 40%, with an overall response rate of 19%. The 5-FU-mitomycin C combination, although less extensively evaluated (Table 6), has similar degrees of efficacy and hematologic toxicity. A recent comparative study by the Southwest Oncology Group, in which random patients received a 96-hour infusion of 5-FU in combination with either methyl CCNU or mitomycin C, showed no difference in response rate and survival time between the two regimens, as indicated by response rates of 16% and 18%, respectively, and median survival times of 43 weeks each (Buroker et al. 1978b).

Addition of antitumor agents to the fluorinated pyrimidine-methyl CCNU or mitomycin C 2-drug regimens did not result in an increase in response rate. The 5-FU-methyl CCNU-vincristine chemotherapy regimen has been the most extensively evaluated 3-drug combination (Table 7). The pilot study from the Mayo Clinic with this regimen reported a response rate of 43%

Table 6. *Reported Response Rates with 5-Fluorouracil-Mitomycin C Combination in Colorectal Cancer*

References	Total No. Pts.	Response No. Pts.	%
(Buroker et al. 1978b)	136	25	18
(Krauss et al. 1979)	24	8	33
(Reitemeier et al. 1970)	17	3	18

Table 7. *Reported Response Rates with 5-Fluorouracil-Methyl CCNU-Vincristine Combination in Colorectal Cancer*

References	Total No. Pts.	Response No. Pts.	%
(Moertel 1978a)	137	37	27
(Kemeny et al. 1980b, 1979)	90	9	10
(Engstrom et al. 1980)	81	10	12
(Joss et al. 1979)	52	6	11
(Falkson and Falkson 1976)	46	17	37
(Ravry 1977)	25	10	40
(Stone et al. 1977)	21	1	5
(Pratt et al. 1976)	9	4	44

Table 8. *Efficacy of Other Fluorinated Pyrimidine-Nitrosourea Containing Regimens in Colorectal Cancer*

Treatment	Total No. Pts.	Response No. Pts.	%	References
5-FU + methyl CCNU + vincristine + streptozotocin	105	34	32	(Kemeny et al. 1980a, 1980b)
Ftorafur + methyl CCNU	91	13	14	(Buroker et al. 1977a, 1978c, Belt and Stephens 1979, Diggs et al. 1977)
5-FU + methyl CCNU + DTIC	83	14	17	(Engstrom et al. 1980)
5-FU + methyl CCNU + DTIC + vincristine	71	11	15	(Engstrom et al. 1980)
5-FU + CCNU + cyclophosphamide	61	9	15	(Bedikian et al. 1978, White et al. 1980)
5-FU + BCNU + DTIC + vincristine	61	19	31	(van Eyben et al. 1976, Falkson et al. 1974)
5-FU + BCNU + vincristine	47	12	26	(Luporini et al. 1980)
Ftorafur + methyl CCNU + methotrexate	38	8	21	(Valdivieso and Mavligit 1978)
5-FU + CCNU + vincristine	35	8	23	(Ratkin et al. 1977)
5-FU + methyl CCNU + Baker's antifol	31	6	19	(Shaw and Heilbrun 1979)
5-FU + BCNU	28	2	7	(Moertel et al. 1976, Lokich and Skarin, 1972)
5-FU + methyl CCNU + daunomycin	27	5	19	(Perry et al. 1978)

(Moertel et al. 1978b). However, with increased patient accrual, the overall response rate fell to 27% (Moertel 1978a). Other investigators using the same schedule of administration of the three drugs have obtained response rates ranging from 10% to 12% (Kemeny et al. 1980b, 1979, Engstrom et al. 1980). In fact, the response rate with this triple-drug regimen has varied from 5% to 44% (Pratt et al. 1976, Stone et al. 1977). Other multiple drug regimens based on 5-FU-methyl CCNU combinations thus far have shown no significant advantage (Table 8). The 5-FU-methyl CCNU-vincristine-streptozotocin combination was based on the observation that methyl CCNU administered in divided doses over five days was associated with a marked reduction of gastrointestinal toxicity, and that streptozotocin, a nitrosourea with little myelosuppressive effect, could safely be given in combination with the three-drug regimen. Overall, two successive studies utilizing the four-drug regimen gave three complete and 31 partial responses in 105 evaluable patients (Kemeny et al. 1980a, 1980b). In addition, the overall duration of survival of patients on the four-drug regimen was significantly longer than that of patients treated with the three-drug regimen by the same investigators, i.e., 11 versus 9 months, respectively ($p = 0.003$). Improvement in the response rate and duration of survival with the 5-FU-methyl CCNU-vincristine-streptozotocin combination awaits confirmation. Similarly, multiple drug regimens based on the 5-FU-mitomycin combination have failed to improve the response rate obtained by the two-drug regimens (Table 9).

These results indicate that progress in the chemotherapy of advanced colorectal cancer will depend on the discovery of new active agents and the judicious use of the available drugs, based on a better understanding of the

Table 9. *Efficacy of Other Fluorinated Pyrimidine-Mitomycin C Containing Regimens in Colorectal Cancer*

Treatment	Total No. Pts.	Response No. Pts.	%	References
5-FU + mitomycin C + Ara C	73	17	23	(De Jager et al. 1976, Ota et al. 1972, Yagoda et al. 1974)
5-FU + mitomycin C + Adriamycin	56	6	11	(Haller et al. 1978, Kessinger et al. 1979)
5-FU + mitomycin C + Adriamycin + Ara C	54	9	17	(Davis and Park 1978)
Ftorafur + mitomycin C	37	8	22	(Buroker 1978c, 1977a)
5-FU + mitomycin C + methotrexate	22	1	5	(Biran and Sulkes 1980)
5-FU + mitomycin C + methotrexate + vincristine	19	8	42	(Beck et al. 1980)

Table 10. *PALA + 5-FU Chemotherapy Study Design*

| | | RANDOMIZE | | |
| | | Single Dose Weekly | | 5 Daily Doses q 4 weeks |
	Dose levels	PALA g/m^2	5-FU mg/m^2	PALA g/m^2/day	5-FU mg/m^2/day
	+1	2.5	600	1.0	500
Initial doses →	—	2.0	480	0.80	400
	−1	1.6	360	0.54	320
	−2	1.0	240	0.40	200

biochemical interactions of the chemotherapeutic agents with neoplastic and normal tissues. The need for systematic evaluation of the new antitumor agents for activity against colorectal cancer does not need further emphasis. Recently, preclinical studies indicated success in enhancing the antitumor activity of 5-FU, as reflected by increased incorporation of 5-FU into RNA when PALA or thymidine is administered with 5-FU (Ardalan et al. 1980, Collins and Stark 1971, Kufe 1980). The efficacy of the modulation of 5-FU activity with metabolites and antimetabolites in man is currently under investigation. Recently, we completed evaluation of a PALA-5-FU combination in patients with colorectal cancer. Fifty previously untreated patients were randomized to receive single doses of PALA and 5-FU either weekly, as long as the patient responded to treatment, or daily for 5 days every 4 weeks. The starting and subsequent doses of both drugs on either regimen were as shown in Table 10. The dose of 5-FU was equivalent on both regimens. During a four-week treatment period, the dose of PALA on the weekly schedule was equal to twice the dose administered on the 5-day schedule. On both schedules, the daily dose of PALA was administered intravenously over 1 hour; the 5-FU was administered intravenously, over 30 minutes, 3 hours after completion of the PALA dose. Unfortunately, the 14% response rate obtained with the PALA-5-FU regimen is very modest and presents no advantage over that seen with 5-FU alone (Table 11). There was no significant difference in duration of

Table 11. *Responses to PALA + 5-FU by Treatment Schedule*

	Weekly	5-Day
No. evaluable patients	24	26
Partial responses	4	3
Stabilization of disease	15	12
Progression of disease	5	11

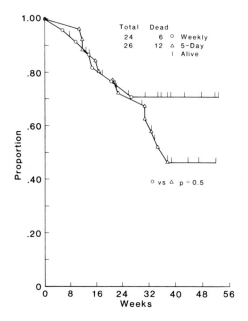

FIG. 1. Duration of survival of patients treated with PALA + 5-FU combination, by treatment schedule.

survival between patients on the weekly regimen and those on the 5-day regimen (Figure 1). Currently, we are evaluating the activity of a PALA-thymidine-5-FU three-drug combination in patients with malignant tumors of the gastrointestinal tract. In view of absence of in vitro and animal tumor models predictive of antitumor activity of drugs against colorectal cancer in humans, there is a need for systematic evaluation of antitumor agents alone or in combination to determine their efficacy against colorectal cancer.

The role of adjuvant chemotherapy after colonic resection has not been well defined to date. In contrast to the positive reports from several investigators, the results of prospective randomized controlled studies have failed to show conclusively that adjuvant chemotherapy in patients with colorectal carcinoma has had any major effect. Perhaps as more effective multidrug regimens for metastatic disease are developed, better results with adjuvant chemotherapy will be obtained.

In summary, this review shows that chemotherapy for colorectal cancer is at an early stage of development. Although a few multidrug regimens have produced tumor regressions in a small fraction of patients, prolongation of survival in responding patients has been short, failing to influence the overall survival to any significant degree. However, occasional patients do obtain substantial benefit. Thus, chemotherapy should be attempted, and there should be systematic trials of new antitumor agents to find regimens capable of favorably influencing patient survival.

ACKNOWLEDGMENTS

This investigation was supported by Contract number NO1-CM-57042 and Grant number CA-05831, awarded by the National Cancer Institute, Department of Health and Human Services.

REFERENCES

Adler, S., S. Lowenbraun, R. Jarrell, A. Bartolucci, P. Arena, and The Southeast Cancer Study Group. 1979. Study of anguidine (A, NSC-141537) by continuous infusion (CI) for treatment of solid tumors. Proc. ASCO 20:306.

Alberto, P., M. Rozenweig, D. Gangji, A. Brugarolas, F. Cavalli, P. Siegenthaler, H. H. Hansen, and R. Sylvester. 1978. Phase II study of anhydro-ara-5-fluorocytidine in adenocarcinoma of gastrointestinal tract, epidermoid carcinoma of lung, head and neck, breast carcinoma and small cell anaplastic carcinoma of lung: A study report of the E.O.R.T.C. early clinical trial cooperative group. Eur. J. Cancer 14:195–201.

Ansfield, F. J. 1975. A randomized phase II study of four dosages of 5-fluorouracil. Preliminary report. AACR 16:224.

Ansfield, F. J., and A. R. Cuerri. 1963. Further clinical comparison between 5-fluorouracil (5-FU) and 5-fluoro-2-deoxyuridine (5-FUDR). Cancer Chemother. Rep. 32:101–105.

Ansfield, F. J., G. Kallas, J. Singson, and B. Uy. 1980. Further phase I–II studies with oral Tegafur (T. Ftorafur). Proc. ASCO 21:347.

Ardalan, B., R. Glazer, T. Kensler, H. Jayaram, D. Cooney, and J. MacDonald. 1980. Biochemical mechanisms for the synergism of 5-fluorouracil (5-FU) and phosphonoacetyl-L-aspartate (PALA) in human mammary carcinoma cells. Proc. ASCO 21:8.

Baker, L. H., R. M. Izbicki, and V. K. Vaitkevicius. 1976a. Phase II study of porfiromycin vs. mitomycin C utilizing acute intermittent schedules. Med. Pediatr. Oncol. 2:207–213.

Baker, L. H., R. W. Talley, R. Matter, D. E. Lehane, B. W. Ruffner, S. E. Jones, F. S. Morrison, R. L. Stephens, G. E. Gehan, and V. K. Vaitkevicius. 1976b. Phase II comparison of the treatment of advanced gastrointestinal cancer with bolus weekly 5-FU vs. methyl CCNU plus bolus weekly 5-FU. Cancer 38:1–6.

Bateman, J., L. Irwin, R. Pugh, F. Cassidy, J. Weiner, and Western Cancer Study Group. 1975. Comparison of intravenous (IV) and oral (PO) administration of 5-fluorouracil (5-FU) for colorectal carcinoma. Proc. AACR 16:242.

Beck, T. M., N. E. Hart, and C. E. Smith. 1980. Treatment of colorectal carcinoma with combination chemotherapy. Proc. ASCO 21:342.

Bedikian, A. Y., R. Staab, R. Livingston, M. Valdivieso, M. A. Burgess, and G. P. Bodey. 1978. Chemotherapy for colorectal cancer with 5-fluorouracil, cyclophosphamide and CCNU. Comparison of oral and continuous IV administration of 5-fluorouracil. Cancer Treat. Rep. 62:1603–1605.

Bedikian, A. Y., M. Valdivieso, G. P. Bodey, W. K. Murphy, and E. J Freireich. 1979a. Phase II evaluation of videsine in the treatment of colorectal and esophageal tumors. Cancer Chemother. Pharmacol. 2:263–266.

Bedikian, A. Y., M. Valdivieso, G. P. Bodey, W. K. Murphy, and E. J Freireich. 1979b. Initial clinical studies with Bruceantin. Cancer Treat. Rep. 63:1843–1847.

Bellet, R. E., P. F. Engstrom, R. B. Castalano, R. H. Creech, and M. J. Mastrangelo. 1976. Phase II study of ICRF-159 in patients with metastatic colorectal carcinoma previously exposed to systemic chemotherapy. Cancer Treat. Rep. 60:1395–1397.

Belt, R. J., and R. Stephens. 1979. Phase I–II study of ftorafur and methyl CCNU in advanced colorectal cancer. Cancer 44:869–872.

Berman, R., G. R. Giles, A. Malhotra, G. G. Bird, P. D. Gajjar, G. A. Bunch, and R. Hall. 1978. Randomized trial of melphalan plus 5-fluorouracil (5-FU) vs. methyl CCNU plus 5-FU in patients with advanced colorectal cancer. Cancer Treat. Rep. 62:457–460.

Biran, H., and A. Sulkes. 1980. FMM:5-fluorouracil (F) methotrexate (MTX) and mitomycin C (MMC). A phase II study in advanced colorectal cancer. Proc. ASCO 21:339.

Blum, R. H., B. R. Wittenburg, G. P. Canellos, R. J. Mayer, A. T. Skarin, I. C. Henderson, L. M. Parker, and E. Frei, III. 1978. A therapeutic trial of maytansine. Cancer Clin. Trials 1:113–117.

Bukowski, R. M., C. B. Vaughn, J. Hampton, and W. J. Stuckey. 1980. Anguidine in gastrointestinal malignancies. SWOG phase II. Proc. ASCO 21:352.

Buroker, T., L. Baker, J. Correa, L. A. Schwartz, and V. K. Vaitkevicius. 1977a. Phase I trial of ftorafur combined with mitomycin C or methyl CCNU in gastrointestinal cancer. Cancer Treat. Rep. 61:463–467.

Buroker, T. R., P. N. Kim, L. Baker, V. Ratanatharathorn, B. Wojtaszak, and V. K. Vaitkevicius. 1978a. Mitomycin C alone or in combination with infused 5-fluorouracil in the treatment of disseminated gastrointestinal carcinomas. Med. Pediatr. Oncol. 4:35–42.

Buroker, T., P. N. Kim, C. Groppe, J. McCracken, R. O'Bryan, F. Panettiere, C. Coltman, R. Bottomley, H. Wilson, J. Bonnet, T. Thigpen, V. K. Vaitkevicius, B. Hoogstraten, and L. Heilbrun. 1978b. 5-FU infusion mitomycin C vs. 5-FU infusion with methyl CCNU in the treatment of advanced colon cancer. Cancer 42:1228–1233.

Buroker, T., A. Miller, L. Baker, M. McKenzie, M. Samson, and V. K. Vaitkevicius. 1977b. Phase II clinical trial of ftorafur in 5-fluorouracil refractory colorectal cancer. Cancer Treat. Rep. 61:1579–1580.

Buroker, T., F. Padilla, C. Groppe, G. Guy, J. Quagliana, J. McCracken, V. K. Vaitkevicius, B. Hoogstraten and L. Heilbrun. 1979. Phase II evaluation of ftorafur in previously untreated colorectal cancer. Cancer 44:48–51.

Buroker, T., B. Wojtaszak, A. Dindrogru, M. DeMattia, L. Baker, C. Groth and V. K. Vaitkevicius. 1978c. Phase II trial of ftorafur with mitomycin C vs. ftorafur with methyl CCNU in untreated colorectal cancer. Cancer Treat. Rep. 62:689–692.

Carroll, D., R. J. Gralla, and N. Kemeny. 1979. Phase II evaluation of vindesine in patients with colorectal carcinoma. Cancer Treat. Rep. 63:2097–2098.

Carroll, D., R. J. Gralla, and N. E. Kemeny. 1980. Phase II evaluation of N-(phosphonacetyl)-L-aspartic acid (PALA) in patients with advanced colorectal carcinoma. Cancer Treat. Rep. 64:349–351.

Clarysse, A., A. Brugerolas, P. Siegenthaler, R. De Jager, F. Cavalli, P. Alberto, and H. Hansen. 1980. Phase II study of 9-hydroxy-methyl-ellipticinum (9-HME) in advanced solid tumors. Proc. ASCO 21:348.

Collins, K. D., and G. R. Stark. 1971. Aspartate transcarbamylase interaction with transition state analogue N-(phosphonacetyl)-L-aspartate. J. Biol. Chem. 246:6599–6605.

Crooke, S. T., and W. T. Bradner. 1976. Mitomycin C. A Review. Cancer Treat. Rev. 3:121–139.

Davis, S. M., and Y. K. Park. 1978. Chemotherapy for colorectal cancer with combination of 5-fluorouracil, mitomycin C, Adriamycin and cytosine: A pilot study. Cancer Treat. Rep. 62:1557–1559.

De Jager, R., A. Brugarolas, H. Hansen, F. Cavalli, H. Russell, P. Siegenthaler, A. Clarysse, A. Renard, J. Kenis, and P. Alberto. 1979. Dianhydrogalactitol (NSC-132313) Phase II study in solid tumors. Eur. J. Cancer 15:971–974.

De Jager, R. L., G. B. Magill, R. B. Goldbey, and I. H. Krakoff. 1976. Combination chemotherapy with mitomycin C, 5-fluorouracil, and cytosine arabinoside in gastrointestinal cancer. Cancer Treat. Rep. 60:1373–1375.

Diggs, C. H., M. J. Scoltock, and P. H. Wiernik. 1978. Phase II evaluation of anguidine (NSC-141537) for adenocarcinoma of the colon. Cancer Clin. Trials 1:297–299.

Diggs, C. H., P. H. Wiernik, and A. C. Smythe. 1977. IV methyl CCNU and ftorafur with or without methanol extracted residue of BCG for metastatic adenocarcinoma of the colon. Cancer Treat. Rep. 61:1581–1583.

Douglass, H. O., Jr., J. Kaufman, P. F. Engstrom, D. J. Klaassen, and P. P. Carbone for the Eastern Cooperative Oncology Group (ECOG). 1979a. Single agent chemotherapy of advanced colorectal cancer with ICRF-159, Yoshi-864, piperazinedione (PZD), CCNU, actinomycin D (DACT), L-PAM or methotrexate (MTX). Proc. ASCO 20:434.

Douglass, H. O., Jr., P. T. Lavin, A. Mittleman, and P. P. Carbone. 1979b. Phase II evaluation of Diglycoaldehyde, VP-16-213 and combination of methyl CCNU and β-2-Deoxythioguanosine in previously treated patients with colorectal cancer: An Eastern Cooperative Oncology Group Study (EST—1275). Cancer Treat. Rep. 63:1355–1357.

Douglass, H. O., Jr., P. T. Lavin, and C. G. Moertel. 1976. Nitrosoureas: Useful agents for the treatment of advanced gastrointestinal cancer. Cancer Treat. Rep. 60:769–779.

Douglass, H. O., Jr., P. T. Lavin, J. Woll, J. F. Conroy, and P. P. Carbone. 1978. Chemotherapy of advanced measurable colon and rectal carcinoma with oral 5-fluorouracil alone or combination with cyclophosphamide or 6-thioguanine, with intravenous 5-fluorouracil or beta-2-deoxy-thioguanosine or with oral 3(4-methyl-cyclohexyl)-1(2-chloroethyl)-1-nitrosourea. Cancer 42:2538–2545.

Eastern Cooperative Group in Solid Tumor Chemotherapy. 1967. Comparison of antimetabolite in the treatment of breast and colon cancer. JAMA 200:770–778.

Engstrom, P., J. MacIntyre, H. Douglass, Jr., and P. Carbone, for Eastern Cooperative Oncology Group. 1980. Combination chemotherapy of advanced bowel cancer. Proc. ASCO 21:384.

Falkson, G., and H. C. Falkson. 1976. Fluorouracil, methyl CCNU and vincristine in cancer of the colon. Cancer 38:1468–1470.

Falkson, G., E. B. van Eden, and H. C. Falkson. 1974. Fluorouracil, dimethyl triazeno, imidazole carboxamide, vincristine and bis-chlorethyl nitrosourea in colon cancer. Cancer 33:1207–1209.

Fischetti, M. R., R. W. Carey, S. A. Weitzman, S. Kaufman, R. M. Kelley, and W. D. Sohier. 1978. Treatment of advanced colorectal cancer with a combination of 5-fluorouracil and methyl CCNU. Med. Pediatr. Oncol. 4:271–278.

Friedman, M. A., V. A. Levin, and S. K. Carter. 1980. Phase I toxicity and pharmacology study of PCNU. Proc. ASCO 21:184.

Hahn, R. G., C. G. Moertel, A. J. Schutt, and H. H. Bruckner. 1975. A double blind comparison of intensive course 5-fluorouracil by oral versus intravenous route in the treatment of colorectal carcinoma. Cancer 35:1031–1035.

Haller, D. G., P. V. Woolley, J. S. Macdonald, L. F. Smith, Jr., and P. S. Schein. 1978. Phase II trial of 5-fluorouracil, Adriamycin and mitomycin C in advanced colorectal cancer. Cancer Treat. Rep. 62:563–565.

Hartman, H. A., Jr., A. Kessinger, H. M. Lemon, and J. F. Foley. 1979. 5-day continuous infusion of 5-fluorouracil for advanced colorectal, gastric and pancreatic adenocarcinoma. J. Surg. Oncol. 11:227–238.

Hoth, D., T. Butler, S. Winokur, A. Kales, P. Woolley, and P. Schein. 1978. Phase II study of chlorozotocin. Proc. ASCO 19:381.

Issell, B. F., and S. T. Crooke. 1979. Etoposide (VP-16-213). Cancer Treat. Rep. 6:107–124.

Issell, B. F., A. W. Prestayko, R. L. Comis, and S. T. Crooke. 1979. Zinostatin (neocarzinostatin). Cancer Treat. Rev. 6:239–249.

Joss, R. A., R. S. Goldberg, and J. W. Yates. 1979. Combination chemotherapy of colorectal cancer with 5-fluorouracil, methyl 1,3-cis(2-chloroethyl)-1-nitrosourea and vincristine. Med. Pediatr. Oncol. 7:251–255.

Kane, R. C., M. R. Cashdollar, and A. M. Bernath. 1978. Treatment of advanced colorectal cancer with methyl CCNU plus 5-day 5-fluorouracil infusion. Cancer Treat. Rep. 62:1521–1525.

Kemeny, N., A. Yagoda, D. Braun, Jr., and R. Goldbey. 1979. A randomized study of two different schedules of methyl CCNU (meCCNU), 5-fluorouracil (5-FU) and vindesine (VCR) for metastatic colorectal carcinoma. Cancer 43:78–82.

Kemeny, N., A. Yagoda, D. Braun, and R. Goldbey. 1980a. Therapy for metastatic colorectal carcinoma with combination of methyl-CCNU, 5-fluorouracil, vincristine and streptozotocin (MOF-strep). Cancer 45:876–888.

Kemeny, N., A. Yagoda, and J. H. Burchanal. 1978. Phase II study of 2,2′anhydro-1-β-arabinofuranosyl-5-fluorocytosine in advanced colorectal carcinoma. Cancer Treat. Rep. 62:463–464.

Kemeny, N., A. Yagoda, and R. A. Goldbey. 1980b. Prospective randomized study of methyl CCNU 5-fluorouracil and vincristine (MOF) plus streptozotocin (MOF-strep) in patients with metastatic colorectal cancer. Proc. ASCO 21:417.

Kessinger, M. A., J. F. Foley, and H. M. Lemon. 1979. Adriamycin, mitomycin C and 5-fluorouracil in combination for advanced colorectal adenocarcinoma previously treated with 5-fluorouracil. Cancer Clinical Trials 2:317–319.

Killen, J., D. Hoth, F. P. Smith, P. S. Schein, and P. V. Woolley. 1980. Methyl gloxal bis-guanyl hydrazone (NSC-32946) (Methyl GAG) phase II experience and clinical pharmacology. Proc. ASCO 21:368.

Knight, W. A., R. B. Livingston, J. Costanzi, and R. Pague. 1980. Methyl-gloxal bis-guanyl hydrazone (Methyl-GAG, MCBG) in advanced colon carcinoma. Proc. ASCO 21:164.

Kovach, J. S., C. G. Moertel, A. J. Schutt, R. G. Reitemeier, and R. G. Hahn. 1973. Phase II study of cis-diamminechloroplatinum (NSC-1198/5) in advanced carcinoma of the large bowel. Cancer Chemother. Rep. 57(1):357–359.

Krauss, S., T. Sonoda, and A. Solomon. 1979. Treatment of advanced gastrointestinal cancer with 5-fluorouracil and mitomycin C. Cancer 43:1598–1603.

Kufe, D. 1980. Metabolic enhancement of 5-fluorouracil (5-FU) incorporation into human cell RNA. Proc. AACR 21:265.

Leichman, L., T. R. Buroker, R. M. O'Bryan, and L. H. Baker. 1980. A phase II trial of AMSA in disseminated adenocarcinoma of the colon and rectum. Proc. ASCO 21:355.

Lokich, J. J., and A. T. Skarin. 1972. Combination therapy with 5-fluorouracil (5-FU) and 1,3,bis(2-chloroethyl)1-1-nitrosourea (BCNU) for disseminated gastrointestinal carcinoma. Cancer Chemother. Rep. 56:653–657.

Lokich, J. J., A. T. Skarin, R. J. Mayer, and E. Frei, III. 1977. Lack of effectiveness of combined 5-fluorouracil and methyl CCNU therapy in advanced colorectal cancer. Cancer 40:2792–2796.

Luporini, G., R. Labianca, P. Fraschini, and L. Tedeschi. 1980. Evaluation of combination with BCNU, vincristine and 5-fluorouracil in the treatment of disseminated neoplasia of the large intestine. Minerva Med. 41(10):773–779.

Lynch, G., N. Kemeny, R. Gralla, V. Currie, and C. Young. 1980. Phase II trial of metoprine in patients with colorectal carcinoma and non-small cell lung carcinoma. Proc. ASCO 21:351.

Macdonald, J. S., D. F. Kisner, T. Smythe, P. V. Woolley, L. Smith, Jr., and P. S. Schein. 1976. 5-Fluorouracil (5-FU), methyl CCNU, and vincristine in the treatment of advanced colorectal cancer: phase II study utilizing weekly 5-FU. Cancer Treat. Rep. 60:1597–1600.

Mario, J. R., R. Ravry, and M. Moore. 1979. Randomized comparison of 5-fluorouracil (FU) and semustine (S) vs. 5-fluorouracil, and DTIC in advanced gastrointestinal cancer (GICA). Proc. ASCO 20:277.

McCreary, R. H., C. G. Moertel, A. J. Schutt, M. J. O'Connell, R. G. Hahn, and R. J. Reitemeier. 1977. A phase II study of triazinate (NSC-139105) in advanced colorectal carcinoma. Cancer 40:9–13.

McNamee, R., J. C. Ruckdeschel, and J. Horton. 1980. Treatment of advanced large bowel cancer with M-AMSA. A GITSC pilot study. Proc. ASCO 21:420.

Moertel, C. G. 1975a. Clinical management of advanced gastrointestinal cancer. Cancer 36:675–682.

Moertel, C. G. 1978a. Current concepts in cancer chemotherapy of gastrointestinal cancer. N. Engl. J. Med. 299:1049–1052.

Moertel, C. G. 1978b. Cancer of the large bowel. Topics in Cancer. New York, Physicians Program Inc. Lesson 15, pp. 1–8.

Moertel, C. G., and R. J. Reitemeier, Eds. 1969. Advanced Gastrointestinal Cancer: Clinical Management and Chemotherapy. Harper and Row, New York, pp. 86–118.

Moertel, C. G., R. J. Reitemeier, and R. G. Hahn. 1970. Oral methotrexate therapy of gastrointestinal carcinoma. Surg. Gynecol. Obstet. 130:292–294.

Moertel, C. G., A. J. Schutt, R. G. Hahn, and R. J. Reitemeier. 1975b. Therapy of advanced gastrointestinal cancer with a combination of 5-FU, methyl-1,3-cis(2-chloroethyl)-1-nitrosourea and vincristine. J. Natl. Cancer Inst. 54:69–71.

Moertel, C. G., A. J. Schutt, R. J. Reitemeier, and R. G. Hahn. 1976. Therapy of gastrointestinal cancer with the nitrosoureas alone and in combination. Cancer Treat. Rep. 60:729–732.

Moore, G. E., I. D. J. Bross, and R. Ausman. 1968. Effects of 5-fluorouracil (NSC-19893) in 390 patients with cancer. Cancer Chemother. Rep. 52:641–653.

Murphy, W. K., M. A. Burgess, M. Valdivieso, and G. P. Bodey. 1978. Anguidine: An early phase II study in colorectal adenocarcinoma. Proc. ASCO 19:411.

Nadler, S. H., and G. E. Moore. 1968. A clinical study of fluorouracil. Surg. Gynecol. Obstet. 127:1210–1214.

Ota, K., S. Kurita, M. Nashimura, M. Ogawa, Y. Kamei, K. Imai, Y. Ariyoshi, K. Kataoka, M. Murakami, A. Oyama, A. Hoshino, H. Amo, and T. Kato. 1972. Combination therapy with mitomycin C (NSC-26980), 5-fluorouracil (NSC-19893) and cytosine arabinoside (NSC-63878) for advanced cancer in man. Cancer Chemother. Rep. 56(3):373–385.

Padilla, F., J. Correa, T. Buroker, and V. K. Vaitkevicius. 1978. Phase II study of Baker's antifol in advanced colorectal cancer. Cancer Treat. Rep. 62:553–554.

Paul, A. R., P. F. Engstrom, and R. B. Catalano. 1979. Phase III trial of Roxane (ICRF-159) vs. 5-fluorouracil (5-FU) in advanced metastatic colorectal carcinoma. Proc. ASCO 21:311.

Perry, M. C., C. G. Moertel, A. J. Schutt, R. J. Reitemeier, and R. G. Hahn. 1976. Phase II studies of dianhydrogalactitol and VP-16-213 in colorectal cancer. Cancer Treat. Rep. 60:1247–1250.

Perry, M. C., L. White, and C. Kardinal. 1978. 5-Fluorouracil, methyl CCNU and daunomycin in advanced colorectal adenocarcinoma. Proc. ASCO 19:328.

Posey, L. E., and L. R. Morgan. 1977. Methyl CCNU vs. methyl CCNU and 5-fluorouracil in carcinoma of the large bowel. Cancer Treat. Rep. 61:1453–1458.

Pratt, C. B., W. Terrell, and W. Shouks. 1976. Carcinoma of the colon in adolescents: Treatment with vincristine, methyl CCNU and 5-fluorouracil. Proc. ASCO 17:25.

Radice, P. A., P. A. Bunn, Jr., and D. C. Ihde. 1979. Therapeutic trial with VP-16-213 and VM 26. Active agents in small cell lung cancer, non-Hodgkin's lymphomas, and other malignancies. Cancer Treat. Rep. 63:1231–1240.

Ratkins, G., C. A. Presant, and J. L. Zeffren. 1977. Combination chemotherapy with 5-FU infusion in metastatic colorectal carcinoma. Proc. ASCO 18:322.

Ravry, M. J. R. 1977. Three different schedules of methyl CCNU (MMU) plus 5-fluorouracil (5-FU). Proc. ASCO 18:298.

Ravry, M. J., S. Lowenbraun, and R. Birch. 1980. A broad phase II evaluation of maytansine (MTS) in advanced solid tumors. Proc. ASCO 21:154.

Reitemeier, R. J., and C. G. Moertel. 1962. Comparison of rapid and slow intravenous administration of 5-fluorouracil in treating patients with adyanced carcinoma of the large intestine. Cancer Chemother. Rep. 30:1425–1428.

Reitemeier, R. J., C. G. Moertel, and R. G. Hahn. 1970. Combination chemotherapy in gastrointestinal cancer. Cancer Res. 30:1425–1428.

Rossof, A. H., G. Chandra, J. Wolter, and J. Showel. 1979. Phase II trial of vindesine (desacetyl vinblastine amide sulfate, VND) in advanced metastatic cancer. Proc. AACR 20:146.

Seifert, P., L. H. Baker, M. L. Reed, and V. K. Vaitkevicius. 1975. Comparison of continuously infused 5-fluorouracil with bolus injection in the treatment of patients with colorectal adenocarcinoma. Cancer 36:123–128.

Shaw, M. T., and L. K. Heilbrun. (For Southwest Oncology Group) 1979. Baker's antifol (BAF) in combination with methyl-CCNU and 5-fluorouracil (5-FU) for the treatment of metastatic colorectal cancer. Proc. ASCO 20:300.

Silverberg, E. 1979. Cancer statistics. CA 29:6–21.

Slavik, M. 1976. Clinical studies with DTIC (NSC-45388) in various malignancies. Cancer Treat. Rep. 60:213–214.

Somal, B., V. Vainutis, A. Singhakowinta, R. O'Bryan, T. Buroker, M. Samson, and L. Baker. 1978. Cis-diamminedichloroplatinum (CDDP) in advanced breast and colorectal carcinomas. Proc. ASCO 19:347.

Stambaugh, J. E. 1980. Vindesine (DVA) in the treatment of patients with advanced neoplastic disease. Proc. ASCO 21:344.

Stewart, D. J., R. S. Benjamin, M. Leavens, M. Valdivieso, M. A. Burgess, E. McKelvey, and G. P. Bodey. 1980. Phase I study of 1-(2-chloroethyl)-3-(2,6-dioxo-3-piperidyl)-1-nitrosourea (PCNU NSC-95466). Proc. ASCO 21:168.

Stone, L., T. M. Hoeltgen, C. P. Perlia, and J. Wolter. 1977. Combination chemotherapy of disseminated gastrointestinal adenocarcinoma with vincristine (VCR), methyl-CCNU, and 5-fluorouracil (5-FU). Proc. ASCO 18:326.

Sullivan, R. D., E. Miller, W. Z. Zurek, R. A. Oberfield, and Y. Ojima. 1967. Reevaluation of methotrexate as an anticancer drug. Surg. Gynecol. Obstet. 125:819–824.

Talley, R. W., R. W. Brownlee, L. H. Baker, N. A. Oberhauser, and K. Pitts. 1979. Chlorozotocin (CTZ) (NSC-178248), Phase II trial. Proc. ASCO 20:440.

Taylor, S. G., W. D. Dewys, C. P. Perlia, J. Wolter, R. E. Slayton, L. A. Kosoven, and J. D. Khandeker. 1979. A randomized comparison of two dosage schedules for methyl CCNU three-week versus six-week treatments. Cancer 44:824–830.

Valdivieso, M., and G. M. Mavligit. 1978. Chemotherapy and immunotherapy of colorectal cancer: Role of carcinoembryonic antigen. Surg. Clin. North Am. 58:619–631.

Van Echo, D. A., C. H. Diggs, M. Scoltock, and P. H. Wiernik. 1980. Phase II evaluation of N-(phosphonacetyl)-L-aspartic acid (PALA) in metastatic adenocarcinoma of the colon and rectum. Cancer Treat. Rep. 64:339–342.

Van Eyben, F. E., V. Larsen, and H. Pedersen. 1976. 5-Fluorouracil, DTIC, BCNU, and vincristine in advanced colorectal cancer. Cancer Treat. Rep. 60:21–32.

White, D. R., F. Richards, H. B. Muss, M. R. Cooper, and C. L. Spurr. 1980. Therapy of advanced colorectal carcinoma with 5-fluorouracil and cyclophosphamide in combination with either CCNU or methotrexate. Cancer 45:662–665.

Yagoda, A., A. Lippman, R. Winn, A. Rosenberg, and P. Schulman. 1974. Mitomycin C, 5-FU and cytosine arabinoside (miFuCa) in adenocarcinomas. Proc. ASCO 15:190.

Young, C. W., R. R. Ellison, R. D. Sullivan, S. N. Levick, R. Kaufman, E. Miller, I. Woldow, G. Escher, M. C. Li, D. A. Karnofsky, and J. L. Burchenal. 1960. The clinical evaluation of 5-fluorouracil and 5-fluoro-2′ deoxyuridine in solid tumors in adults. Cancer Chemother. Rep. 6:17–20.

Gastrointestinal Cancer, edited by
John R. Stroehlein and
Marvin M. Romsdahl.
Raven Press, New York © 1981.

Experience With A Two-Layer Soft Agar System for Growing Gastrointestinal Tumors

Matilda Perkins, M.D.,* and Daniel D. Von Hoff, M.D.†

*Departments of *Surgery, and †Medicine (Division of Oncology),
The University of Texas Health Science Center at San Antonio, San Antonio, Texas*

INTRODUCTION

In 1977 Hamburger and Salmon reported the use of a two-layer soft agar system to support the growth of human tumor stem cells in culture (Hamburger and Salmon 1977a, b). Their work followed previous success by Park et al. (1971) in culturing murine myeloma and that of other investigators working with tumors in pediatric patients (McAllister and Reed 1968, Altman et al. 1975). Since the initial report of Hamburger and Salmon, a variety of human tumors, including myeloma, ovarian carcinoma, neuroblastoma, melanoma, breast carcinoma, and lung carcinoma, have been shown to form colonies in this two-layer agar system (Von Hoff et al. 1980, Pollard et al. 1980, Sandbach et al. 1980, Meyskens and Salmon 1980, Hamburger et al. 1978). In retrospective studies using this system to assay chemosensitivity of human tumors, there has been a 70% accuracy for positive prediction (sensitivity) and a 94% accuracy for negative prediction (specificity) between in vitro responses and responses in patients (Von Hoff 1980, Salmon et al. 1978). This paper describes the growth of a variety of gastrointestinal tumors in the two-layer soft agar system.

MATERIALS AND METHODS

From September 1978 to September 1980, 93 pathologically proven tumor specimens originating from the gastrointestinal tract were evaluated. Of the 93 specimens, 50 were colorectal, 14 pancreatic, 13 gastric, seven hepatic, three esophageal, and one biliary. In addition, there were five miscellaneous, nonmalignant specimens. Specimens were obtained during routine diagnostic and therapeutic procedures in multiple hospitals within a 90-mile radius of the cloning laboratory. The specimens were secured by means of surgical excision, thoracentesis, or paracentesis and were handled with usual sterile techniques. Specimens of solid tumors were placed in a transport medium containing McCoy's 5a enriched medium with 10% fetal calf serum. Fluid specimens were collected in a variety of containers to which 100 units of preservative-free heparin was added per milliliter of fluid. Specimens arrived at the cloning laboratory within eight hours of collection and were handled and evaluated by personnel who had no prior knowledge of the pathologic determination or staging. Solid tumor specimens were processed and plated the same day, whereas the fluid specimens were processed and plated the following day.

Solid specimens were mechanically dissociated using iris scissors, a 0.3-mm sieve, and final passage through a 25 gauge needle until a single cell suspension was obtained. Fluid specimens were centrifuged to collect the cellular component. If bloody, fluids were washed with lysing buffer (containing ammonium chloride, potassium bicarbonate, and ethylenediaminotetraacetate (EDTA)) to remove red blood cells. All specimens were then washed and resuspended in Hank's balanced salt solution (HBSS). Cell counts were done using a hemocytometer. Viability was determined using tryphan blue dye exclusion. Viability was from zero to 100% (median 30%, mean 39%).

Cells were cultured as described by Hamburger and Salmon (1977a, b), but without the use of medium conditioned by adherent spleen cells of mineral oil primed BALB/c mice. Cells were suspended in 0.3% agar in enriched CMRL 1066 medium (Grand Island Biological Co.) supplemented with 15% horse serum, penicillin (100 units/ml), streptomycin (2 mg/ml), glutamine (2 mM), calcium chloride (4 mM), and insulin (3 units/ml). Immediately before plating, this medium was enriched with asparagine (0.6 mg/ml), DEAE-dextran (0.5 mg/ml) (Pharmacia Fine Chemical, Division of Pharmacia, Inc., Piscataway, N.J.), and 2-mercaptoethanol (final concentration 50 uM prepared within seven days). The final concentration of cells was 5×10^5 viable cells per milliliter of agar medium mixture, but not more than 2.5×10^6 total cells per milliliter in specimens with low viability. One milliliter of this cell-agar medium mixture was pipetted into 35–mm Petri dishes onto a previously made feeder layer. The feeder layer consisted of McCoy's 5a medium plus 15% heat-inactivated fetal calf serum and a variety of nutrients as described by Pike and Robinson (1970). Immediately before it was used, 40 ml of enriched McCoy's medium was further enriched with 10 ml of 3% tryptic soybroth (Grand Island Biological Co.), 0.6 ml asparagine, and 0.3 ml DEAE-dextran. Agar (0.5% final concentration) completed the ingredients for the feeder layer. After preparation of both layers, plates were incubated at 37°C in a 7.5% carbon dioxide 100% humidified atmosphere. All control specimens and drug-treated specimens were plated in triplicate.

Testing of drug sensitivity required specimens with a cell count of 3×10^6 or greater. One milliliter of cells with an optimal concentration of 1.5×10^6 viable cells/ml HBSS were incubated for one hour at 37°C with 0.15 ml of drug and 0.85 ml of HBSS. The final concentrations of drugs were those corresponding to one tenth of the attainable serum concentrations based on current clinical pharmacology data. At the end of one hour cells were washed with HBSS and plated as described above. Controls were incubated with 1 ml HBSS only.

Tamoxifen and vinblastine were not washed off after incubation and were therefore in continuous association with cells in culture.

At two to four weeks postplating, cultures were examined with a Zeiss inverted phase microscope at magnifications of 30, 75, and 120. Spherical aggregates of cells measuring more than 70 microns in diameter (greater than 20 cells) were considered colonies.

The histologic characteristics of the colonies growing in soft agar were assessed by means of slides prepared according to the method of Salmon and Buick (1979).

Whether or not carcinoembryonic antigen (CEA) was secreted by cloned cells was determined in colonies mechanically removed from the plates after final counting. Colonies were plucked using micropipettes and 27-gauge needles. Slides were made by fixing the cells in methanol. To allow observation of CEA, the slides were incubated with rabbit anti-human CEA (provided by Dr. Charles Todd, City of Hope National Medical Center, Duarte, California) for 45 minutes at 37°C in a humidified atmosphere. After three washings with phosphate buffered saline (PBS), the slides were incubated with fluorescein tagged goat anti-rabbit immunoglobulin G (IgG) (Cappel Laboratories, Cochranville, Pa.) for 30 minutes at 37°C in a humidified atmosphere. After being washed eight times with PBS, the slides were examined microscopically with a 540-nm ultraviolet source. To dissolve the agar the slides were soaked in xylene, ethanol, or 60-degree water from two to twenty minutes.

Plating efficiencies were determined by the following equation:

$$\left(\frac{\text{Number of colonies}}{\text{Total number of cells plated}} \times 100 \right)$$

Viable plating efficiencies were determined by the following equation:

$$\left(\frac{\text{Number of colonies}}{\text{Number of viable cells plated}} \times 100 \right)$$

Colorectal tumors were staged according to the classification of Dukes (1932). Growth was considered present if the average number of colonies in a control plate was five or more. Drug sensitivity was considered reliable if an average of 30 colonies or greater was present in control plates. Drugs were considered to be effective in vitro if there was a 70% or greater reduction in colonies in drug-treated plates compared to controls (Von Hoff 1980).

RESULTS

Colorectal Adenocarcinoma

Fifty specimens were evaluated; 41 (82%) grew and three (6%) were contaminated. Of the 50 specimens, 40 were solid tumors. Twenty-four specimens (48%) had an average of 30 or greater colonies per control plate and one or more drugs tested, i.e., were evaluable for drug sensitivity. Table 1

Table 1. *Correlation Between Origin of Tumor and Growth in Soft Agar*

Category	Origin of Tumor					
	Colorectal	Gastric	Pancreas	Hepatic	Esophagus	Biliary
Plated	50	13	14	7	3	1
Grew (>5 colonies)	41 (82%)	9 (69%)	10 (71%)	7 (100%)	2 (66%)	1 (100%)
Evaluable (>30 colonies and drugs tested)	24 (48%)	4 (30%)	6 (42%)	3 (42%)	2 (66%)	1 (100%)
Solid tumors	40	13	10	6	3	0
Grew (>5 colonies)	36 (90%)	9	7 (70%)	6 (100%)	2 (66%)	—
Evaluable (>30 colonies and drugs tested)	21 (52%)	4	4 (40%)	3 (50%)	2 (60%)	—
Fluid tumors	10	0	4	1	0	1
Grew (>5 colonies)	5 (50%)	—	3 (75%)	1 (100%)	—	1 (100%)
Evaluable (>30 colonies and drugs tested)	3 (30%)	—	2 (50%)	0	—	1 (100%)
Mean drugs evaluable	4.2	4.0	6.0	2.0	6.0	—
Median drugs evaluable	4	3	3	2	—	—

details the relationship between origin of specimens and growth. In four specimens the drugs were effective in vitro, i.e., there was a 70% or greater reduction in colonies compared with controls. Table 2 outlines specific drugs tested. The mean number of drugs evaluable per tumor specimen was 4.2, and the median, four.

Table 2. *In Vitro Results of Drug Testing in Colorectal Tumor Specimens*

Drug	mcg/ml Tested	In Vitro Responses/Number Tested
Conventional Agents		
Adriamycin	0.04	0/6
BCNU*	0.10	1/13
Cis-platinum†	0.20	0/1
5-Fluorouracil	6.0	2/19
Mitomycin C	0.10	0/12
6-Thioguanine	20.00	0/1
Tamoxifen	0.18	0/1
Vinblastine	0.05	0/1
Vincristine	0.01	0/1
Investigational Agents		
AMSA‡	0.50	0/2
CL216942§	0.01	0/8
DHAD//	0.05	0/7
ICRF187#	0.50	0/1
Interferon	1000.00+	1/16
MGBG"	10.00	0/1

*BCNU = 1,3-bis (β-chloroethyl)-1-nitrosourea; †Cis-platinum = cis-diamminedichloroplatinum II; ‡AMSA = 4'- ((9-acridinyl) amino) methane sulfon-in-anisidine; §CL216942 = anthracenedicarboxaldehyde derivative; //DHAD = dihydroxyanthracenedione; #ICRF187 = 2, 6-piperazinedione, 4,4' (1-methyl-1, 2 ethanediyl); "MGBG = methyl-GAG or methylglyoxalbisguanhydrazone; +Units per cc.

Gastric Adenocarcinoma

Thirteen solid specimens were evaluated. Nine (69%) grew. All of the specimens that did not grow had less than 0.24×10^6 viable cells per plate. Four specimens could be evaluated for drug sensitivity but in no specimen was the drug-induced decrease in colony count 70% or more. The mean number of drugs evaluable was four and the median, three. Table 3 notes the drugs tested for effectiveness against gastric tumors.

Pancreatic Adenocarcinoma and Islet Cell Carcinoma

Fourteen specimens were evaluated. Ten (71%) grew; seven of the 10 solid tumors grew and three of the four fluid specimens grew. Of the four that did not grow, three had less than 0.09×10^6 viable cells per plate. Six specimens were evaluable for drug sensitivity. In three different specimens one drug resulted in a 70% or greater colony reduction. Table 4 lists the drugs tested. The mean number of drugs evaluated was six and the median, three.

Hepatoma

Seven specimens were evaluated; six were solids and all grew. Three (43%) were evaluable for drug sensitivity. No drugs reduced the colony count by 70%. The mean and median drugs evaluable were two. The drugs that were evaluated are noted in Table 5.

Esophageal Squamous Cell Carcinoma

Three solid specimens were evaluated; two (66%) grew. Both specimens that grew were evaluable for drug sensitivity, but no drug was effective. The mean number of drugs evaluated in the two specimens was six. Conventional

Table 3. *In Vitro Results of Drug Testing in Gastric Tumor Specimens*

Drug	mcg/ml Tested	In Vitro Responses/Number Tested
Conventional Agents		
Adriamycin	0.04	0/2
BCNU	0.10	0/4
5-Fluorouracil	6.00	0/2
Mitomycin C	0.10	0/2
Vinblastine	0.05	0/1
Investigational Agents		
CL216942	0.01	0/1
DHAD	0.05	0/1
Interferon	1000.00*	0/1
MGBG	10.00	0/2

*Units per ml.

Table 4. *In Vitro Results of Drug Testing in Pancreatic Tumor Specimens*

Drug	mcg/ml Tested	In Vitro Responses/Number Tested
Conventional Agents		
Adriamycin	0.04	0/3
Bleomycin	0.20	0/3
BCNU	0.10	0/2
Cis-platinum	0.20	0/1
Chlorambucil	0.10	0/2
5-Fluorouracil	6.00	0/5
Methotrexate	0.30	0/1
Mitomycin C	0.10	0/3
Investigational Agents		
AMSA	0.50	0/4
AT-125*	10.00	0/2
CC1065†	.0005	1/1
DHAD	0.05	0/2
MGBG	10.00	1/4
Interferon	1000.00+	1/2
PALA‡		0/1

*AT-125 = acivicin; †CC1065 = a glutamine antagonist; ‡PALA = PALA disodium or L-aspartic acid, N-(phosphonoacetyl)-disodium; +units per ml.

agents tested were cis-diamminedichloroplatinum II, bleomycin, methotrexate, vinblastine, and mitomycin C. Investigational drugs tested were dihydroxyanthracenedione (DHAD), CL216942 (an anthracene dicarboxaldehyde derivative) and CC1065 (a glutamine antagonist).

Biliary Adenocarcinoma (Extrahepatic)

One peritoneal fluid specimen was evaluated and grew. Three conventional agents [Adriamycin, 5-fluorouracil, and 1, 3-bis(β-chloroethyl)-1-nitrosourea (BCNU)] and one investigational agent [methyl-GAG or methyl-glyoxal-bis-guanylhydrazone (MGBG)] were tested. None of these drugs was effective in vitro.

Nonmalignant Specimens

Three colon specimens (diverticulitis, submucosal abscess of the cecum, active Crohn's disease) were plated and none grew. Two pleural fluids from patients with advanced abdominal disease but negative pleural fluid cytologic examinations did not grow.

Proof of the Malignant Nature of the Colonies

The malignant nature of myeloma cells, neuroblastoma cells, and ovarian carcinoma cells grown in this two-layer soft agar system has been previously demonstrated using light microscopy, tumor marker determinations, and karyotyping (Von Hoff and Johnson 1979, Von Hoff et al. 1980, Hamburger et

Table 5. *In Vitro Results of Drug Testing in Hepatoma Specimens*

Drug	mcg/ml Tested	In Vitro Responses/Number Tested
Conventional Agents		
Adriamycin	0.04	0/3
BCNU	0.10	0/1
5-Fluorouracil	6.00	0/3
Investigational Agents		
MGBG	10.00	0/1

al. 1978). In the present study, the morphologic characteristics of colonies of colorectal carcinoma, gastric carcinoma, pancreatic carcinoma, and hepatoma were identical to those characteristics of the original human tumors. Figures 1A and 1B show the colony and corresponding histologic characteristics of cells in a pancreatic carcinoma colony growing in soft agar.

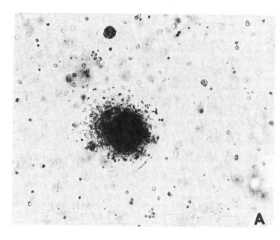

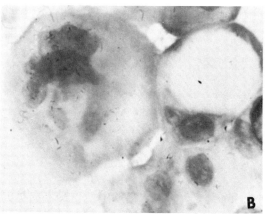

FIG. 1. A. Pancreatic carcinoma colony (160X). **B.** Detail of light microscopy of this colony on permanent slide (1000X).

Carcinoembryonic Antigen

Von Hoff and Johnson have shown that cells growing in the two-layer agar system secrete tumor markers (Von Hoff and Johnson 1979). Despite strenuous efforts at mechanical removal and/or physical dissolution of agar, the agar could not be completely removed from the plucked colonies. Fluorescence was seen around the agar-containing colonies of colorectal carcinoma and around agar from the same plates without colonies. No fluorescence was seen if the anti-human CEA was omitted. Presumably the anti-human CEA was attaching to CEA excreted by the cells into the agar. Further attempts to quantitate CEA production by radioimmunoassay are under way. Additional studies of note would be chromosomal analysis and tumor production in nude mice. Preliminary results of these studies are encouraging.

DISCUSSION

In this paper we have reported the growth of a number of gastrointestinal tumors in a soft agar system. Buick et al. (1980) described their experience with the system applied to colon carcinoma. They reported growth of colonies from three effusions and no growth with four solid tumor specimens. We have shown that solid specimens can be processed to a single cell suspension and grown reproducibly in our laboratory (Table 1). Our overall success with growth of gastrointestinal malignant tumors reported here is 79%; it is 83% with solid specimens and 62% with fluids.

From a limited amount of data presented here, the soft tissue agar system appears to be specific for growth of malignant cells. In this blind study, five of five nonmalignant lesions did not form colonies in vitro.

Evaluation of one or more chemotherapeutic agents was possible in 47% of the specimens. The mean number of drugs that could be evaluated was 4.3. One or more drugs were efficacious in only 11% of the specimens evaluated for drug sensitivity. The likelihood of finding useful adjuvant or primary therapy for gastrointestinal tumors among our current chemotherapeutic agents is poor. Nevertheless, despite the pessimism of these figures, the cloning assay correlates well with what we already know about the insensitivity of gastrointestinal tumors to conventional single agents. Thus the assay may be a useful method for screening new agents for use in treating patients with gastrointestinal cancer.

ACKNOWLEDGMENTS

This investigation was supported by American Cancer Society Grant CH162 and by the Clinical Cancer Education Grant CA26047, awarded by The National Cancer Institute, Department of Health and Human Services.

REFERENCES

Altman, A. J., F. G. Crussi, W. J. Rierden, and B. L. Baehner. 1975. Growth of rhabdomyosarcoma colonies from pleural fluid. Cancer Res. 35:1809–1812.

Buick, R. N., S. E. Fry, and S. E. Salmon. 1980. Application of in vitro soft agar techniques for growth of tumor cells to the study of colon cancer. Cancer 45:1238–1242.

Dukes, C. E. 1932. The classification of cancer of the rectum. J. Pathol. Bacteriol. 35:323–332.

Hamburger, A. W., and S. E. Salmon. 1977a. Primary bioassay of human tumor stem cells. Science 197:461–463.

Hamburger, A. W., and S. E. Salmon. 1977b. Primary bioassay of human myeloma stem cells. J. Clin. Invest. 60:846–854.

Hamburger, A. W., S. E. Salmon, M. B. Kim, J. M. Trent, B. J. Soehnlen, D. Alberts, and H. J. Schmidt. 1978. Direct cloning of human ovarian carcinoma cells in agar. Cancer Res. 38:3438–3443.

McAllister, R. M., and G. Reed. 1968. Colonial growth in agar of cells derived from neoplastic and non-neoplastic tissues of children. Pediatr. Res. 2:356–360.

Meyskens, F. L., Jr., and S. E. Salmon. 1980. Regulation of human melanoma clonogenic cell expression in soft agar by follicle stimulating hormone, nerve growth factor, and melatonin (Abstract). Proc. Am. Assoc. Cancer Res. and ASCO 21:199.

Park, C. H., D. E. Bergsagel, and E. A. McCulloch. 1971. Mouse myeloma tumor stem cells: A primary cell culture assay. J. Natl. Cancer Inst. 46:411–422.

Pike, B. L., and W. A. Robinson. 1970. Human bone marrow colony growth in agar-gel. J. Cell. Physiol. 76:77–81.

Pollard, E. B., F. Tio, J. P. Whitecar, C. A. Coltman, Jr., and D. D. Von Hoff. 1980. Utilization of a soft agar system to moniter for marrow involvement with small cell carcinoma of the lung (Abstract). Proc. Am. Assoc. Cancer Res. and ASCO 21:192.

Salmon, S. E., B. J. Soehnlen, B. G. M. Durie, D. S. Alberts, and T. E. Moon. 1978. Quantitation of differential sensitivity of human tumor stem cells to anti-cancer drugs. N. Engl. J. Med. 298:1321–1327.

Salmon, S. E., and R. N. Buick. 1979. Preparation of permanent slides of intact soft agar colony cultures of hematopoietic and tumor stem cells. Cancer Res. 39:1133–1136.

Sandbach, J., M. O'Brien, D. Welch, S. C. Cohen, D. H. Gordon, V. Rodriguez, J. P. Whitecar, Jr., and D. D. Von Hoff. 1980. Assay for clonogenic cells in human breast cancer (Abstract). Proc. Am. Assoc. Cancer Res. and ASCO. 21:139.

Von Hoff, D. D. 1980. Clinical correlations of drug sensitivity in tumor stem cell assay (Abstract). Proc. Am. Assoc. Cancer Res. and ASCO 21:134.

Von Hoff, D. D., J. Casper, E. Bradley, J. M. Trent, A. Hodach, C. Reichert, R. Makuch, and A. Altman. 1980. Direct cloning of human neuroblastoma cells in agar: A potential assay for diagnosis, response and prognosis. Cancer Res. 40:3591–3597.

Von Hoff, D. D., and G. E. Johnson. 1979. Secretion of tumor markers in the human tumor stem cell assay system (Abstract). Proc. Am. Assoc. Cancer Res. and ASCO 20:51.

Gastrointestinal Cancer, edited by
John R. Stroehlein and
Marvin M. Romsdahl.
Raven Press, New York © 1981.

New Approaches to the Treatment of Dukes' C Colorectal Carcinoma and Metastatic Colorectal Carcinoma Confined to the Liver

Y. Z. Patt, M.D., A. Y. Bedikian, M.D., V. P. Chuang, M.D.,*
S. Wallace, M.D.,* R. Fuqua, R.N., and G. M. Mavligit, M.D.

*Departments of Developmental Therapeutics and *Diagnostic Radiology,
The University of Texas System Cancer Center
M. D. Anderson Hospital and Tumor Institute, Houston, Texas*

INTRODUCTION

It is estimated that there will be 114,000 new cases of colorectal carcinoma and that 53,000 patients in the United States will succumb to the disease in 1980 (Silverberg 1980). Considering the high incidence of colorectal carcinoma and the high death rate associated with it, it is not surprising that utmost efforts have been undertaken in an attempt to control this disease.

The median disease-free interval from surgery in Dukes' stage C colorectal cancer is 21 months; the median survival is 42 months. It is not surprising therefore that this group of patients was the target of various surgical adjuvant studies (Mavligit et al. 1977, Mavligit et al. 1980). Liver metastases in colorectal carcinoma patients tend to be regionally confined for a prolonged period of time and determine the prognosis, independent of extrahepatic metastases (Jaffe 1968). Attempts at controlling regional disease by local measures such as arterial infusion of chemotherapy (Ansfield et al. 1975, Oberfield et al. 1979, Patt et al. 1980, Petrek and Minton 1979), tumor ischemia (Nillson 1966, Wallace 1976), tumor resection (Stehlin et al. 1974), radiotherapy, or combinations thereof (Webber et al. 1978) have been previously reported. Liver metastases could be identified in a significant proportion of patients, at their first presentation with colorectal carcinoma (Stehlin et al. 1974). The liver has therefore become one of the targets of adjuvant treatment of colon cancer.

This paper will deal with our approach to the treatment of metastatic colorectal carcinoma confined to the liver and the adjuvant treatment of Dukes' stage C colorectal carcinoma.

Table 1. *Hepatic Arterial Infusion of Mitomycin C + FUDR Treatment Plan*

	Days of Cycle*	Mode of Administration
Mitomycin C 10–15 mg/m²	1	Two-Hour Infusion
FUDR 100 mg/m²	1–5	Continuous Infusion

*Cycles repeated every 4 to 5 weeks

MATERIALS AND METHODS

Hepatic Arterial Infusion (HAI) of FUDR and Mitomycin C for Colorectal Carcinoma Confined to the Liver

Fifty-five patients with metastatic colorectal carcinoma confined to the liver were treated with hepatic arterial infusion of FUDR + mitomycin C. The treatment plan is shown in Table 1. Mitomycin C at a dose of 10–15 mg/m² was given in 400 ml of normal saline with 2,000 units of heparin over two hours. This was followed by FUDR at a dose of 100–150 mg/m²/day given by continuous infusion in 1,000 ml D-5-1/2 normal saline plus 15,000 units of heparin daily for five days. All drugs were administered with a Sigma Motor 4002 infusion pump (Sigma Corp., Middleport, New York) or with an IMED 922 Volumetric infusion pump (IMED Corp., San Diego, California), as previously described (Patt et al. 1980). Characteristics of the patients entered in this study are described in Table 2.

Table 2. *Comparability of Colorectal Carcinoma Patients with Liver Metastases Treated with HAI of FUDR + MMC or IV Chemotherapy*

Prognostic Variable	HAI N = 55 (%)	IV N = 56 (%)	P Value χ^2
Performance Status (Karnofsky < 70%)	6 (10.9)	23 (41.0)	<.01
Liver Involvement State III–IV	37 (63.3)	26 (46.4)	.04
Liver Function Tests (Bilirubin > 1.0) (Alkaline Phosphatase > 200)	26 (47.3)	21 (37.5)	N.S.
Pretreatment CEA (> 100 ng/ml)	33 (60.0)	21 (37.5)	.03
Stage at Initial Presentation (Dukes' D)	30 (54.5)	31 (55.3)	N.S.
Sex (male)	39 (70.9)	34 (60.7)	N.S.

Fifty-six colorectal carcinoma patients with metastatic disease confined to the liver were selected as controls. Treatment specifics of this group of patients are described in Table 3. All patients were given 5-FU or ftorafur IV and additional drugs as shown in the table. Comparability to patients treated with hepatic arterial infusion of FUDR and mitomycin C is described in Table 2.

Response was evaluated by physical examination and imaging techniques including radionuclide scan, computerized tomography (CT), sonography, and hepatic angiography. In addition, response by imaging techniques was correlated with serum levels of CEA. The duration of response was calculated from initiation of therapy to the first rise in CEA level. Complete remission (CR) was defined as disappearance of all evidence of disease on all imaging tests. Partial remission (PR) was defined as a decrease of more than 50% in the sum of multiplication of two perpendicular diameters of all the visible lesions in the imaging tests. This was usually measured on the hepatic angiogram.

Adjuvant Chemoimmunotherapy of Dukes' C Colorectal Carcinoma

Only patients with Dukes' C carcinoma of the large bowel (involvement of the regional lymph nodes without invasion of adjacent structures or distant organs), whose adjuvant treatment could be started within 4–8 weeks from

Table 3. *Chemotherapy Combinations Given to Control Patients*

Chemotherapy*	Dose Schedule	Number Patients
Sequential 5-FU/BAF or MTX ± Levamisole	5-FU 500 mg/m²/dx5 q 6 wks	9
	OR MTX 15 mg/m²/dx3 q 6 wks BAF 250 mg/m²/dx3 q 6 wks	
5-FU + VDS + MeCCNU	5-FU 400 mg/m²/dx4 ⎫ VDS 4 mg/m²/d ⎬ q 4 wks MeCCNU 100 mg/m²/d ⎭	7
Ftorafur + MTX + MeCCNU ± BCG	Ftorafur 2 mg/m²/dx5 ⎫ MTX 30 mg/m²/d, days 1,8,15 ⎬ q 4 wks MeCCNU 100 mg/m²/d ⎭	21
5-FU + CCNU + Cyclophosphamide	5-FU 800 mg/m²/dx5 q 4 wks CCNU 40 mg/m²/dx4 wks CTX 200 mg/m²/dx q 4 wks	7
5-FU + PALA	5-FU 480 mg/m²/d weekly OR PALA 2 g/m²/d weekly 5-FU 400 mg/m²/dx5 q 4 wks PALA 800 mg/m²/dx5 q 4 wks	12
Total		56

*5-Fluorouracil (5-FU), Baker's Antifol (BAF), Vindesine (VDS), Methyl CCNU (MeCCNU), Methotrexate (MTX), Cyclophosphamide (CTX).

surgery, were entered on three consecutive trials of adjuvant therapy between 1973 and 1980.

5-FU + BCG

One hundred and twenty-one patients were entered in this study. The treatment consisted of immunotherapy with BCG by scarification, or the combination of BCG immunotherapy with oral 5-FU as previously described (Mavligit et al. 1976). Details of the randomization to various treatment arms and the criteria for exclusion from this study have been discussed at length in previous publications on this study (Mavligit et al. 1976, 1977, 1980). Treatment evaluation in terms of disease-free interval and overall survival were compared to those of a consecutive series of comparable patients with Dukes' C colorectal carcinoma treated with surgery alone at M. D. Anderson Hospital between 1963 and 1973.

After informed consent was obtained, patients were categorized according to the number of positive lymph nodes (<5 vs. >5) and were randomized to receive either BCG alone or BCG in combination with oral 5-FU. The lyophilized Pasteur strain of BCG was administered by a scarification method, in a dose of 6×10^8 viable organisms, weekly for three months and every other week thereafter. 5-FU was given orally in a dose of 100 mg/m^2 four times a day for five days and repeated every four weeks during a period of two years. The patients who were randomized to receive 5-FU received BCG on days 7, 14, and 21 of each course during the first three courses and on days 7 and 21 thereafter.

5-FU, BCG, and C. parvum *with or without Radiation Therapy*

Thirty-three patients with Dukes' stage C colorectal carcinoma were treated with 5-FU, *C. parvum,* and BCG between 1976 and 1978. 5-FU was given intravenously at a dose of 400 mg/m^2 daily for five days. On cycles 1, 6, and 12, *C. parvum* at a dose of 0.5–5 mg/m^2 was added daily for 10 days following 5-FU administration. BCG was given on days 7, 14, and 21 of the first three cycles, or weekly during radiation therapy and every other week thereafter to complete three years of treatment. Additionally, patients with primary lesions of the rectosigmoid who underwent anterior resection received 5,100 rads of radiation therapy to the pelvis. Those who underwent abdominoperineal resection received 4,500 rads to the pelvis plus 1,000 rads to the perineal area (Table 4).

Arterial Infusion of Chemotherapy

Twelve patients have been entered so far in the protocol utilizing adjuvant treatment with hepatic arterial infusion of FUDR and mitomycin C with BCG immunotherapy or hepatic arterial infusion, and pelvic arterial infusion of FUDR and mitomycin C with XRT and BCG. The outlines of this program are

Table 4. *Treatment of Dukes' Stage C Colorectal Carcinoma with 5-FU, BCG, and C. Parvum with or without Radiation Therapy (XRT) to the Pelvis*

Treatment Modality	Site of Primary Lesion	
	Ascending, Transverse, and Descending Colon	Rectosigmoid
5-FU	IV 400 mg/m²/d × 5/q 4 wks Cycles 1–12	IV 400 mg/m²/d × 5 Cycle 1 and Cycles 3–12
C. parvum	IV 0.5–5.0 mg/m²/d × 10 on cycles 1, 6, 12	IV 0.5–5.0 mg/m²/d × 10 on cycles 1, 6, 12
XRT		5100 r to the pelvis in patients with anterior resection. 4500 r to the pelvis + 1000 r to the perineum in those with abdomino-perineal resection.
BCG	6 × 10⁸ organisms wkly × 12 and every other week for 3 years	6 × 10⁸ organisms weekly, day 17–52 (during XRT) and every other week for 3 years

shown in Table 5. Basically the patients were treated with four cycles of hepatic arterial infusion of mitomycin C and FUDR. BCG scarifications were administered weekly for one month and every other week thereafter, to complete two years of treatment. Patients with primary lesions in the rectosigmoid area (less than 18 cm from the anal orifice) were treated with one cycle of hepatic arterial infusion of mitomycin C and FUDR followed by radiation therapy to the pelvis and a repeated hepatic arterial infusion with mitomycin C and 5-FU. This was followed by one cycle of iliac arterial infusion of

Table 5. *Adjuvant Therapy for Dukes' C Colorectal Cancer January 1979*

Rectosigmoid Primary	Other Sites	Comment
Hepatic Arterial × 1 Infusion (per Cutan.)	Hepatic Arterial Infusion (per Cutan.)	5 FUDR 100 mg/m² daily × 5 cont. Mitomycin C 10 mg/m² × 1
↓ ↓ ↓ ↓ ↓	↓ ↓ ↓	
	Q 30 days × 4 ↓	
XRT ↓ ↓	↓	XRT—4500 R
Hepatic Arterial Infusion × 1 ↓	BCG for 2 years	
Pelvic Infusion × 1 ↓ ↓ ↓ ↓		5-FU 500 mg/m² daily × 5 cont. Mitomycin C 10 mg/m² × 1
BCG for 2 years		

mitomycin C and 5-FU. These patients were also subsequently treated with BCG to complete two years of treatment.

RESULTS

Hepatic Arterial Infusion of FUDR and Mitomycin C for Liver Metastases

The response rates observed in the two treatment groups, HAI and IV, are shown in Table 6. Complete and partial remissions were observed in 5.4% and 38.0%, respectively, among patients receiving hepatic arterial infusion (HAI) as opposed to 1.8% and 14.3% complete and partial remissions, respectively, in those receiving intravenous therapy (IV). The overall response rate was 43.4% for the HAI group and 14.3% for the IV group ($p < 0.01$). The median time interval from beginning of HAI chemotherapy to relapse, as judged by an increasing CEA, was six months. A good correlation was again noted between the decrease in size of the metastases in the HAI group and the decline in serum CEA levels in the HAI group, as previously described (Patt et al. 1980, 1981). The median overall survival of the patients treated with chemotherapy given intravenously or by the hepatic arterial route was not significantly different (10 and 11 months, respectively). Survival among responders to HAI chemotherapy was double that of nonresponders, with medians of 16 and 8 months, respectively ($p < 0.01$) (Figure 1). This survival difference between responders and nonresponders was unique to the HAI-treated group and not to the IV-treated patients. The 14.3% responders to IV chemotherapy did not live significantly longer than the nonresponders (11 and 10 months median survival, respectively). The difference in survival of nonresponding HAI-treated patients (8 months) and nonresponding IV-treated ones (10 months) was not significant.

In 24 of the 55 patients treated with HAI, an occlusion of the hepatic arterial circulation was effected. It occurred inadvertently in 13 patients as a result of physical trauma to the vessel wall, or by chemical arteritis infrequently induced by mitomycin C, or both. In 11 additional patients, arterial occlusion was intentional and achieved by using Gelfoam or Ivalon coil as previously described (Chuang and Wallace 1980). In two of those, hepatic arterial flow

Table 6. *Response Rates in Patients with Liver Metastases*

Evaluable	HAI N = 55 (%)	IV N = 56 (%)	P Value χ^2
C.R.	3 (5.4)	1 (1.8)	
P.R.	21 (38.0)	7 (12.5)	
<P.R.	9 (16.3)	8 (14.2)	
Stable	14 (25.4)	23 (41.0)	
P.D.	8 (14.5)	17 (30.3)	
C.R. + P.R.	43.4%	14.3	<.01

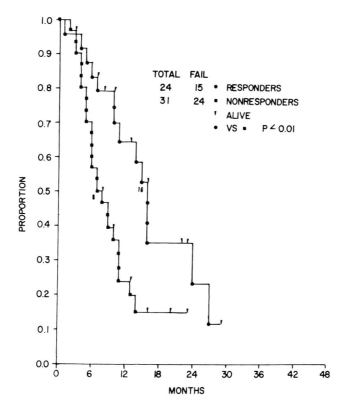

FIG. 1. Survival of responding and nonresponding patients to HAI chemotherapy.

redistribution was necessary to optimize the arterial administration of chemotherapy into the tumor-bearing area and to avoid untoward side-tracking. In the remaining nine patients, hepatic arterial occlusion was performed primarily after maximum benefit from arterial chemotherapy had already been achieved. Survival among responding patients (CR, PR, and <PR) with arterial occlusion (16 patients) was 16 months as opposed to only 11 months among responding patients who had no arterial occlusion ($p = 0.01$) (Figure 2).

Adjuvant Treatment of Dukes' C Colorectal Carcinoma

BCG ± 5-FU P.O. (BCG Group)

Since oral administration of 5-FU did not alter the prognosis of Dukes' C colorectal carcinoma patients, all 121 patients have been analyzed together and compared to the control group.

The effect of this treatment on disease-free interval is shown in Figure 3. Twenty-five percent of the patients have relapsed, at 11 months if not treated and at 16 months if given BCG. Fifty percent of the patients have relapsed at 23 months in the control group and at 36 months if given BCG ($p = 0.02$). Figure 4

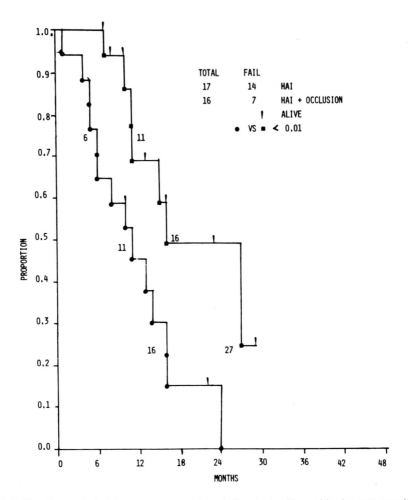

FIG. 2. The effects of arterial occlusion on survival of all patients with an objective response (CR, PR, and <PR).

depicts the effect of BCG treatment on the survival of these patients. Median survival of the BCG-treated group was 62 months, versus 46 months for the control group ($p = 0.02$).

IV 5-FU, BCG, and *C. parvum*, and Radiotherapy (XRT) (*C. parvum* Group)

Figure 5 shows the disease-free interval among 35 patients treated with this regimen as compared to that of 121 patients treated with BCG alone. The addition of *C. parvum*, IV 5-FU, and XRT offered no advantage in terms of disease-free interval (Figure 5) or survival (Figure 6). A subgroup of patients with primary lesions of the rectosigmoid included 15 of 35 patients in the *C.*

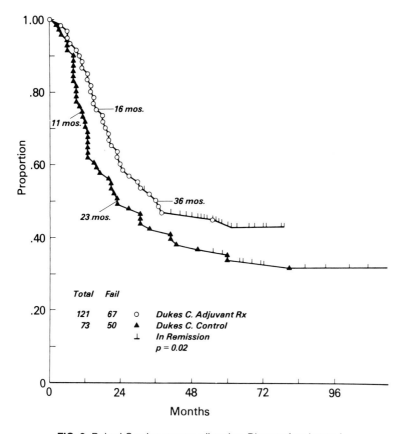

FIG. 3. Dukes' C colon cancer, all nodes. Disease-free interval.

parvum group, 84 of 121 in the BCG group, and 31 of 73 in the historical control group. There were no local relapses among 15 patients treated with *C. parvum* + XRT as opposed to 22 of 84 in the BCG group, and 10 of 31 in the control group.

Arterial Infusion of Chemotherapy

Only 13 patients have so far received the new adjuvant treatment protocol utilizing HAI of FUDR + MMC or HAI of FUDR + MMC, XRT, and pelvic infusion of 5-FU + MMC. None of these patients has experienced a recurrence. Long-term effects will have to be analyzed in a few years.

DISCUSSION

These results suggest that colorectal carcinoma patients with liver metastases can gain additional palliation from hepatic arterial infusion of FUDR and mitomycin C, particularly when supplemented by some form of arterial occlusion (Patt et al. 1981).

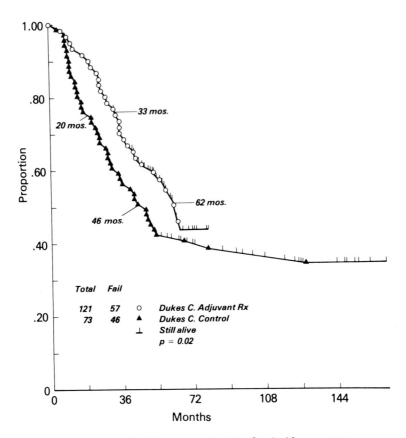

FIG. 4. Dukes' C colon cancer, all nodes. Survival from surgery.

Although overall survival among HAI- and IV-treated groups was similar, prolongation of survival was unique to responding HAI patients and not to responding IV patients. The fact that nonresponding HAI patients did not have a significantly shorter survival than nonresponding IV patients (8 vs. 10, respectively) means that hepatic arterial infusion of FUDR and mitomycin C did not result in the earlier demise of nonresponding patients. When some form of response to chemotherapy (CR, PR, and <PR) was supplemented by arterial occlusion, survival was further prolonged, as shown in Figure 2.

The basic assumptions supporting the advantage of intra-arterial infusion of chemotherapy over the intravenous route include the following: (1) The achievement of a higher drug concentration in the tumor-bearing region due to a more efficient drug delivery. (2) The potential for an uptake of a substantial amount of the drug by the tumor-bearing organ during its first passage. This would result in significant drug elimination and perhaps a reduction in its excessive peripheral toxicity (Chen and Gross 1980). These theoretical con-

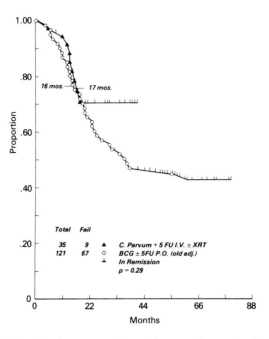

FIG. 5. Dukes' C colon cancer adjuvant therapy. Disease-free interval.

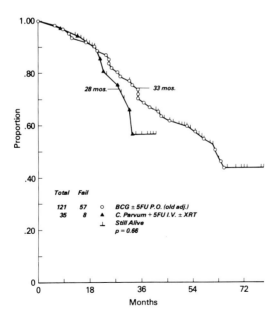

FIG. 6. Dukes' C colon cancer adjuvant therapy. Survival from surgery.

siderations were clearly confirmed in practice by clinical pharmacology data with 5-FU (Ensminger et al. 1978) and mitomycin C (Hashimoto 1978), while increments in tissue concentrations following infusion with methotrexate (Anderson et al. 1970) or Adriamycin (Kraybill et al. 1977) were only moderate.

Our study suggests that maximal benefit from arterial infusion of chemotherapy can be further supplemented by arterial occlusion (Patt 1981), which demonstrated antitumor effects by virtue of causing necrotic changes resulting from ischemia (Nillson 1966, Wallace 1976). Transient arterial occlusion during arterial administration of BCNU resulted in enhanced uptake of the drug by the tumor-containing liver (Ensminger et al. 1980). This could possibly be the mechanism of increased survival in some of the patients with inadvertant arterial occlusion. Our current protocol for the treatment of Dukes' C colorectal carcinoma patients calls for hepatic arterial infusion of FUDR and mitomycin C and scarifications with BCG. Pelvic irradiation as well as pelvic infusion of 5-FU and mitomycin C have been added to the treatment of patients with primary tumors of the rectosigmoid (Table 5). The introduction of HAI of FUDR and mitomycin C was based on the effective antitumor effect that this regimen had on patients with established liver metastases (Patt 1980, Patt 1981). A similar successful approach was reported previously (Taylor et al. 1977). In that study drugs were administered into the portal vein. This method can be utilized only in patients who have had a catheter introduced into the portal vein at time of their initial surgery, while our treatment regimen can be given to any patient who qualifies for adjuvant treatment of Dukes' C colorectal carcinoma. The addition of BCG to this treatment program is based on previously reported results (Figures 3 and 4) (Mavligit et al. 1976, 1977, 1980).

Administration of *C. parvum* did not alter the prognosis of Dukes' C colorectal carcinoma patients (Figures 5 and 6). The addition of radiation therapy, however, has altered the pattern of relapse in patients with primary lesions of the rectosigmoid. Since none of the patients in this group had a local recurrence, it would seem justified to add pelvic irradiation to the adjuvant treatment of any patients with a primary lesion of that region.

A rational approach to the treatment of Dukes' C colorectal carcinoma has thus been developed. The ingredients incorporated were taken from previous protocols that showed positive results. We hope in this way to be able to change the natural course of the disease.

REFERENCES

Anderson, L. L., G. J. Collins, Y. Ojima, and R. D. Sullivan. 1970. A study of the distribution of methotrexate in human tissues and tumors. Cancer Res. 30:1344–1348.

Ansfield, F. J., G. Ramirez, H. L. Davis, Jr., G. W. Wirtanem, R. O. Johnson, G. T. Bryan, F. B. Manalo, E. C. Bordon, T. E. Davis, and M. Esmaili. 1975. Further clinical studies with intrahepatic arterial infusion with 5-fluorouracil. Cancer 36:2413–2417.

Chen, H. A. G., and J. F. Gross. 1980. Intra-arterial infusion of anti-cancer drugs: Theoretic aspects of drug delivery and review of response. Cancer Treat. Rep. 64:3–40.

Chuang, V. P., and S. Wallace. 1980. Hepatic arterial redistribution for intra-arterial infusion of hepatic neoplasms. Radiology 135:295–299.

Ensminger, W. D., S. Dakhill, and K. Cho. 1980. Improved regional selectivity of hepatic arterial bischlorethylnitrosourea plus degradable starch microspheres. Clin. Res. 28:742.

Ensminger, W. D., A. Rosowsky, V. Raso, D. C. Levin, M. Glode, S. Come, G. Steele, and E. Frei, III. 1978. A clinical pharmacological evaluation of hepatic arterial infusion of 5-fluorouracil. Cancer Res. 38:3784–3792.

Hashimoto, Y. 1978. Fundamental investigations on local chemotherapy for local cancer. Arch. Jpn. Chir. 47:302–318.

Jaffe, B. M., W. L. Donegan, F. Watson, and J. D. Spratt, Jr. 1968. Factors influencing survival in patients with untreated hepatic metastases. Surg. Gynecol. Obstet. 127:1–11.

Kraybill, W. G., M. Harrison, T. Sasaki, and W. S. Fletcher. 1977. Regional intra-arterial infusion of Adriamycin in the treatment of cancer. Surg. Gynecol. Obstet. 144:335–338.

Mavligit, G. M., J. U. Gutterman, M. A. Burgess, N. Khankhanian, G. B. Seibert, J. F. Speer, A. V. Jubert, E. A. Gehan, and E. M. Hersh. 1976. Prolongation of postoperative disease-free interval and survival in human colorectal cancer by BCG or BCG + 5-fluorouracil. Lancet 1:871–876.

Mavligit, G. M., J. U. Gutterman, M. A. Malahy, M. A. Burgess, C. M. McBride, A. Jubert, and E. M. Hersh. 1977. Adjuvant immunotherapy and chemoimmunotherapy in colorectal cancer (Dukes' class C). Prolongation of disease-free interval and survival. Cancer 40:2726–2730.

Mavligit, G. M., M. A. Malahy, M. A. Burgess, C. M. McBride, and E. M. Hersh. 1980. Systemic adjuvant therapy with BCG versus BCG + 5-FU in colorectal cancer Dukes' class C updated critical analysis. Prog. Exp. Tumor Res. 25:275–292.

Nillson, L. A. 1966. Therapeutic hepatic artery ligation in patients with secondary liver tumors. Rev. Surg. 5:374–376.

Oberfield, R. A., J. A. McCaffrey, J. Polio, M. E. Clouse, and T. Hamilton. 1979. Prolonged and continuous percutaneous intra-arterial hepatic infusion chemotherapy in advanced metastatic liver adenocarcinoma from colorectal primary. Cancer 44:414–423.

Patt, Y. Z., V. P. Chuang, S. Wallace, E. M. Hersh, E. J Freireich, and G. M. Mavligit. 1981. The palliative role of hepatic arterial infusion and arterial occlusion in colorectal carcinoma metastatic to the liver. Lancet 1:349–351.

Patt, Y. Z., G. M. Mavligit, V. P. Chuang, S. Wallace, S. Johnson, R. S. Benjamin, M. Valdivieso, and E. M. Hersh. 1980. Percutaneous hepatic arterial infusion (HAI) of mitomycin C and floxuridine (FUDR): An effective treatment for metastatic colorectal carcinoma in the liver. Cancer 46:261–265.

Petrek, J. A., and J. P. Minton. 1979. Treatment of hepatic metastases by percutaneous hepatic arterial infusion. Cancer 43:2182–2188.

Silverberg, E. 1980. Cancer statistics 1980. Cancer 30:23–38.

Stehlin, J. S., L. Hotstrom, and P. J. Greefi. 1974. Experience with infusion and resection in cancer of the liver. Surg. Gynecol. Obstet. 138:855–863.

Taylor, I., P. Brooman, and T. T. Rowling. 1977. Adjuvant liver perfusion in colorectal cancer: Initial result of a clinical trial. Br. Med. J. 2:1320–1322.

Webber, B. M., C. H. Soderberg, Jr., L. A. Leone, V. B. Rege, and A. S. Glicksman. 1978. A combined approach to management of hepatic metastases. Cancer 42:1087–1095.

Wallace, S. 1976. Interventional radiology. Cancer 37:517–531.

Gastrointestinal Cancer, edited by
John R. Stroehlein and
Marvin M. Romsdahl.
Raven Press, New York © 1981.

Directions for Future Research and Prospects for Control of Gastrointestinal Cancer

R. Lee Clark, M.D.

President Emeritus, The University of Texas System Cancer Center
M. D. Anderson Hospital and Tumor Institute, Houston, Texas

In 1965, M. D. Anderson Hospital and Tumor Institute convened the 10th Annual Clinical Conference, and the subject discussed was the same as that of the present conference, *Cancer of the Gastrointestinal Tract.* In the introduction to that conference, I stated that cancer of the digestive organs and peritoneum was the cause of more than 50% of the total deaths from cancer at the turn of the century. By 1965, digestive tract cancers were responsible for 34.4% of total deaths from cancer. During those years, the incidence of lung cancer began increasing, and the incidence of gastric cancer decreased. Today, *The American Cancer Society Facts and Figures* (1980) estimates that gastrointestinal cancers account for approximately 25% of the total deaths from cancer. Since 1970, incidence decreased for cancers of the stomach, rectum, and esophagus, but there was a slight increase of cancers of the colon and a 20% increase in pancreatic cancers. The reasons for these changes are not known.

As you will hear in detail in the subsequent talks, there are numerous areas in which more progress can be made in controlling gastrointestinal cancers. As has always been true for all cancers, earlier detection is essential. We must give the members of the medical profession easier and quicker methods for detecting cancers along the gastrointestinal tract, since especially for esophageal, pancreatic, and liver cancers, the symptomatology is too non-specific and occurs too late to depend on it for assisting in early detection.

Several types of serum assays and guaiac testing for fecal occult blood show potential for alerting physicians to the possibility of the presence of cancer. Flexible fiberoptic endoscopes reveal preneoplastic changes, and combined with brush cytology and/or biopsy (needle aspiration or excisional) and laparoscopy (for examination of the liver), small malignant tumors can be diagnosed. There are not, however, a sufficient number of physicians who are trained to use these instruments skillfully.

Computerized tomographic, radiologic, and sonographic scanning equipment (used with isotopic materials when appropriate) is becoming more sensitive and is capable of revealing small lesions, but once again, skilled interpretation is essential. Arteriograms, cholangiograms, and the old standby, air-contrast barium studies, add significantly to the diagnostic tool kit for identifying primary and metastatic lesions. Immunobiological assays, including hybridoma clones and the monoclonal antibodies they produce, show potential for distinguishing malignant from normal cells, which can be exploited diagnostically and therapeutically.

Our best bet, however, still lies in the prevention of malignant disease, and we are making progress along several lines. There are some risk factors that have been identified over which some control can be exercised. Examples include the well-known precancerous conditions of chronic ulcerative colitis, familial polyposis coli, Gardner's syndrome, chronic gastric ulcers, and leukoplakia of the esophagus. Other individuals at high risk of developing esophageal and liver cancer are those who inhale smoke from 20 to 50 cigarettes each day and/or drink large quantities of alcohol.

Prevention can lower the incidence of tumors in the liver related to epidemiological associations of hepatomas and hepatocellular carcinoma occurring in some patients receiving androgen therapy or long-term oral contraceptive steroids and in those tumors related to the increasing numbers found in Western countries who have alcoholic cirrhosis. There is also evidence that in many patients the progression of events leading to primary hepatic carcinoma may include infection with hepatitis B virus, development of hepatitis B, progression of hepatitis to chronic hepatitis, and postnecrotic cirrhosis. Consequently, management of high-risk populations, for instance in African nations, for the future may well involve vaccination against hepatitis B virus.

Cytogeneticists are revealing more hereditary and genetic conditions that predispose individuals to the development of malignant disease. Identification of such individuals and prophylactic measures or close long-term follow-up studies can either prevent cancer or control it in its earliest stages.

Of little consequence in this country but of major consequence in large populations elsewhere in the world is the contamination of improperly stored grains and nuts with *Aspergillus flavus,* producing carcinogenic aflatoxins, and other predisposing conditions such as viral diseases, parasites, and ingestion of fern bracken, which lead to high incidences of liver, esophageal, or stomach cancers.

Research is ongoing with regard to the carcinogenic potential of other dietary factors believed to be involved in the etiology of a majority of gastrointestinal cancers in the Western hemisphere, such as high levels of beef fat, and the interaction of their metabolites with intestinal microflora and biliary products. Concurrent with this research are studies identifying chemopreventive substances that inhibit tumor formation or slow tumor growth in animals and that have the potential for similar action against human tumors and preneoplastic cells. Such substances are antioxidants, retinoids, vitamins C and E, protease inhibitors, selenium compounds, prostaglandins, and cyclic nucleotides. More detailed investigations of molecular mechanisms regulating cell division in normal and malignant cells certainly open up possibilities for better therapeutic control as well as for prevention.

Transplantable tumors and normal and malignant cell cultures have made possible the evaluation of the biochemical effects of new and presently available anticancer agents used alone or in combinations. Some of the drugs being studied include nitrosourea derivatives, fluorinated pyrimidines, and quinazoline analogs of folic acid. The thermosensitivity of human colon adenocarcinoma cells has been investigated and, especially when coupled with some drugs such as cis-platinum (II) and mitomycin C, demonstrates a level of lethality that indicates the need for clinical trials using regional and total body hyperthermia alone and in combination with active drugs.

Immunological control of gastrointestinal tumors is becoming a distinct possibility. An example is a study conducted here at M. D. Anderson Hospital since 1973, coupling BCG with subtoxic doses of 5-fluorouracil, which is achieving longer disease-free intervals for Dukes' class C colorectal cancer. The possible effectiveness of transfer factor is being investigated.

Radiotherapy has been used very selectively for all gastrointestinal tumors except esophageal tumors, because of the potential for residual long-term adverse effects. Animal studies are being conducted to determine if tumor-localizing antibodies combined with a neutron-capturing agent, such as boron, can make cancers selectively sensitive to irradiation with slow neutrons.

Systemic metastatic disease has always been the primary challenge for oncologists. Studies of the mechanisms of the metastatic process eventually will tell us why malignant cells separate from the primary tumor, what type of environment is essential for eventual implantation of a small minority of those cells, and even why certain types of malignant cells metastasize preferentially to specific organ tissues. Until our increasingly better screening and diagnostic techniques and equipment and our preventive measures have significantly reduced the number of patients presenting at initial diagnosis with systemic disease, and until our therapeutic measures succeed in reducing to a minimum the incidence of recurrent disease in the gastrointestinal tract, we must continue to mobilize our every resource in every possible combination to control the processes of dissemination and recurrence without inducing iatrogenic second primary disease.

Numerous reports have been published advocating surgical resection of solitary and even multiple liver metastases and indicating significant extension of survival time as compared to survival of patients who have had resection of the primary tumor only. It is anticipated that the use of this type of extended surgical management will become more frequent in the future.

For supportive therapy, hyperalimentation is enhancing responses to chemotherapy and radiation therapy and is decreasing mortality rates significantly, especially following total gastrectomy and pancreatectomy. For inoperable esophageal cancer, Celestin's esophageal prostheses are enabling a majority of patients to eat soft and even regular diets until the time of their deaths.

There is little need to further delay information to be presented to you in considerably more detail than this brief summary, which of necessity omits more than it reveals. We consider ourselves fortunate to learn about risk factors from our good friend from Cornell University College of Medicine, Professor Martin Lipkin; about site-specific metastatic determinates from Professor Garth Nicolson, whom we have had the good fortune to welcome to our staff recently; about the pharmacologic possibilities for more specific cancer drugs from Daniel Griswold, Doctor of Veterinary Medicine at The Southern Research Institute; about carcinogenic assays from our good neighbor to the immediate South, Dr. Marvin Legator with The University of Texas Medical Branch in Galveston; and about the increasingly more hopeful and exciting prospects for cancer prevention and better control from Professor Lee Wattenberg of The University of Minnesota.

Gastrointestinal Cancer, edited by
John R. Stroehlein and
Marvin M. Romsdahl.
Raven Press, New York © 1981.

Individuals at Risk for Cancer of the Large Intestine: Memorial Sloan-Kettering Cancer Center Program of Surveillance

Martin Lipkin, M.D., Paul Sherlock, M.D., and Sidney J. Winawer, M.D.

Gastroenterology Service and Diagnostic Gastrointestinal Unit, Department of Medicine, and Laboratory of Gastrointestinal Cancer Research, Memorial Sloan-Kettering Cancer Center, New York, New York

INTRODUCTION

Improved methods of surveillance have been considered among recent approaches to the early detection and control of large bowel neoplasia. For programs of surveillance to be most efficient, improvements must be made in the identification of those population groups at increased risk of developing colorectal cancer, as well as those at average risk. In addition, programs of intervention with physical and chemical means are being considered to inhibit the origin and progression of colorectal neoplasms in populations at increased risk.

Studies of cell proliferation in the colon of human beings have contributed to these approaches, mainly because the boundaries of the cell proliferation and maturation compartments within the colonic mucosa have been demarcated. In recent years these findings, together with related parameters, have been applied to the study of early indices of susceptibility in human population groups at high risk for gastrointestinal cancer. The following sections describe the major population groups in the Memorial Sloan-Kettering registry of subjects at high risk of developing cancer of the large intestine, which are contributing to the development of these indices. The high risk populations that have been studied to date are those with a hereditary predisposition to colorectal cancer. Current findings are leading to the development of risk factor profiles for these populations, and for individuals with varying degrees of susceptibility to cancer of the large intestine. These findings, together with our current approach to the surveillance of these subjects, are summarized below.

MEMORIAL SLOAN-KETTERING REGISTRY OF POPULATION GROUPS AT HIGH RISK FOR CANCER OF THE LARGE INTESTINE

Individuals who are at increased risk for colon cancer and who have been patients at Memorial Hospital have been identified with the development of the population registries described in this section. This has been described recently (Lipkin et al. 1980a), and major points are summarized. In each population group, individuals who have had cancer of the large intestine, and diseases predisposing to it, are currently involved in this activity. Additional subjects, including members of the familial aggregates who are symptomatic and asymptomatic, as well as spouses and other controls, also are available. Information on each of the population groups follows:

Hereditary Polyposis Syndromes (Familial Polyposis and the Gardner Syndrome)

At present, in our Memorial Hospital registry, 31 families with familial polyposis are available for measurement of risk parameters. These include 71 symptomatic individuals, 325 asymptomatic individuals at risk, and 71 spouse family members.

Familial polyposis is distinguished from colon cancer in the general population by a number of criteria (Morson and Bussey 1970, Bussey 1975, Gardner 1951, Gardner and Richards 1953, Smith 1959). It is a disease which has an

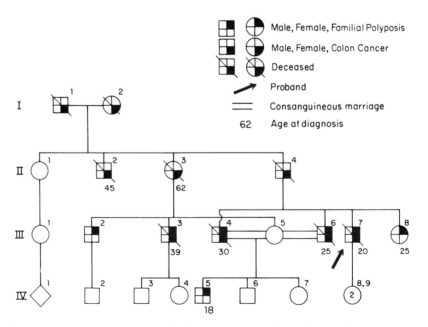

FIG. 1. Typical pattern of inheritance in familial polyposis, together with ages of onset of polyposis in family members (Lipkin et al. 1980a).

autosomal dominant mode of inheritance, and it is characterized by the development of large numbers of adenomatous polyps throughout the entire colon and rectum. In this disease, carcinomas eventually develop in virtually all individuals affected. These occur with highest frequency in the distal colon, similar to the appearance of colorectal cancer in the general population. The pattern of inheritance of a familial aggregate with familial polyposis is shown in Figure 1.

In addition to neoplasms of the large intestine, tumors in other organs are also likely to develop. For example, in individuals with familial polyposis in Japan, high frequencies of gastric and duodenal polyps also have been noted. This is in contrast to observations made in western countries. In the pathogenesis of these neoplasms, the possibility of cells highly susceptible to neoplastic transformation interacting with intraintestinal compounds having carcinogenic or promotor activity has been considered.

One of the criteria by which the onset of cancer in individuals with familial polyposis can be distinguished from the onset of cancer in the general population is the early age at appearance. This is illustrated in Figure 2, which shows the cumulative percentage of incident cases having familial polyposis at various ages, compared to the incident cases of colorectal cancer in other population groups. The latter include familial colon cancer-prone groups without polyposis, and colon and rectal cancer in the general population in the United States and Japan.

In our population registry at Memorial Hospital, numerous familial aggregates demonstrate manifestations of the Gardner's syndrome (Gardner 1951, Gardner and Richards 1953, and Bussey 1975) in addition to those of familial polyposis. In the Gardner's syndrome, an autosomal dominant mode of inheritance and a high degree of penetrance are present. As in familial polyposis, Gardner's syndrome is characterized by adenomatous polyposis of the colon and, in addition, soft tissue abnormalities including fibroblast and desmoid tumors, epidermal and sebaceous cysts, and bone abnormalities. Adenomas and carcinomas also have been observed in the small intestine; these often occur in the region of the ampulla of Vater, where bile and pancreatic juice flow into the intestine.

The age distribution at onset of colonic polyps and the progression to colon cancer are similar to familial polyposis.

Colon Cancer-Prone Familial Aggregates without Polyposis

Our population registry of familial groups having high frequencies of colon cancer without familial polyposis includes 15 families with mainly site-specific colon cancer, 41 affected family members, and 178 asymptomatic individuals at risk. In addition, 12 families with high frequencies of colonic and other cancers, with 30 affected and 209 at-risk individuals, are available. The pedigree of a typical familial aggregate is shown in Figure 3. These individuals do not have the extensive colonic polyposis that characterizes familial polyp-

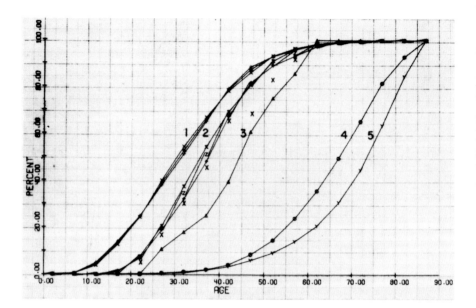

FIG. 2. Computer printout illustrating cumulative percent of incident cases at various ages having familial polyposis, compared to cumulative age incidence of colon cancer in other population groups. Curve 1 shows the onset of nonmalignant polyposis and Curve 2 the onset of cancer in familial polyposis, both derived from data of 655 cases obtained from Dr. R. Bussey, St. Marks Hospital, London (males, females, and males and females combined). (x) shows cumulative incidence of colon cancer in 13 polyposis cases in Memorial Hospital series. Curve 3 shows early age of onset of cancer in 28 affected individuals from Memorial Hospital series who have familial colon cancer-prone disease without polyposis. Curve 4 illustrates the age of onset of colon and rectal cancer in the general population of the United States, from the Third National Cancer Survey, NCI, and includes white and black males and females combined. Curve 5 illustrates the onset of colon and rectal cancer in males and females in Japan from data supplied by Dr. T. Hirayama (Lipkin et al. 1980a).

osis, and they are believed to have a hereditary form of colon cancer with an autosomal dominant mode of inheritance (Lynch 1976, Anderson et al. 1977, Fraumeni 1977). The early age of onset of cancer of the large intestine also is shown in Figure 2. Systematic surveillance has recently been started at Memorial Hospital to detect additional pedigrees of familial cancer. We are now able to identify new familial groups and continually enlarge our registry at this hospital.

Multiple Cancers Including Colorectal

We now have a population registry of subjects at Memorial Hospital of 324 individuals who have had colorectal plus other primary tumors. The latter include breast (21%), gynecological (16%), genitourinary (11%), and other regions of the gastrointestinal tract (9%). The early age of onset of colorectal cancer in these individuals with colorectal plus other primary tumors is shown in Figure 4. Three subgroups are present.

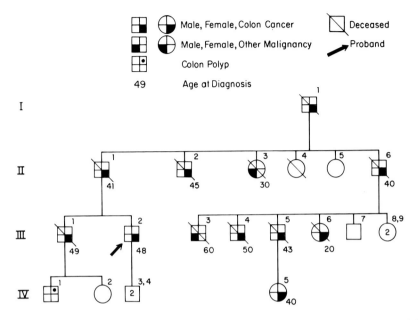

FIG. 3. Typical pattern of inheritance of cancer in a Memorial Hospital familial aggregate highly predisposed to colon cancer without polyposis, together with ages of onset of cancer in some family members (Lipkin et al. 1980a).

1. Individuals having a familial history of colorectal cancer: Individuals in this subgroup have colorectal cancer, a second primary tumor, and a familial history of colorectal cancer. The age distribution differs significantly from the U.S. general population (Figure 4, curve 4), revealed by the logrank analysis ($p < .05$). Thirty familial aggregates are present in this registry.

2. Individuals having a familial history of cancer other than colorectal: This group includes 131 individuals with colorectal cancer, a second primary tumor, and a familial history of cancer other than colorectal. The age distribution in this group (Figure 4) also appears slightly earlier than the age distribution in the U.S. general population, with a significant difference present ($p < .05$).

3. Individuals with no family history of cancer: This group includes 163 individuals with colorectal cancer, a second primary tumor, and a negative family history of cancer. The cumulative age incidence in this group (Figure 4) also differs significantly from the U.S. general population.

Single and Multiple Colorectal Adenomas

The presence of one or more adenomas occurs in 5% to 10% of all individuals in the general population, and is associated with the development of adenocarcinomas. Kindreds have also been reported showing an association of single and multiple adenomas with adenocarcinoma, with an apparent

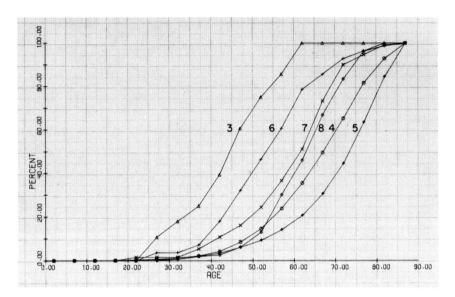

FIG. 4. Computer printout of cumulative percent of incident cases having multiple cancers, including colorectal, from Memorial Hospital series. Curves 3, 4, and 5 show the same population groups seen in Figure 2. Curve 6 shows the onset of colorectal cancer in individuals with multiple primary cancers and family history of colorectal cancer. Curve 7 shows the onset of colorectal cancer in individuals with multiple primary cancers and family history of cancer other than colorectal. Curve 8 shows onset of colorectal cancer in individuals with multiple primary cancers and no family history of cancer (Lipkin et al. 1980a).

genetic susceptibility (Woolf 1955). It has been estimated that 5% of all of these adenomas become malignant, and the development of villous characteristics in the adenomas is associated with increased frequency of malignancy. Colonic adenomas also appear with a peak incidence five to ten years earlier than colon cancer in the general population. These adenomatous polyps have an epidemiologic distribution similar to colon cancer (Morson and Bussey 1970, Correa 1978). Our registry of single and multiple adenomas now includes 634 individuals; we are developing age-incidence data for the appearance of multiple adenomas in these individuals.

Primary Colorectal Cancer in the General Population

Individuals in this category, who have had colorectal cancer without other malignant disease, also are available for comparison with the aforementioned population groups. At present, our registry at Memorial Hospital also has been subdivided into three categories: 1. individuals with primary colorectal cancer plus a familial history of colorectal cancer; 2. individuals with a familial history of cancer other than colorectal cancer; and 3. individuals with no family history of cancer. These are shown in Fig. 5. The age-incidence

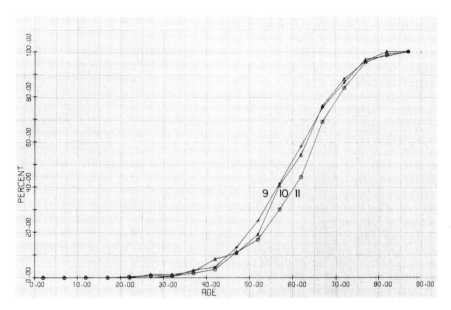

FIG. 5. Computer printout of cumulative percent of incident cases in Memorial Hospital series having primary colorectal cancer without a second tumor. Curve 9 shows primary colorectal cancer and family history of cancer other than colorectal. Curve 10 shows primary colorectal cancer and family history of colon cancer. Curve 11 shows primary colorectal cancer and no family history of cancer (Lipkin et al. 1980a).

distributions in these groups are closer to the age incidence of colon cancer in the general population of the U.S. and Japan. Our population registry now consists of 374 individuals having primary colorectal cancer; 59 have a family history of colorectal cancer, 123 have a family history of cancer other than colorectal, and 192 have no family history of cancer. Further subdivisions are being made for individuals with colon cancer and for those with rectal cancer. In several studies it has been shown that familial associations of colorectal cancer among index cases of colorectal cancer in the general population are higher than in control groups. Environmental as well as inherited factors could be associated with the development of neoplasms in these groups.

Familial Aggregates Cancer-Free for Two and More Generations

Familial aggregates with 41 individuals cancer-free for two and more generations also have been identified and are available for this study. In addition, spouses of individuals in the population groups mentioned and medical student volunteers also are available as control subjects. Measurements have also been begun on populations at low risk for colorectal cancer in geographic areas that include Medellin, Colombia, South America, and various regions in

Japan, for further comparison with the high risk population groups in the Memorial Sloan-Kettering registry.

The development of these population registries has enabled us to call up individuals and familial aggregates in the above categories for measurements of phenotypic abnormalities associated with high frequency and early age of development of colorectal cancer. Verification is made of individual and family history of previous colorectal cancer and other pathological findings by obtaining pathology records and death certificates and by consulting physicians of record of family members affected.

PROLIFERATIVE ABNORMALITIES IN COLONIC EPITHELIAL CELLS OF INDIVIDUALS WITH FAMILIAL POLYPOSIS

Studies of cell proliferation have aided our understanding of events that develop during neoplastic transformation of colonic cells, in the hereditary diseases leading to large bowel cancer, and in the sporadic large bowel cancers believed to be caused mainly by environmental or endogenously produced carcinogens. In familial polyposis, colonic epithelial cells predestined to develop neoplasia show characteristic proliferative changes. During progressive stages of abnormal development, cell phenotypes appear in which epithelial cells gain an increased ability to proliferate and to accumulate in the mucosa (Deschner et al. 1963, Cole and McKalen 1963, Lipkin 1977, Bleiberg et al. 1972, and Iwana et al. 1977). This finding has been observed in normal-appearing colonic epithelial cells of subjects with familial polyposis before as well as after the cells develop adenomatous changes and begin to accumulate as polyps. It has been noted in over 80% of random biopsy specimens (Lipkin 1978) and has now been shown to occur with higher frequency than in population groups at low risk of developing colorectal cancer (Lipkin et al. 1980b).

Current observations in our laboratory also have indicated a significantly higher frequency of abnormal proliferative activity of this type in colon cancer-prone families without familial polyposis (Lipkin et al. 1980b). In our ongoing studies we are continuing to quantitate several proliferative abnormalities as they are observed in the colonic mucosa of high- and low-risk population groups, to further analyze their discriminatory value in pointing to colon cancer risk in subjects in different geographic regions.

A failure of colonic epithelial cells to repress DNA synthesis also occurs in other diseases of man including ulcerative colitis (Eastwood and Trier 1973). In ways similar to diseases of the colon, in atrophic gastritis, a condition associated with the development of gastric cancer, epithelial cells also fail to repress DNA synthesis and undergo abnormal maturation as they migrate through the gastric mucosa (Winawer and Lipkin 1969, Deschner et al. 1972). A similar event occurs in precancerous disease of the cervical epithelium in human beings (Wilbanks et al. 1967) and in cervix of rodents after exposure to a chemical carcinogen (Hasegawa et al. 1976). Thus, during the development of neoplasms in other organs as well as in the colon, persistent DNA synthesis occurs in cells that normally would be terminal or end cells. Associated pathological changes accompany this development leading to atypias, dysplasias, and malignancy, as also occurs in familial polyposis.

In familial polyposis, as colonic epithelial cells which do not repress proliferative activity undergo abnormal maturation and accumulate in the mucosa, they develop the morphological changes characteristic of adenomas; these further develop the tubular or villous structures noted above. In terms of cell proliferation kinetics, we have estimated that most epithelial cells in these adenomas are extruded, while only a minor fraction are retained to proliferate and induce growth (Lightdale and Lipkin 1975). Carcinomas develop with increasing frequency as these adenomatous excrescences enlarge (Morson 1976).

We believe that a sequence of events leads to malignancy in inherited polyposis (Lipkin 1978). Cells having the germinal mutation fail to repress DNA synthesis (phase 1 proliferative lesion) (Lipkin 1974). Additional events then occur, giving rise to new clones from the original cell population. An early event leads to the development of the well-known adenomatous cells that proliferate and accumulate near the surface of the mucosa (phase 2 proliferative lesion) (Lipkin 1974). In familial polyposis, according to this concept, an additional event then occurs in the cells giving rise to invasive malignancy. This concept allows for a contribution of endogenous or exogenous carcinogenic or promotor elements to interact with the cells having a hereditary predisposition to neoplasia. It also allows for the introduction of preventive measures to block the steps leading to malignant transformation of cells.

CEA IN COLONIC LAVAGE OF INDIVIDUALS AT HIGH RISK OF LARGE BOWEL CANCER

In addition to abnormal proliferative activity in colonic epithelial cells of familial polyposis, identifiable at an early stage before the development of visible adenomas, increased CEA also has been noted in colonic lavage specimens obtained from members of polyposis family aggregates (Poleski et al. 1978). Plasma CEA has been disappointing as an indicator of early lesions; however, elevated CEA concentrations have been shown in colonic lavage specimens from individuals with large adenomas and cancer, compared to specimens from individuals without evidence of colonic disease (Winawer et al. 1977). A recent study was carried out to measure CEA concentrations in colonic lavage of hereditary polyposis families, nonpolyposis colon cancer-prone families, and control subjects without evidence of colonic disease or familial predisposition to colon cancer. Current findings have indicated a significant elevation of CEA in colonic lavage of many of the individuals in familial polyposis aggregates who do not have visible adenomas (Poleski et al. 1978). The reasons for the CEA elevation are unknown at present, but they may be associated with early hyperplasia of the cells or other inflammatory changes that develop within the mucosa in familial polyposis.

STUDIES OF CUTANEOUS CELLS OF INDIVIDUALS WITH FAMILIAL POLYPOSIS

Recent studies also have indicated that phenotypic expressions of the genetic defect leading to familial polyposis can be detected in cutaneous cells. Increased heteroploidy in cutaneous epithelial cells derived from individuals with Gardner's syndrome has been reported. It was also noted that cutaneous fibroblasts derived from individuals previously diagnosed as having familial polyposis, or Gardner's syndrome, have abnormal growth characteristics. Recent studies have shown differences in the distribution of the cytoskeletal protein actin within cultured cells from individuals with familial polyposis compared to normals (Kopelovich et al. 1980). In order to determine the specificity of these observations, additional measurements are presently being carried out on cutaneous cells from larger control groups at low risk for large bowel cancer and from additional families with various patterns of inherited polyposis and large bowel cancer.

IMMUNOLOGIC STUDIES

Recently, an immunologic abnormality has been reported in individuals from colon cancer-prone families without polyposis (Berlinger et al. 1977). When cancer-free individuals from families predisposed to large bowel cancer, but without familial polyposis, were studied to determine the nature of their cell-mediated immune capacities, 44% demonstrated an apparent perturbation of adherent cell function which manifested itself as an inappropriate suppression of potentially normal lymphocyte ability to respond to an allogeneic stimulus. This in vitro defect in recognitive immunity that had developed in these individuals was the same defect demonstrated in individuals with established malignant diseases. Several patients with Gardner's syndrome also showed the deficit of recognitive immunity (Berlinger et al. 1977). These studies also are being extended to asymptomatic individuals in additional familial aggregates having the various disorders leading to large bowel cancer; they offer the possibility of a new immunological approach to the early detection of susceptible population groups.

EXAMINATION OF FECAL CONTENTS

In familial polyposis and related disorders, still other studies are in progress to identify those constituents of fecal contents that may be abnormal, and to examine their potential carcinogenic activity on cells of the colon. The bile acids and their bacterial conversion products are a group of compounds currently under examination. Several recent reports have analyzed and compared the fecal neutral sterols and bile acids in patients with familial polyposis and controls other than relatives (Reddy et al. 1976, Drasar et al. 1975, Lipkin et al. 1981). Individuals with familial polyposis excreted higher amounts of cholesterol and lower levels of the degradation products of cholesterol: coprostanol and coprostanone. Nondegradation of cholesterol also has been found in familial colon cancer-prone aggregates without polyposis (Lipkin et al. 1981) and in a minor fraction of individuals in the general population (Wilkins and Hackman 1974) whose background and related characteristics have not been defined.

Current results also have suggested differences in metabolic activity of fecal microflora in members of familial polyposis aggregates, compared to age- and sex-matched controls who consumed similar western style diets. Differences in metabolic activity of fecal microflora have previously been shown in population groups at increased risk for large bowel neoplasia. Further studies also are in progress to extend these findings to individuals in the familial colon cancer-prone groups in order to assess the utility of these variations in metabolic activity of fecal microflora and in cholesterol and its metabolites. Findings of this type may contribute to the screening of polyposis family siblings for disease, and could point to mechanisms of initiation or promotion during large bowel carcinogenesis.

Recently, an additional and potentially important lead in the identification of factors involved in colon cancer development was provided by detection of mutagenic activity in the feces of human beings (Varghese et al. 1977, Land and Bruce 1978). It was suspected that a nitroso group exchange reaction occurred by transfer from nitrosamine to an amide moiety, resulting in the generation of highly reactive nitrosamide compounds in feces (Mandel et al. 1977), and that endogenous nitrates in humans might lead to formation of carcinogens (Tannenbaum et al. 1978). In current work, patients in the familial polyposis and hereditary large bowel cancer-prone (nonpolyposis) aggregates are under study; this topic remains an interesting one for further development. We now have a variety of approaches to the analysis of fecal contents of individuals in high- and low-risk categories underway, including the above parameters.

These findings have led to the development of the risk factor profiles shown in Figures 6 and 7 which now serve as working models for the study of population groups with increased susceptibility to colorectal cancer, and for individuals within these high risk populations (Lipkin et al. 1980c).

CURRENT APPROACHES TO THE SURVEILLANCE OF INDIVIDUALS WITH INCREASED SUSCEPTIBILITY TO COLORECTAL CANCER

In view of these and related observations that have been made on the identification of subjects with increased susceptibility to colorectal neoplasia, can reasonable approaches be developed to attempt to improve the sur-

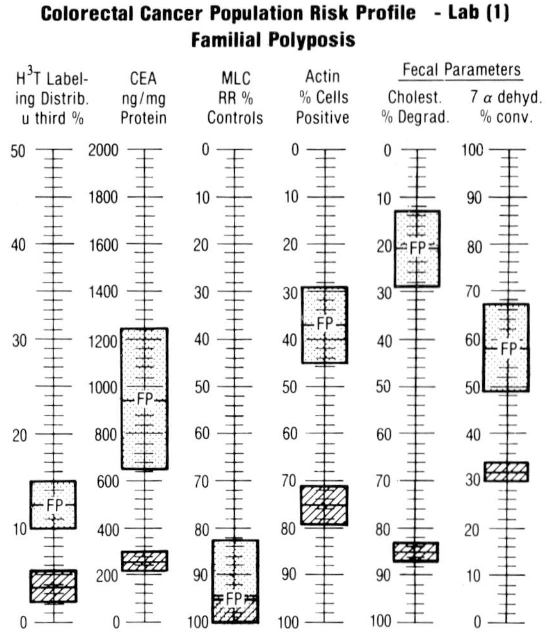

FIG. 6. Laboratory portion of the colorectal cancer risk profile currently being developed to quantitate the occurrence of phenotypic attributes in population groups having increased suscep- tibility to cancer of the large intestine. The frequency (mean ± 1SE) of each characteristic in the familial polyposis symptomatic group is shown (dotted segments) compared to its control group (segments with diagonal lines). Column 1: percent of ^{3}TdR-labeled epithelial cells in upper third of colonic crypt, in random biopsy specimens of flat colonic mucosa. Column 2: amount of CEA in colonic lavage specimens (ng/mg protein). Column 3: mixed leukocyte response, RR (relative response as percent of control group). Column 4: percent of cutaneous fibroblasts having normal pattern of actin. Fecal parameters are given in Columns 5–6: percent of undegraded cholesterol in stool specimens; and 7α dehydroxylase (% cholic acid converted to deoxycholic acid). In mea- surements underway, observed differences between means of FP and respective control groups are statistically significant (t test, p < .01), for ^{3}HTdR labeling, CEA, actin and fecal cholesterol degradation (Lipkin et al. 1980c).

veillance of these subjects efficiently enough to reduce the onset and progres- sion of lesions? In support of this possibility are several studies in which surveillance programs relying on proctosigmoidoscopic examination (Gilbertsen, 1974) or family history of cancer (Anderson 1977) have begun to increase the efficiency with which early lesions can be identified. In our current studies, we are attempting to develop the risk factor profiles in all of the population groups with increased susceptibility to cancer of the large intestine in the Memorial Hospital registry noted previously. Affected mem- bers of polyposis families also are recommended for prophylactic colectomy, and asymptomatic members undergo flexible sigmoidoscopy or colonoscopy every 2–3 years. For the ongoing surveillance of the other groups at the present, the approaches outlined in Figures 8–10 have been developed.

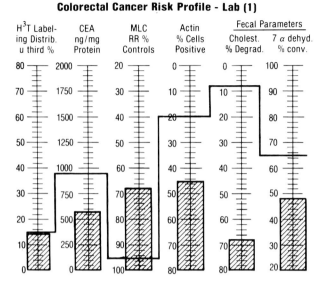

FIG. 7. Laboratory portion of the colorectal cancer risk profile currently being developed to quantitate the occurrence of the phenotypic attributes in individuals with varying degrees of susceptibility to colorectal neoplasia. Columns 1–6 have the same parameters as in Figure 1. Shaded areas show tentative normal ranges with upper limits at 2SD from mean values in control groups. Horizontal line shows test results in an individual with symptomatic familial polyposis (Lipkin et al. 1980c).

With regard to surveillance for gastrointestinal neoplasms as conventionally carried out in medical practice today, most patients with colorectal cancer seek medical attention after symptoms have occurred. When this delay is sufficiently prolonged, morbidity and mortality are significantly increased (Miller 1976). Although the presence of symptoms in patients with

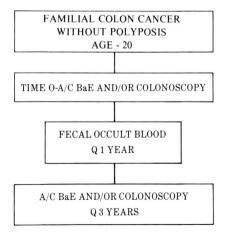

FIG. 8. Proposed algorithm for screening patients with a family history of the non-polyposis inherited colon cancer. Since fecal occult blood testing appears to have low sensitivity for detecting adenomas, the colon must be cleared of premalignant adenomas by direct visualization. The value of the barium enema has been questioned because of the young age at which screening begins, with possible periodic accumulative radiation exposure during repeated screening. The barium enema could be justified along with the colonoscopy initially on the basis that initially the screening is for cancers as well as adenomas (A/C indicates air-contrast). (Winawer et al. 1981.)

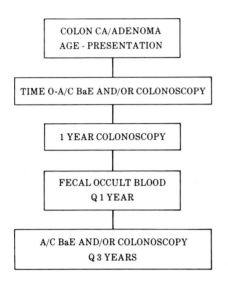

FIG. 9. Proposed algorithm for screening average risk patients. There is controversy as to whether screening should begin at age 40 or 50. Sigmoidoscopy is not necessary more often than every 3–5 years since several years are necessary for a new adenoma to arise de novo from a normal mucosa and grow to a premalignant size of 1 cm. Some physicians feel that both the barium enema and colonoscopy should be done, whereas others feel that colonoscopy alone is adequate. (A/C indicates air-contrast.) (Winawer et al. 1981.)

colorectal cancer leads to a less favorable prognosis, the symptoms that arise also may be associated with one of the premalignant lesions, e.g., adenomas, particularly in the familial syndromes where these occur with high frequency. The major age risk in individuals at standard risk in the general population begins in men and women at about age 40 and begins to rise more steeply at age 50. The age of onset can be modified strongly by familial history. Individuals who have a strong family history of colorectal cancer may begin to have an

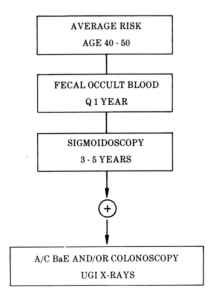

FIG. 10. Proposed algorithm for screening patients who have had removal of a colon cancer or adenoma. Follow-up surveillance should begin when their risk is identified, regardless of age. The value of the air-contrast barium enema in addition to the colonoscopy every three years has been questioned since the lesion primarily being searched for is an adenoma, for which the barium enema has low sensitivity. The initial barium enema could be justified on the basis that initially the screening is for synchronous cancers, as well as synchronous adenomas (Winawer et al. 1981.)

increased cancer risk at a much younger age, beginning in the 20's (Figures 1-4). For reasons unknown, a very young age of onset of colorectal cancer also can occur in individuals with no family history of cancer.

Individuals who have had an adenoma of the colon also are at increased risk for colorectal cancer both at the time the adenoma developed and also at later periods (Winawer et al. 1976). Similarly, patients who have had colorectal cancer successfully resected are at increased risk for the development of another cancer of the colon (Morson 1976). The probability of having a simultaneous second adenoma (synchronous lesion) following the discovery of a single adenoma is about 0.50, while the probability of having a synchronous colorectal cancer with a single cancer of the colon is somewhere between 0.015 and 0.05. The probability of having a metachronous adenoma at a later time after a single adenoma has been removed is about 0.30 while a second or metachronous colorectal cancer occurs with a probability of 0.05-0.10.

In these various groups, the frequencies of appearance of early lesions at given ages in family members are being measured to analyze the rate at which new lesions appear in these groups. These programs are accompanied by evaluations of the efficiency with which lesions can be detected and the economic impact of the measurements. Thus, in asymptomatic subjects at average risk of developing colorectal cancer who are over 40 years of age, fecal occult blood tests carried out once a year and a flexible sigmoidoscopy done every three to five years are currently recommended for this ongoing evaluation. Fecal occult blood tests have been shown to be feasible, with a low false-positive rate of about 2%, and with a "predictive value" for neoplasia of about 50% in individuals with a positive screening test. Approximately 38% of persons with a positive fecal occult blood test will have an adenoma, and 12% will have a cancer (Winawer 1979). These cancers have been mainly of the Dukes' A and B type with high probability of cure as a result of surgery. The fecal occult blood test screening programs with the best results have used the method of Greegor, with a high-fiber, meat-free diet, and with six specimens examined (two per day for three days in patients who are totally asymptomatic) (Greegor 1967). One positive slide from the six collected is sufficient for a diagnostic investigation. Flexible sigmoidoscopy has given a higher yield than rigid sigmoidoscopy, and is a much more comfortable examination for the patient. It is very likely in the future that flexible sigmoidoscopy with a 30-35 cm instrument, in addition to the fecal occult test, will replace rigid sigmoidoscopy for periodic screening (Winawer et al. 1977).

The population groups at higher risk for colorectal cancer should at present be screened with different programs, generally with colonoscopy, whether or not barium enema is done. A major principle in screening high-risk groups involves the direct and clear visualization of the colon for the detection of underlying premalignant as well as malignant lesions at intervals sufficiently short to accomplish the desired result, despite lesion regrowth that is likely to occur. For the groups with familial forms of colon cancer, and for subjects with a prior adenoma or colorectal cancer, the suggested interval for routine surveillance is about three years for repeat colonoscopy, including the right side of the colon, after initially clearing the colon of adenomas.

REFERENCES

Anderson, D. E., and M. M. Romsdahl. 1977. Family history: A criterion for selective screening, *in* Genetics of Human Cancer, J. J. Mulvihill, R. W. Miller, and J. F. Fraumeni, Jr., eds. Raven Press, New York, pp. 257–262.

Berlinger, N. T., C. Lopez, J. Vogel, M. Lipkin, and R. A. Good. 1977. Defective recognitive immunity in family aggregates of colon carcinoma. J. Clin. Invest. 59:761–769.

Bleiberg, H., P. Mainguet, and P. Galand. 1972. Cell renewal in familial polyposis: Comparison between polyps and adjacent healthy mucosa. Gastroenterol. 63:240–245.

Bussey, H. J. R. 1975. Familial Polyposis Coli. The Johns Hopkins University Press, Baltimore, 104 pp.

Cole, J. W., and A. McKalen. 1963. Studies on the morphogenesis of adenomatous polyps in the human colon. Cancer 16:998–1002.

Deschner, E. E., C. M. Lewis, and M. Lipkin. 1963. In vitro study of human rectal epithelial cells. I. Atypical zone of H3 thymidine incorporation in mucosa of multiple polyposis. J. Clin. Invest. 42:1922–1928.

Deschner, E. E., S. Winawer, and M. Lipkin. 1972. Patterns of nucleic acid and protein synthesis in normal human gastric mucosa and atrophic gastritis. J. Natl. Cancer Inst. 48:1567–1574.

Drasar, B. S., E. S. Bone, M. F. Hill, and C. G. Marks. 1975. Colon cancer and bacterial metabolism in familial polyposis. Gut 16:824–825.

Eastwood, G. L., and J. S. Trier. 1973. Epithelial cell renewal in cultured rectal biopsies in ulcerative colitis. Gastroenterology 64:383–390.

Fraumeni, J. F., Jr. 1977. Clinical patterns of familial cancer, *in* Genetics of Human Cancer, J. J. Mulvihill, R. W. Miller, and J. F. Fraumeni, Jr., eds. Raven Press, New York, pp. 223–235.

Gardner, E. J. 1951. A genetic and clinical study of intestinal polyposis: A predisposing factor for carcinoma of the colon and rectum. Am. J. Hum. Genet. 3:167–176.

Gardner, E. J., and R. C. Richards. 1953. Multiple cutaneous and subcutaneous lesions occurring simultaneously with hereditary polyposis and osteomatosis. Am. J. Hum. Genet. 5:139–147.

Gilbertson, V. A. 1974. Proctosigmoidoscopy and polypectomy in reducing the incidence of rectal cancer. Cancer 34:936–939.

Greegor, D. H. 1967. Diagnosis of large-bowel cancer in the asymptomatic patient. JAMA 201:943–945.

Hasegawa, I., Y. Matsumira, and S. Tojo. 1976. Cellular kinetics and histological changes in experimental cancer of the uterine cervix. Cancer Res. 36:359–364.

Iwana, T., J. Utsunomiya, and J. Sasaki. 1977. Epithelial cell kinetics in the crypts of familial polyposis of the colon. Jpn. J. Surg. 7:230–234.

Kopelovich, L., M. Lipkin, W. Blattner, J. F. Fraumeni, Jr., H. Lynch, and R. Pollack. 1980. Organization of actin-containing cables in cultured skin fibroblasts from individuals at high risk of colon cancer. Int. J. Cancer 26:301–307.

Land, P. C., and W. R. Bruce. 1978. Fecal mutagens: A possible relationship with colorectal cancer. (Abstract) Proc. A.A.C.R. 19:167.

Lightdale, C., and M. Lipkin. 1975. Cell division and tumor growth, *in* Cancer, F. F. Becker, ed., vol. 3. Plenum Publishing Co., New York, pp. 201–215.

Lipkin, M. 1974. Phase 1 and phase 2 proliferative lesions of colonic epithelial cells in diseases leading to colon cancer. Cancer 34:878–888.

Lipkin, M. 1977. Growth kinetics of normal and premalignant gastrointestinal epithelium, *in* Growth Kinetics and Biochemical Regulation of Normal and Malignant Cells. Williams and Wilkins, Co., Baltimore, pp. 562–589.

Lipkin, M. 1978. Susceptibility of human population groups to colon cancer. Adv. Cancer Res. 27:281–304.

Lipkin, M., B. S. Reddy, J. W. Weisburger, and L. J. Schechter. 1981. Nondegradation of fecal cholesterol in subjects at high risk for cancer of the large intestine. J. Clin. Invest. 67:304–307.

Lipkin, M., S. Scherf, L. Schechter, and D. Braun. 1980a. Memorial Hospital Registry of populations at high risk for cancer of the large intestine: Age at onset of neoplasms. Prev. Med. 9:335–345.

Lipkin, M., E. E. Deschner, W. Blattner, J. F. Fraumeni, Jr., and H. Lynch. 1980b. Tritiated thymidine incorporation into colonic epithelial cells of subjects in colon cancer prone families. (Abstract) Proc. A.A.C.R. 21:188.

Lipkin, M., P. Sherlock, and J. DeCosse. 1980c. Risk factors and preventive measures in the control of cancer of the large intestine. Curr. Probl. Cancer 4:1–57.

Lynch, H. T. 1976. Cancer Genetcs. Charles C Thomas Co., Springfield, Ill., 639 pp.

Mandel, M., D. Ichinotsubo, and H. Mower. 1977. Nitroso group exchange as a way of activation of nitrosamines by bacteria. Nature 267:248–249.

Miller, D. G. 1976. The early diagnosis of cancer, *in* Physiopathology of Cancer, F. Hombarger, ed. Basel, S. Karger, pp. 5–64.

Morson, B. C. 1976. Genesis of colorectal cancer. Clin. Gastroenterol. 5:505–525.

Morson, B. C., and H. R. J. Bussey. 1970. Predisposing causes of intestinal cancer, *in* Current Problems in Surgery, Year Book Medical Publishers, Inc., Chicago, pp. 1–50.

Poleski, M. H., W. A. Blattner, M. Chait, S. W. Winawer, M. Fleischer, M. D. Schwartz, J. F. Fraumeni, Jr., and M. Lipkin. 1978. CEA in colonic lavage of individuals at high risk for large bowel cancer. Gastroenterol. 74:1140.

Reddy, B. S., A. Mastromarino, C. Gustafson, M. Lipkin, and E. L. Wynder. 1976. Fecal bile acids and neutral stools in patients with familial polyposis. Cancer 38:1694–1698.

Smith, W. G. 1959. Desmoid tumors in familial multiple polyposis. Mayo Clin. Proc. 34:31–38.

Tannenbaum, S. R., D. Fett, V. R. Young, P. D. Land, and W. R. Bruce. 1978. Nitrite and nitrate are formed by endogenous synthesis in human intestine. Science 200:1487–1489.

Varghese, A. J., P. Land, R. Furrer, and W. R. Bruce. 1977. Evidence for the formation of mutagenic N-nitroso compounds in the human body. (Abstract) Proc. A.A.C.R. 18:80.

Wilbanks, G. D., R. M. Richart, and J. Y. Terner. 1967. DNA content of cervical intraepithelial neoplasms studied by two wave length Feulgen cytophotometry. Am. J. Obstet. Gynecol. 98:792–799.

Wilkins, T. D., and A. S. Hackman. 1974. Two patterns of neutral steroid conversion in the feces of normal North Americans. Cancer Res. 34:2250–2254.

Winawer, S. J. 1979. Progress report of controlled trial of screening with fecal occult blood testing, *in* Screening and Early Detection of Colorectal Cancer, D. Brodie, ed. NIH Publication No. 80:2075.

Winawer, S. J., M. Fleischer, S. Green, D. Bhargava, S. D. Leidner, C. Boyle, P. Sherlock, and M. K. Schwartz. 1977. Carcinoembryonic antigen in colonic lavage. Gastroenterol. 73:719–722.

Winawer, S. J., and M. Lipkin. 1969. Cell proliferation kinetics in the gastrointestinal tract of man. J. Natl. Cancer Inst. 42:9–17.

Winawer, S. J., and P. Sherlock. 1981. Screening for premalignant and malignant diseases of the colon, *in* Harrison's Textbook of Medicine (in press).

Winawer, S. J., P. Sherlock, D. Schottenfield, and D. G. Miller. 1976. Screening for colon cancer. Gastroenterol. 70:783–789.

Gastrointestinal Cancer, edited by
John R. Stroehlein and
Marvin M. Romsdahl.
Raven Press, New York © 1981.

The Use of Animal Tumor Models to Study the Metastatic Process

Garth L. Nicolson, Ph.D.

*Department of Tumor Biology, The University of Texas System Cancer Center
M. D. Anderson Hospital and Tumor Institute, Houston, Texas*

INTRODUCTION

Although metastasis is one of the most important events in the pathogenesis of cancer, there have been surprisingly few comprehensive studies of this process in man or in experimental models. Important inroads in this area have been made through the development of transplantable tumors, tissue culture, and sophisticated biochemical, immunological, genetic, and ultrastructural techniques, and we now know far more about the pathogenesis of tumor metastasis. Metastasis involves a complex series of sequential steps whereby malignant cells invade adjacent tissues and penetrate into the lymphatic and circulatory systems, detach from the primary tumor mass, spread to near and distant sites, arrest and invade at these secondary sites, and finally proliferate to form new metastatic colonies (Weiss 1977, Fidler and Nicolson 1981, Fidler et al. 1978, Sugarbaker 1979, Poste and Fidler 1980). That metastasis is the end result of several highly selective sequential steps whereby fewer and fewer tumor cells eventually survive to form secondary colonies is an important concept in the pathogenesis of metastasis (Poste and Fidler 1980, Fidler and Nicolson 1981). This concept suggests that the actual cells that are capable of forming metastases represent only a very minor subpopulation of the cells that comprise the primary tumor mass.

Metastasis usually begins when a tumor mass extends or invades surrounding tissues; this loss of proper cell positioning and cell-cell interactions characterizes the malignant state (Nicolson and Poste 1976). Invasion is thought to occur by mechanical extension (Eaves 1973) or enzymatic destruction of extracellular tissue matrix (Dresden et al. 1972, Hashimoto et al. 1973), or both.

Invading malignant cells can detach and be transported away from the original tumor mass. The far more important routes in this process are the blood vessels and the lymphatics where penetrating tumor cells can be released and circulated as single cells or as multiple cell emboli. The release of such emboli into the blood is known to be affected by venous pressure, blood flow, and trauma due to surgery or other manipulations (Fisher et al. 1967). However, the presence of malignant cells or cell emboli in the blood is not a good indicator that subsequent distant metastasis will form (Salsbury 1975). This observation is probably because most tumor cells die rapidly in the circulation, and only a very small fraction finally survive to form secondary tumors (Fidler et al. 1978).

During transport in the blood, malignant cells undergo cellular interactions with themselves, other circulating host cells, soluble blood components, and the vascular cell endothelium. Cellular interactions that affect tumor cell arrest and subsequent survival include homotypic adhesion of tumor cells to form multicell emboli (Fidler 1973a, Liotta et al. 1976, Winkelhake and Nicolson 1976), heterotypic adhesion such as that of tumor cells to platelets (Gasic et al. 1973, Warren 1973), lymphocytes (Fidler 1975, Fidler and Bucana 1977) or endothelial cells and their subendothelial matrix (Kramer and Nicolson 1979, Kramer et al. 1980), and interaction of tumor cells with blood components such as fibrinogen or fibrin (Warren 1973, Chew et al. 1976). Although mechanical factors such as tumor emboli size and capillary deformability modify lodgment properties in the first capillary bed encountered (Zeidman and Buss 1952, Sato and Suzuki 1976), malignant cells often pass through capillaries after their initial arrest and recirculate to other sites (Zeidman and Buss 1952, Fidler and Nicolson 1976, 1977, Fisher and Fisher 1967a).

An examination of the blood-borne tumor cell arrest and survival patterns of various malignant neoplasms indicates that mechanical considerations alone are insufficient to explain nonrandom metastatic colonization. In man there are numerous examples where tumors tend to metastasize to particular secondary locations (Salsbury 1975, del Regato 1977, Sugarbaker 1979). In addition, many experimental animal tumor systems show organ preference of secondary tumor colonization (Dunn 1954, Sugarbaker 1952, Potter et al. 1957, Kinsey 1960, Fidler and Nicolson 1976, 1977, Brunson and Nicolson 1978, Hart and Fidler 1980), suggesting that metastasis is influenced by unique tumor cell and/or host properties. Recognition of unique capillary vascular endothelial cell surface determinants by circulating malignant cells could result in implantation at specific sites (Nicolson and Winkelhake 1975, Nicolson et al. 1976), or the subsequent growth of arrested site-dependent cells (Hart and Fidler 1980).

Extravasation or secondary invasion of the endothelium and its underlying basement membrane is the next most common step after implantation of blood-borne tumor cells in the microcirculation. This process may (Wood 1964, Chew et al. 1976) or may not (Fisher and Fisher 1967b, Ludatsher et al. 1967) involve deposition and dissolution of a fibrin matrix around the arrested tumor cells. Penetration of the vascular endothelium may in some cases occur by diapedesis or intracellular penetration (Dingemans 1973), but the usual route appears to be penetration at the sites of endothelial cell retraction (Ludatsher et al. 1967, Kramer and Nicolson 1979, 1981). The retraction of vascular endothelial cells caused by tumor cell–endothelial cell interactions and exposure of underlying basement membrane allows malignant cells to move to the basement membrane surface. This occurs because of an adhesive gradient from the endothelial cell surface to the basement membrane and results in the net movement of the malignant cells to the basement membrane (Kramer et al. 1980). Subsequent invasion is probably determined by cell surface or secreted enzymes (Strauch 1972, Dresden et al. 1972, Sylvén 1973, Hashimoto et al. 1973, Koono et al. 1974). Tissue damage or tumor cell secretion of angiogenesis factors (Folkman 1974) is probably responsible for vascularization of the secondary tumor colony, an event that appears to be important for rapid tumor growth.

ANIMAL MODELS AND METASTASIS

In order to study the role of tumor cell properties in the metastatic process it is useful to have available animal tumor models that mimic human metastatic disease. Since animal tumor cell lines exist that share common genetic backgrounds but differ in their metastatic phenotypes, certain aspects of metastasis may be traceable to identifiable tumor cell characteristics. Koch (1939) was the first to attempt to study the cellular characteristics important in metastasis by selecting tumor cell variants for their malignant properties. One of the more useful techniques for obtaining malignant cells of common genetic origin and differing metastatic properties was developed by Fidler (1973b). By sequential selection of variant tumor cell sublines for enhanced ability to form blood-borne experimental pulmonary metastases in syngeneic hosts, Fidler (1973b) was able to develop a series of variant B16 melanoma cell sublines that showed increasing lung colonization potentials. Several types of in vivo

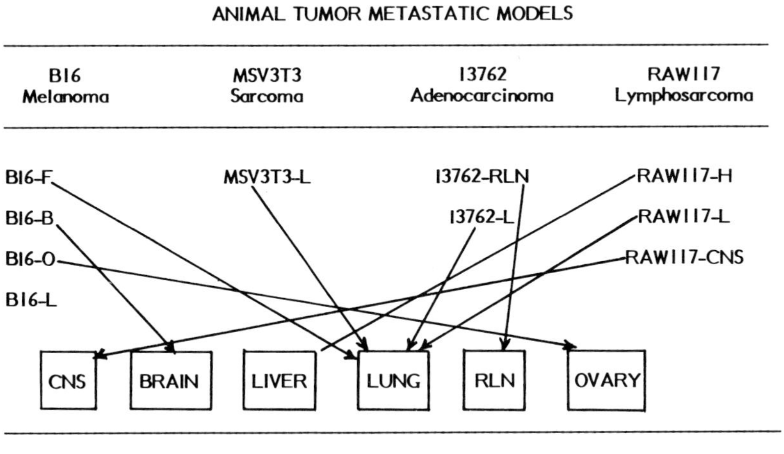

FIG. 1. In vivo selection for organ site colonization.

selections have now been performed utilizing the B16 melanoma, and sublines are available that show enhanced abilities to colonize lung, liver, ovary, or brain. In Figure 1, the various metastatic models, either developed or under development in our laboratory, are shown with the in vivo selection site for organ preference of colonization. Some of these in vivo selections were performed by implanting tumor cells subcutaneously and allowing the implanted cells to spontaneously metastasize (13762 adenocarcinoma metastasis to regional lymph nodes or lung) while others were developed using the blood-borne route. In addition to these models, a number of other in vivo selections for altered metastatic behavior exist and are available (Table 1). When similar selections were attempted without the requirement for blood-borne or lymphatic tumor cell arrest, variants with enhanced metastatic properties were not obtained. Brunson and Nicolson (1980) attempted to sequentially adapt B16 melanoma cells for brain survival and growth by direct intra-cerebral implantation. After ten adaptations for brain survival and growth, the resulting cell line was analyzed for its blood-borne brain implantation, survival, and growth characteristics and found to be no different in its metastatic properties than the original cell line from which it was adapted. This result is consistent with other data (see below) that strongly suggest that metastasis is a process of selection, not simply of gradual adaptation to the environment at a new secondary site.

An alternative method for the selection of metastatic variant tumor cell lines, based upon selection in vitro for particular cell surface properties, has also had some success. For example, it has been possible to select in vitro for

Table 1. *Animal Tumor Metastatic Models and Their Sites of Colonization*

Tumor Type	Selection for Site of Metastasis	References
Carcinoma	Lung	Koch 1939
Carcinoma	Lung	Klein 1955
Undifferentiated	Liver, Lung	Kerbel et al. 1978
Melanoma	Lung	Fidler 1973b
Melanoma	Brain	Brunson et al. 1978
Melanoma	Brain	Raz and Hart 1980
Melanoma	Brain	Nicolson et al. 1981
Melanoma	Ovary	Brunson and Nicolson 1979
Melanoma	Liver	Tao et al. 1979
Lymphoma	Liver	Schirrmacher et al. 1979
Sarcoma	Lung	Nicolson et al. 1978
Sarcoma	Lung	Salk and Lanza 1979
Lymphosarcoma	Liver	Brunson and Nicolson 1978
Lymphosarcoma	Lung	Belloni and Nicolson unpublished observations
Adenocarcinoma	Lung, RLN	Neri et al. 1979
Adenocarcinoma	Ascites, lung	Takahashi et al. 1978
Adenocarcinoma	Lung	Talmadge et al. 1979

Table 2. *Animal Tumor Cell Models Selected In Vitro for Altered Metastatic Behavior*

Cell Type	Mode of Selection	References
B16 melanoma	Resistance to lymphocyte killing	Fidler et al. 1976
B16 melanoma	Detachment from plastic	Briles and Kornfeld 1978
B16 melanoma	Resistance to lectin Toxicity	Tao and Burger 1977
B16 melanoma	Attachment to collagen	Liotta et al. 1978
B16 melanoma	Invasion of tissue	Poste et al. 1980
B16 melanoma	Invasion of bladder	Hart 1979
RAW117 lymphosarcoma	Loss of lectin binding	Reading et al. 1980a

tumor cell properties such as loss of sensitivity to lymphocyte-mediated cytotoxicity (Fidler et al. 1976), decreased sensitivity to toxic doses of lectins (Tao and Burger 1977), decreased binding to immobilized lectins (Reading et al. 1980a), increased invasiveness of tissue (Hart 1979) or veins (Poste et al. 1980), as well as other cellular properties (Table 2). Often these selections have resulted in concomitant modifications in the metastatic properties of the selected cell sublines (Table 2). In the examples presented in Table 2, some variant sublines were eventually obtained with altered in vivo metastatic properties, indicating that successful selections of the highly metastatic phenotype do not require in vivo selection procedures. These results have implications for the eventual selection of human tumor cell sublines with altered metastatic potentials.

HOST PROPERTIES AND METASTASIS

Tumor metastasis is also dependent upon the status of the host. In many clinical and experimental tumor situations, endocrine state appears to play an important role in metastasis. Analogous to the situation with human malignant melanoma (Cochran 1973), Proctor et al. (1976) found that B16 melanoma grew more slowly and metastasized less often in female than in male mice. However, these differences were abrogated by ablation of female hormonal systems. Traumatization, inflammation, or damage of host tissues can lead to increased arrest and survival of blood-borne tumor cells to form distant metastases (Fisher et al. 1967). One of the more interesting host characteristics is the immunological recognition and destruction of metastatic tumor cells. Although some experimental animal metastatic models are susceptible to immunodestruction (Castro 1978, Fidler and Nicolson 1981), the mere fact that metastasis occurs is thought to be an indication that host antitumor immunity is insufficient in many cases to prevent this process. Experimental studies on the role of host immunity in metastasis have not yet yielded a clear-cut answer to the importance of host immunity in metastasis. In some cases host immune status appears to be linked to the incidence of metastasis such that depression of an antitumor immune state resulted in enhanced metastasis (Alexander 1976), while in others the abrogation of host immune status had no effect (Fidler et al. 1979), or even a negative effect on metastasis (Fidler and Nicolson 1978, Vaage 1978). In cases where there is a clear-cut immunological difference between cells of high and low metastatic potential (Reading et al. 1980b) and the host is capable of responding against these specific immunological determinants, immunological parameters seem to be important. Reading et al. (1980b) found that malignancies of RAW117 lympho-sarcoma variant cell sublines and their abilities to colonize liver were related to specific cell surface properties including: quantities of lectin-binding sites, RNA tumor virus antigens, exposure of specific cell surface glycoproteins, and quantities of certain cell surface glycoproteins visualized in gels with ^{125}I-labeled lectins or antibodies. In several RAW117 sublines and cell clones derived from these sublines the amounts and exposures of gp70 in sublines and clones were correlated with metastasis, and enhanced malignancy and metastasis to liver was always accompanied by decreases in the cell surface exposure of gp70. In this system the host immunity may eliminate individual pre-existent cells with strong viral antigens, allowing only subpopulations of cells to survive that have lowered amounts of expression of gp70. Indeed, when macrophage function was abrogated in hosts by a variety of treatments known to kill macrophages or lessen their ability to respond, even the lowly metastatic sublines or clones were highly metastatic, suggesting that anti-tumor immune surveillance based on macrophages can control metastasis in model systems. However, in general, there is no simple relationship between host immunity and metastasis, and much more information is necessary in order to understand these complex tumor-host relationships.

HETEROGENEITY OF MALIGNANT TUMOR CELLS

Metastasis is thought to be a highly selective phenomenon such that only a small fraction of the total cells at a primary lesion are probably able to complete the entire process (Fidler 1978). It has been proposed that as a tumor progresses, cell variants arise within the lesion, and these variants are sub-jected to host selection pressures, resulting in the overall emergence of rare sublines with enhanced malignant potential (Nowell 1976). The fact that metastatic variant sublines can be selected using in vitro or in vivo procedures is consistent with this proposal, but the most convincing data have come from cloning experiments. Among the first to clone tumors such as the B16 melanoma were Fidler and Kripke (1977). They compared individual clones for their metastatic potentials and found that experimental metastasis in animals receiving melanoma cells intravenously varied widely among the different clones, and also when compared to the parental B16 melanoma line. It was concluded that cell subpopulations with high metastatic potential existed in the parental B16 tumor and were not produced by the cloning techniques. Heterogeneity in tumor cell subpopulations with respect to metastatic potential and malignant phenotype has been seen in a variety of neoplasms of widely different origin and type (Table 3). If tumors are, indeed, monoclonal in origin, this suggests that heterogeneity could have resulted from random phenotypic drift. There is some evidence for phenotypic drift in the metastatic properties of cell clones of B16 melanoma (Fidler and Nicolson 1981), 13762 adenocarcinoma (Neri and Nicolson, unpublished observations), and RAW117 lymphosarcoma (unpublished observations), suggesting that an important property of malignant tumor cells might be their abilities to change or drift phenotypically at much higher rates than normal or benign cells.

The existence of heterogeneous cell subpopulations has important implications for the treatment of cancer. The success of antitumor therapy could well depend upon the abilities of various treatments to eliminate the rare, highly metastatic cell subpopulations that exist within a tumor. However, heterogeneous properties, with respect to radiation sensitivity (Revesz and Norman 1963) and susceptibility to cytotoxic (Fuji and Mihich 1975, Heppner et al. 1978, Nicolson et al. 1981) or cytostatic (Lotan and Nicolson 1979, 1980) drugs, as well as differences in immunogenicity (Pimm and Baldwin 1977) or antigen content (Reading et al. 1980b), may pose serious problems for cancer management if highly metastatic variant subpopulations, refractory to various treatment strategies, persist after the treatments are terminated (Goldin and Johnson 1977, Olsson and Ebbesen 1979).

Table 3. *Heterogeneity and Malignancy of Animal Tumor Models*

Tumor Type	Characteristic	Experiment	References
Melanoma	Metastasis	Clones	Fidler and Kripke 1977
Mammary tumor	Metastasis	Clones	Dexter et al. 1978
Fibrosarcoma	Metastasis	Clones	Suzuki et al. 1978
Sarcoma	Metastasis	Clones	Nicolson et al. 1978
Lymphosarcoma	Metastasis	Clones	Reading et al. 1980b
Carcinoma	Metastasis	Clones	Talmadge et al. 1979
Fibrosarcoma	Metastasis	Clones	Kripke et al. 1978
Melanoma	Drug response	Sublines/clones	Lotan and Nicolson 1979
Melanoma	Metastasis/ pigmentation	Clones/sublines	Miner et al. 1981 Brunson and Nicolson 1979
Hepatoma	Drug response	Sublines	Barranco et al. 1978
Melanoma	Drug response	Sublines	Barranco et al. 1972
Carcinoma	Metastasis/drug response	Sublines	Dexter et al. 1978
Carcinoma	Metastasis/drug response	Sublines	Heppner et al. 1978
Carcinoma	Antigens	Sublines	Fogel et al. 1979
Sarcoma	Antigens	Sublines	Pimm and Baldwin 1977
Sarcoma	Antigens	Sublines	Byers and Johnston 1977
Carcinoma	Radiation sensitivity	Sublines	Revesz and Norman 1963

IN VITRO STUDIES OF THE METASTATIC PROCESS

The cell surface seems to be crucial in at least certain steps of the metastatic process. That the ability of B16 melanoma sublines to arrest in the microcirculation and survive is determined in part by cell surface properties has been demonstrated in membrane transfer experiments where the plasma membrane components of highly metastatic cells have been transferred to cells of low metastatic potential (Poste and Nicolson 1980). To transfer cell membrane components we took advantage of the fact that B16 melanoma cells spontaneously shed closed vesicles of plasma membrane in vivo or in vitro. These vesicles can be harvested, purified, and subsequently fused with the plasma membranes of homologous or heterologous cells to introduce vesicle plasma membrane components into the surface membranes of other cells. When vesicles from highly metastatic B16 cells were fused into the cell surfaces of B16 sublines of low metastatic potential, the ability of the vesicle-modified B16 cells to localize in lung and form metastases was significantly increased. Similarly, sensitivity to cell-mediated cytotoxicity could be transferred to a B16 subline resistant to cytotoxicity by using vesicles from sensitive B16 cells. The vesicle-modified B16 cells were sensitive to the cytotoxic action of these cells, but the vesicle-induced changes were transient and correlated with the cell membrane tumor properties (Poste and Nicolson 1980).

Cell surface differences in metastatic sublines of B16 melanoma and RAW117 lymphosarcoma have been correlated with organ site specificity of colonization. Although surface labeling techniques did not differentiate between cells or high or low lung implantation potential, they were able to differentiate between B16 sublines selected for ovary or brain colonization. Consistent differences were found in the surface labeling patterns of ovary-selected B16-O and brain-selected B16-B lines which correlated with their in vivo properties; these differences were an increase in exposure of glycoproteins of approximately 155,000 mol. wt. (B16-O ovary-selected sublines) or approximately 100,000 mol. wt. (B16-B brain-selected sublines) compared to the parental B16 lines (Brunson et al. 1978, Nicolson et al. 1978, Nicolson 1978). In the RAW117 lymphosarcoma metastatic model, dramatic differences were found in two cell surface components of approximate mol. wt. 135,000 and 70,000. Sublines selected for liver colonization showed a dramatic increase in the 135,000 mol. wt. glycoprotein species, as well as loss of the 70,000 mol. wt. viral glycoprotein (gp70) (Reading et al. 1980b).

Several aspects concerning the adhesive properties of metastatic cells and tumor spread have been known for some time to be important (Coman 1954, Weiss 1976). Cell detachment from the primary site and aggregation of tumor cells during transport are obviously important. When we examined the homotypic rates of adhesion of the B16 sublines in qualitative or quantitative (Nicolson et al. 1976, Winkelhake and Nicolson 1976) assays, the highly metastatic B16 sublines always aggregated or adhered at faster rates than the less metastatic lines. The heterotypic rates of adhesion of B16 sublines to platelets (Gasic et al. 1973), lymphocytes (Fidler 1975) indicate that the highly metastatic B16 sublines adhere at greater rates to circulating host cells. In experiments designed to test the hypothesis that organ cell recognition and adhesion may determine, at least in part, the organ specificity of blood-borne arrest, lung-selected B16-F melanoma sublines were mixed with purified, suspended organ cells, and cell aggregation was scored shortly thereafter. Within minutes the highly metastatic B16-F lines aggregated lung cells into a single clump, whereas the parental B16 line caused only slight lung cell aggregation (Nicolson and Winkelhake 1975). Other suspended organ cells from nontarget tissue such as spleen and kidney were not aggregated above control levels by any of the B16 sublines, suggesting that target organ recognition may occur through cell surface adhesive interactions.

The possible recognition of endothelium by circulating metastatic cells could be due to tissue-specific determinants on the endothelial cell surface. Evidence for organ-specific determinants on vascular endothelial cells has been obtained by Pressman and Yagi (1964) using cross-absorbed antiorgan antibodies. That endothelial cells from specific organs can be recognized by B16 variant sublines has been shown in a recent experiment where the adherence of B16-B sublines to mouse brain endothelial cells was measured. In this system the B16-B brain-selected lines adhered at faster rates than the B16-F lung-selected or B16-O ovary-selected sublines to monolayers of brain endothelial cells (Nicolson 1981). The morphologic aspects of metastatic cell interaction with vascular endothelial cells has been studied in vitro utilizing cell monolayers of cultured vascular endothelial cells which synthesize a basolateral extracellular matrix (Kramer and Nicolson 1979, 1981). Highly metastatic tumor cells attach to the endothelial cell monolayers and cause morphologic changes such as rupture of endothelial cell–endothelial cell interactions leading to retraction of endothelial cells and exposure of extracellular matrix (Figure 2). Once the extracellular matrix is exposed, the metastatic cells adhere with much greater avidity to the extracellular matrix (Kramer et al. 1980). Eventually the metastatic cells spread on the underlying extracellular matrix and invade under neighboring endothelial cells between the extracellular matrix and the dorsal endothelial cell surface (Figure 2). Within a few hours the endothelial cell monolayers reform and eventually reestablish extensive intercellular junctions, resulting in a walling off of the migrating metastatic cells. Similar observations have been made in vivo by Ludatsher et al. (1967) who found tumor cells enveloped between resealed endothelial cells and basement membrane.

The major polypeptide of the isolated endothelial extracellular matrix has been determined to be fibronectin (Birdwell et al. 1978, Kramer et al. 1980). Other components in addition to fibronectin are associated with the vascular endothelial extracellular matrix, including collagen (Vlodavsky et al. 1979), laminin (Timple et al. 1979), and glycosaminoglycans (Gamse et al. 1978).

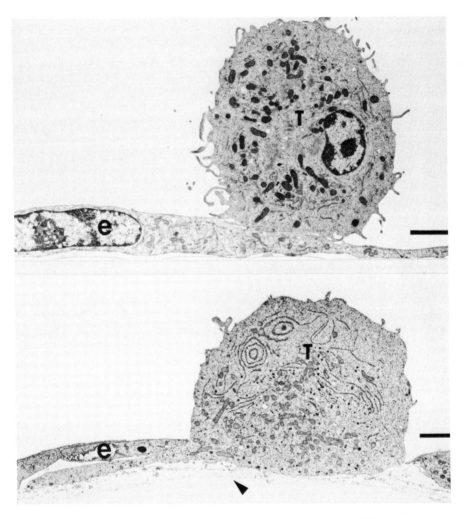

FIG. 2. Electron microscopic examination of the attachment and invasion of B16 melanoma cells on a vascular endothelial monolayer. In the upper panel the monolayer was fixed after 30 minutes of incubation. The lower panel shows a melanoma cell underlapping an adjacent vascular endothelial cell; it was fixed after one hour of incubation and prepared for transmission electron microscopy.

Fibronectin appears to be responsible, at least in part, for preferential tumor cell adhesion to the endothelial extracellular matrix. Metastatic tumor cells such as B16 melanoma will attach at the same rate to polyvinyl-immobilized fibronectin compared to the endothelial extracellular matrix (Kramer et al. 1980). Since fibronectin is not located on the apical surfaces of endothelial cells in monolayer culture (Birdwell et al. 1978), these results suggest that fibronectin may mediate the higher rate of adhesion of metastatic cells to basolateral matrix. Eventually metastatic cells induce the solubilization of the extracellular matrix similar to malignant cells breaching the basement membrane and gaining access to extravascular tissues in vivo. Similar observations have been made with human adenocarcinoma, melanoma, and giant cell sarcoma seeded onto monolayers of human endothelial cells in vitro. These results suggest that animal tumor models and in vitro assays for certain aspects of the metastatic process may be useful for elucidating mechanisms of cancer cell arrest and extravasation.

ACKNOWLEDGMENTS

This investigation was supported by grant numbers RO1-CA-28867, RO1-CA-29571, and RO1-CA-28844 awarded to Dr. G. L. Nicolson from the U.S.P.H.S. National Cancer Institute.

REFERENCES

Alexander, P. 1976. Dormant metastases which manifest on immunosuppression and the role of macrophages in tumours, *in* Fundamental Aspects of Metastasis, L. Weiss, ed. North-Holland Publishing Co., Amsterdam, pp. 227–239.

Barranco, S. C., B. R. Haenelt, and E. L. Gee. 1978. Differential sensitivities of five rat hepatoma cell lines to anticancer drugs. Cancer Res. 38:656–660.

Barranco, S. C., D. H. W. Ho, B. Drewinko, M. M. Romsdahl, and R. M. Humphrey. 1972. Differential sensitivities of human melanoma cells grown in vitro to arabinosylcytosine. Cancer Res. 32:2733–2736.

Birdwell, C. R., D. Gospodarwociz, and G. L. Nicolson. 1978. Identification, localization and the role of fibronectin in cultured bovine endothelial cells. Proc. Natl. Acad. Sci. U.S.A. 75:3273–3277.

Briles, E. G., and S. Kornfeld. 1978. Isolation and metastatic properties of detachment variants of B16 melanoma cells. J. Natl. Cancer Inst. 60:1217–1222.

Brunson, K. W., G. Beattie, and G. L. Nicolson. 1978. Selection and altered tumour cell properties of brain-colonising metastatic melanoma. Nature 272:543–545.

Brunson, K. W., and G. L. Nicolson. 1978. Selection and biologic properties of malignant variants of a murine lymphosarcoma. J. Natl. Cancer Inst. 61:1499–1503.

Brunson, K. W., and G. L. Nicolson. 1979. Selection of malignant melanoma variant cell lines for ovary colonization. J. Supramol. Struct. 11:517–528.

Brunson, K. W., and G. L. Nicolson. 1980. Experimental brain metastasis, *in* Brain Metastasis, L. Weiss, H. Gilbert, and J. B. Posner, eds. G. K. Hall and Co., Boston, pp. 50–65.

Byers, V. S., and J. O. Johnston. 1977. Antigenic differences among osteogenic sarcoma tumor cells taken from different locations in human tumors. Cancer Res. 37:3173–3183.

Castro, J. E., ed. 1978. Immunologic Aspects of Cancer. University Park Press, Baltimore.

Chew, E. E., R. L. Josephson, and A. C. Wallace. 1976. Morphologic aspects of the arrest of circulating cancer cells, *in* Fundamental Aspects of Metastasis, L. Weiss, ed. North-Holland Publishing Co., Amsterdam, pp. 121–150.

Cochran, A. J. 1973. A review of ten years' experience in Glasgow, Scotland. Cancer 23:1190–1199.

Coman, D. R. 1954. Cellular adhesiveness in relation to the invasiveness of cancer: Electron microscopy of liver perfused with a chelating agent. Cancer Res. 14:519–521.

del Regato, J. A., Jr. 1977. Pathways of metastatic spread of malignant tumors. Semin. Oncol. 4:33–38.

Dexter, D. L., H. M. Kowalski, B. A. Blazar, Z. Fligiel, R. Vogel, and G. H. Heppner. 1978. Heterogeneity of tumor cells from a single mouse mammary tumor. Cancer Res. 38:3174–3181.

Dingemans, K. P. 1973. Behavior of intravenously injected malignant lymphoma cells: A morphologic study. J. Natl. Cancer Inst. 51:1883–1897.

Dresden, M. H., S. A. Heilman, and J. D. Schmidt. 1972. Collagenolytic enzymes in human neoplasms. Cancer Res. 32:993–996.

Dunn, T. B. 1954. Normal and pathologic anatomy of the reticular tissue in laboratory mice, with a classification and discussion of neoplasms. J. Natl. Cancer Inst. 14:1281–1433.

Eaves, G. 1973. The invasive growth of malignant tumors as a purely mechanical process. J. Pathol. 109:233–237.

Fidler, I. J. 1973a. The relationship of embolic homogeneity, number, size and viability to the incidence of experimental metastasis. Eur. J. Cancer 9:223–227.

Fidler, I. J. 1973b. Selection of successive tumor lines for metastasis. Nature New Biol. 242:148–149.

Fidler, I. J. 1975. Biological behavior of malignant melanoma cells correlated to their survival in vivo. Cancer Res. 35:218–224.

Fidler, I. J. 1978. Tumor heterogeneity and the biology of cancer invasion and metastasis. Cancer Res. 38:2651–2660.

Fidler, I. J., and C. Bucana. 1977. Mechanism of tumor cell resistance to lysis by syngeneic lymphocytes. Cancer Res. 37:3945–3956.

Fidler, I. J., D. M. Gersten, and M. B. Budman. 1976. Characterization in vivo and in vitro of tumor cells selected for resistance to syngeneic lymphocyte-mediated cytotoxicity. Cancer Res. 36:3160–3165.

Fidler, I. J., D. M. Gersten, and I. R. Hart. 1978. The biology of cancer invasion and metastasis. Adv. Cancer Res. 28:149–250.

Fidler, I. J., D. M. Gersten, and M. L. Kripke. 1979. The influence of immunity on the metastasis of three murine fibrosarcomas of differing immunogenicity. Cancer Res. 39:3816–3821.

Fidler, I. J., and M. L. Kripke. 1977. Metastasis results from pre-existing variant cells within a malignant tumor. Science 197:893–895.

Fidler, I. J., and G. L. Nicolson. 1976. Organ selectivity for implantation, survival and growth of B16 melanoma variant tumor lines. J. Natl. Cancer Inst. 57:1199–1202.

Fidler, I. J., and G. L. Nicolson. 1977. Fate of recirculating B16 melanoma metastatic variant cells in parabiotic syngeneic recipients. J. Natl. Cancer Inst. 58:1867–1872.

Fidler, I. J., and G. L. Nicolson. 1978. Tumor cell and host properties affecting the implantation and survival of blood-borne metastatic variants of B16 melanoma. Israel J. Med. Sci. 14:38–50.

Fidler, I. J., and G. L. Nicolson. 1981. The immunobiology of experimental metastatic melanoma. Cancer Biol. Rev. 2:1–53.

Fisher, B., and E. R. Fisher. 1967a. The organ distribution of disseminated ^{51}Cr-labeled tumor cells. Cancer Res. 27:412–420.

Fisher, B., and E. R. Fisher. 1967b. Anticoagulants and tumor cell lodgment. Cancer Res. 27:241–245.

Fisher, B., E. R. Fisher, and N. Feduska. 1967. Trauma and the localization of tumor cells. Cancer 20:23–30.

Fogel, M., E. Gorelik, S. Segal, and M. Feldman. 1979. Differences in cell surface antigens of tumor metastases and those of local tumor. J. Natl. Cancer Inst. 62:585–588.

Folkman, J. 1974. Tumor angiogenesis. Adv. Cancer Res. 19:331–358.

Fuji, H., and E. Mihich. 1975. Selection for high immunogenicity in drug-resistant sublines of murine lymphomas demonstrated by plaque assay. Cancer Res. 35:946–952.

Gamse, G., H. G. Fromne, and H. Kress. 1978. Metabolism of sulfated glycosaminoglycans in cultured endothelial cells and smooth muscle cells. Biochim. Biophys. Acta 544:514–528.

Gasic, G. J., T. B. Gasic, N. Galanati, T. Johnson, and S. Murphy. 1973. Platelet-tumor cell interaction in mice. The role of platelets in the spread of malignant disease. Int. J. Cancer 11:704–718.

Goldin, A., and R. K. Johnson. 1977. Resistance to antitumor agents, *in* Recent Advances in Cancer Treatment, H. J. Tagnon and M. J. Staquet, eds. Raven Press, New York, pp. 155–169.

Hart, I. R. 1979. The selection and characterization of an invasive variant of B16 melanoma. Am. J. Pathol. 97:587–600.

Hart, I. R., and I. J. Fidler. 1980. The role of organ selectivity in the determination of metastatic patterns of B16 melanoma. Cancer Res. 40:2282–2287.

Hashimoto, K., Y. Yamanishi, E. Maeyens, M. K. Dabbous, and T. Kanzaki. 1973. Collagenolytic activities of squamous cell carcinoma of the skin. Cancer Res. 33:2790–2801.

Heppner, G. H., D. L. Dexter, T. DeNucci, F. R. Miller, and P. Calabresi. 1978. Heterogeneity in drug sensitivity among tumor cell subpopulations of a single mammary tumor. Cancer Res. 38:3758–3763.

Kerbel, R. W., R. R. Twiddy, and D. M. Robertson. 1978. Induction of a tumor with greatly increased metastatic H-2 heterozygous tumor cell line into an H-2 incompatible parental strain. Int. J. Cancer 22:583–594.

Kinsey, D. L. 1960. An experimental study of preferential metastasis. Cancer 13:674–676.

Klein, E. 1955. Gradual transformation of solid into ascites tumors. Evidence favoring the mutation-selection theory. Exp. Cell Res. 8:188–212.

Koch, F. E. 1939. Zur fragoder metastasenbildung bei impflumorin. Krebsforsch. 48:495–507.

Koono, M., K. Ushijima, and H. Hayashi. 1974. Studies on the mechanisms of invasion in cancer. III. Purification of a neutral protease of rat ascites hepatoma cell associated with production of chemotactic factor for cancer cells. Int. J. Cancer 13:105–115.

Kramer, R. H., R. Gonzalez, and G. L. Nicolson. 1980. Metastatic tumor cells adhere preferentially to the extracellular matrix underlying vascular endothelial cells. Int. J. Cancer (in press).

Kramer, R. H., and G. L. Nicolson. 1979. Interactions of tumor cells with vascular endothelial cell monolayers: A model for metastatic invasion. Proc. Natl. Acad. Sci. U.S.A. 76:5704–5708.

Kramer, R. H., and G. L. Nicolson. 1981. Invasion of vascular endothelial cell monolayers and underlying matrix by metastatic human cancer cells, *in* International Cell Biology 1980–1981, H. G. Schweiger, ed. Springer-Verlag, New York, pp. 794–799.

Kripke, M. L., E. Gruys, and I. J. Fidler. 1978. Metastatic heterogeneity of cells from an ultraviolet light-induced murine fibrosarcoma of recent origin. Cancer Res. 38:2962–2967.

Liotta, L. A., J. Kleinerman, and G. M. Saidel. 1976. The significance of hematogenous tumor cell clumps in the metastatic process. Cancer Res. 36:889–894.

Liotta, L. A., D. Vembu, R. K. Saini, and C. Boone. 1978. In vivo monitoring of the death rate of artificial murine pulmonary micrometastases. Cancer Res. 38:1231–1236.

Lotan, R., and G. L. Nicolson. 1979. Heterogeneity in growth inhibition by β-trans-retinoic acid of metastatic B16 melanoma clones and in vivo-selected cell variant lines. Cancer Res. 39:4767–4771.

Lotan, R., and G. L. Nicolson. 1980. Effects of β-all-trans retinoic acid on the growth and implantation properties of metastatic B16 melanoma cell lines, *in* Molecular Actions and Targets for Cancer Chemotherapeutic Agents, vol. 2, A. C. Sartorelli, J. R. Bertino, and J. S. Lazo, eds. Academic Press, New York, pp. 527–539.

Ludatsher, R. M., S. A. Luse, and V. Suntzeff. 1967. An electron microscopic study of pulmonary tumor emboli from transplanted Morris hepatoma 5123. Cancer Res. 27:1939–1952.

Miner, K. M., R. Lotan, and G. L. Nicolson. 1981. Metastatic and melanogenic properties of in vivo-selected B16 melanoma sublines and their clonal derivatives, *in* Proc. XIth Int. Pigment Cell Conference, M. Selji, A. Oikawa, and T. Takeuchi, eds. University of Tokyo Press, Tokyo (in press).

Neri, A., E. Ruoslahti, and G. L. Nicolson. 1979. Relationship of fibronectin to the metastatic behavior of rat mammary adenocarcinoma cell lines and clones. J. Supramol. Struct. suppl. 3:444.

Nicolson, G. L. 1978. Cell surface proteins and glycoproteins of metastatic murine melanomas and sarcomas, *in* Biological Markers of Neoplasia: Basic and Applied Aspects, R. W. Ruddon, ed. North-Holland Publishing Co., New York, pp. 227–239.

Nicolson, G. L. 1981. Metastatic tumor cell attachment and invasion assay utilizing vascular endothelial cell monolayers. J. Histochem. Cytochem. (in press).

Nicolson, G. L., K. W. Brunson, and I. J. Fidler. 1978. Specificity of arrest, survival and growth of selected metastatic variant cell lines. Cancer Res. 38:4105–4111.

Nicolson, G. L., R. Lotan, and A. Rios. 1981. Tumor cell heterogeneity and the in vitro sensitivities of metastatic B16 melanoma sublines and clones to retinoic acid or BCNU. Cancer Treat. Rep. (in press).

Nicolson, G. L., K. M. Miner, and C. L. Reading. 1981. Tumor cell heterogeneity and blood-borne metastasis, *in* Fundamental Mechanisms in Human Cancer Immunology. Elsevier/North Holland, Inc., New York (in press).

Nicolson, G. L., and G. Poste. 1976. The cancer cell: Dynamic aspects and modifications in cell-surface organization. New Engl. J. Med. 250:197–203 and 253–258.

Nicolson, G. L., and J. L. Winkelhake. 1975. Organ specificity of blood-borne tumour metastasis determined by cell adhesion? Nature 255:230–232.

Nicolson, G. L., J. L. Winkelhake, and A. C. Nussey. 1976. An approach to studying the cellular properties associated with metastasis: Some in vitro properties of tumor variants selected in vivo for enhanced metastasis, *in* Fundamental Aspects of Metastasis, L. Weiss, ed. North-Holland Publishing Co., Amsterdam, pp. 291–303.

Nowell, P. C. 1976. The clonal evolution of tumor cell populations. Science 194:23–28.

Olsson, L., and P. Ebbesen. 1979. Natural polyclonality of spontaneous AKR leukemia and its consequences for so-called specific immunotherapy. J. Natl. Cancer Inst. 62:623–627.

Pimm, M. V., and R. W. Baldwin. 1977. Antigenic differences between primary methyl-cholanthrene-induced rat sarcomas and post-surgical recurrences. Int. J. Cancer 20:37–43.

Poste, G., J. Doll, I. R. Hart, and I. J. Fidler. 1980. In vitro selection of murine B16 melanoma variants with enhanced tissue invasive properties. Cancer Res. 40:1636–1644.

Poste, G., and I. J. Fidler. 1980. The pathogenesis of cancer metastasis. Nature 283:139–146.

Poste, G., and G. L. Nicolson. 1980. Arrest and metastasis of blood-borne tumor cells are modified by fusion of plasma membrane vesicles from highly metastatic cells. Proc. Natl. Acad. Sci. U.S.A. 77:399–403.

Potter, M., J. L. Rahey, and H. I. Pilgrim. 1957. Abnormal serum protein and bone destruction in transmissible mouse plasma cell neoplasm (multiple myeloma). Proc. Soc. Exp. Biol. Med. 94:327–333.

Pressman, D., and Y. Yagi. 1964. Chemical differences in vascular beds, *in* Small Blood Vessel Involvement in Diabetes Mellitus, M. D. Siperstein, A. R. Colwell, and K. Meyer, eds. The American Institute of Biological Sciences, Washington, D.C., pp. 177–183.

Proctor, J. W., B. G. Auclair, and L. Stokowski. 1976. Endocrine factors and the growth and spread of B16 melanoma. J. Natl. Cancer Inst. 57:1197–1198.

Raz, A., and I. R. Hart. 1981. Murine melanoma. A model for intracranial metastasis. Br. J. Cancer (in press).

Reading, C. L., P. N. Belloni, and G. L. Nicolson. 1980a. Selection and in vivo properties of lectin-attachment variants of malignant murine lymphosarcoma cell lines. J. Natl. Cancer Inst. 64:1241–1249.

Reading, C. L., K. W. Brunson, M. Torrianni, and G. L. Nicolson. 1980b. Malignancies of metastatic murine lymphosarcoma cell lines and clones correlate with decreased cell surface display of RNA-tumor virus envelope glycoprotein gp70. Proc. Natl. Acad. Sci. U.S.A. 77:5943–5947.

Revesz, L., and L. Norman. 1963. Relationship between chromosome ploidy and radiosensitivity in selected tumor sublines of common origin. J. Natl. Cancer Inst. 25:1041–1063.

Salk, P., and R. P. Lanza. 1979. In vitro growth characteristics, motility and adhesive properties of metastatic variant PW20 cell lines. J. Supramol. Struct. suppl. 3:182.

Salsbury, A. J. 1975. The significance of the circulating cancer cell. Cancer Treat. Rev. 2:55–72.

Sato, H., and M. Suzuki. 1976. Deformability and viability of tumor cells by transcapillary passage, with reference to organ affinity of metastasis in cancer, *in* Fundamental Aspects of Metastasis, L. Weiss, ed. North-Holland Publishing Co., Amsterdam, pp. 311–317.

Schirrmacher, R., G. Shantz, K. Clauer, D. Komitowski, H.-P. Zimmermann, and M.-L. Lohmann-Matthes. 1979. Tumor metastases and cell-mediated immunity in a model system in DBA/2 mice. I. Tumor invasiveness in vitro and metastasis formation in vivo. Int. J. Cancer 23:233–244.

Strauch, L. 1972. The role of collagenases in tumor invasion, *in* Tissue Interactions in Carcinogenesis, D. Tarin, ed. Academic Press, New York, pp. 399–434.

Sugarbaker, E. V. 1952. The organ selectivity of experimentally induced metastasis in rats. Cancer 5:606–612.

Sugarbaker, E. V. 1979. Cancer metastasis: A product of tumor-host interactions. Curr. Probl. Cancer 3:3–59.

Suzuki, M., H. R. Withers, and M. W. Koehler. 1978. Heterogeneity and variability of artificial lung colony-forming ability among clones from a mouse fibrosarcoma. Cancer Res. 38:3349-3351.

Sylvén, B. 1973. Biochemical and enzymatic factors involved in cellular detachment, *in* Chemotherapy of Cancer Dissemination and Metastasis, S. Garattini, and G. Franchi, eds. Raven Press, New York, pp. 129-139.

Takahashi, S., Y. Konishi, K. Nakatanli, S. Inui, K. Kojima, and T. Shiratori. 1978. Conversion of a poorly differentiated human adenocarcinoma to ascites form with invasion and metastasis in nude mice. J. Natl. Cancer Inst. 60:926-927.

Talmadge, J. E., J. R. Starkey, W. C. Davis, and A. L. Cohen. Introduction of metastatic heterogeneity by short-term in vivo passage of a cloned transformed cell line. J. Supramol. Struct. 12:227-243.

Tao, T.-W., and M. M. Burger. 1977. Non-metastasising variants selected from metastasising melanoma cells. Nature 270:437-438.

Tao, T.-W., A. Matter, K. Vogel, and M. M. Burger. 1979. Liver-colonizing melanoma cells selected from B16 melanoma. Int. J. Cancer 23:854-857.

Timple, R., H. Rhode, P. G. Roley, S. I. Rennard, J. M. Joidard, and G. R. Martin. 1979. Laminin-A glycoprotein from basement membranes. J. Biol. Chem. 254:9933-9937.

Vaage, J. 1978. A survey of the growth characteristics of and the host reactions to one hundred C3H/He mammary carcinomas. Cancer Res. 38:331-338.

Vlodavsky, I., L. K. Johnson, and D. Gospodarowitz. 1979. Appearance in confluent vascular endothelial cell monolayers of a specific cell surface protein (CSP-60) not detected in actively growing endothelial cells or in cell types growing in multiple layers. Proc. Natl. Acad. Sci. U.S.A. 76:2306-2310.

Warren, B. A. 1973. Environment of the blood-borne tumor embolus adherent to vessel wall. J. Med. 4:150-177.

Weiss, L., ed. 1976. Fundamental Aspects of Metastasis. North-Holland Publishing Co., Amsterdam.

Weiss, L. 1977. A pathobiologic overview of metastasis. Sem. Oncol. 4:5-19.

Winkelhake, J. L., and G. L. Nicolson. 1976. Determination of adhesive properties of variant metastatic melanoma cells to BALB/3T3 cells and their virus-transformed derivatives by a monolayer attachment assay. J. Natl. Cancer Inst. 56:285-291.

Wood, S., Jr. 1964. Experimental studies of the intravascular dissemination of ascitic V2 carcinoma cells in the rabbit, with special reference to fibrinogen and fibrinolytic agents. Bull. Schweiz. Akad. Med. Wiss. 20:92-121.

Ziedman, I., and J. M. Buss. 1952. Transpulmonary passage of tumor cell emboli. Cancer Res. 12:731-733.

Gastrointestinal Cancer, edited by
John R. Stroehlein and
Marvin M. Romsdahl.
Raven Press, New York © 1981.

Pharmacology and Development of New Therapeutic Agents

Daniel P. Griswold, Jr., D.V.M., Thomas H. Corbett, Ph.D., and Frank M. Schabel, Jr., Ph.D.

Chemotherapy Department, Southern Research Institute, Birmingham, Alabama

INTRODUCTION

Unlike the development and application of antimicrobial therapy where infectious agents, distinct and separate from the host, may be isolated and cultured apart from the host for characterization and determination of sensitivity to various antimicrobial agents—an individual patient's cancer arises from and is an intrinsic extension of some tissue of that patient. Treatment of the etiological agent of an existing cancer is not possible, and the oncologist is thereby forced to use treatments that are aimed at destruction of the end product—cancer. In addition, years of research have identified only one exploitable biochemical difference between normal cells and cancer cells. That is the requirement for asparagine by a limited number of mouse and human leukemias, leading to the use of L-asparaginase (Burchenal 1969, Uren and Handschumacher 1977).

Further complicating this picture is the marked heterogeneity of cancer, even when of the same histologic type, in regard to rates of growth, invasiveness, metastasis, response to treatment, and lethality. Because of these variables it has been impossible to develop a single model that could adequately mimic the behavior and response to treatment of cancer in man. Nevertheless, in spite of the lack of a common identifiable etiologic agent, the lack of exploitable biochemical differences, the heterogeneity that characterizes cancer, and the imprecision of our models, progress has been made.

Today, with the exception of hormonal agents, there are 39 useful and commercially available anticancer agents, and 60 others are in various stages of clinical trial (DeVita and Kershner 1980). DeVita (1980) has listed 12 advanced cancers for which drug treatment has been responsible for some fraction of patients achieving a normal lifespan. Unfortunately, gastrointestinal cancer is not included in that list. Surgical improvement has apparently plateaued (Moertel 1978), and five-year survival rates remain at less than 5% for cancer of the pancreas, 12% for cancer of the stomach, and less than 50% for colorectal cancer (Silverberg 1980). Moertel (1978) recently concluded that there is no chemotherapeutic approach to gastrointestinal carcinoma valuable enough to justify application as standard clinical treatment.

Approaches to New Drug Development

Although faced with this dilemma, the medicinal chemist, the biochemist, the pharmacologist, and the experimental oncologist, whose charge it is to develop new and useful therapies, still have several approaches available. One involves the screening for antitumor activity of randomly selected agents using experimental systems of animal- or human-tumor origin. Another approach involves congener synthesis with the intellectual preparation and selection of candidate agents, drawing from the experience of various disciplines in an effort to develop agents that will have a greater therapeutic index, a broader spectrum of anticancer activity, and other desirable features. Again, such agents must be first evaluated in experimental systems. Tumor models with greater predictive reliability for the drug response of human tumors are clearly needed.

As previously mentioned, little progress has been made in the search for exploitable biochemical differences between cancer and normal tissues. However, a systematic search for any differences that may exist between drug-responsive and nonresponsive cancers has barely begun. One of the greatest enigmas in cancer chemotherapy today relates to the failure of cancers of certain organs to respond to the same chemotherapeutic agents that are effective and sometimes curative when used to treat other forms of cancer. Are these unresponsive cancers inherently insensitive to any cytotoxic agent, have useful agents not been found, or have presently available agents not yet been optimally used?

There is reason to believe that additional useful agents will be found and that currently available agents will be used to better advantage. For example, witness the relatively new entries of Adriamycin with marked activity against breast cancer, and platinum, diamminedichloro-*cis*- (cis DDPt), being particularly useful in the treatment of testicular carcinoma. Also, note the recently reported advantages gained in the treatment of advanced stage Hodgkin's disease with MOPP (Adriamycin, bleomycin, vinblastine, decarbazine) plus ABVD (nitrogen mustard, vincristine, procarbazine, prednisone) (Santoro et al. 1980).

If, then, one is willing to accept that chemotherapeutic progress has been made, it is obvious that still further improvement of methods must be sought while the search for better drugs goes on.

CONCEPTS FOR IMPROVEMENT OF CHEMOTHERAPY

The most simplistic view of the problem suggests two basic means of improving the chemotherapy of gastrointestinal cancer: one, the better use of presently available agents, and, two, the development of more predictive models for new drug selection and for the further development of chemotherapeutic principles.

Better Use of Available Agents

Klaassen (1978) recently reviewed the chemotherapy of colorectal cancer and identified 11 single agents as active against that disease. Patient response rates ranged from 10%–27%, and duration of survival ranged from two to five months. Admittedly, such anticancer agent activity can be considered only marginal at best. It is important to remember, however, that those data resulted from the treatment of patients with advanced disease. Such results, i.e., apparently weak activity, are not unlike those seen following treatment of a variety of very advanced leukemias and solid tumors in experimental animals.

The data presented in Table 1 show the effect of tumor staging on the curability of subcutaneously implanted B16 melanoma. This large body of data resulted from treatment of mice with a maximum tolerated dose of MeCCNU at times when the tumor burden ranged from 10^3 cells to $>10^9$ cells (>1.0 gm tumors). The inverse relationship between tumor burden and curability reinforces the concept derived from many other animal tumor experiments and further points to the need for treatment of patients with subclinical cancer. The necessity for such considerations as well as the hazards involved has recently been reviewed by Weiss and DeVita (1979) and will not be further considered here. It is apparent, however, that, with the current state of the art, presently available drugs, used singly or in combination, cannot be expected to eradicate very large solid tumor masses. That fact plus recent successes through the use of multimodality therapy for certain human cancers suggests the need for consideration of surgical adjuvant chemotherapy of

Table 1. *Effect of Tumor Staging on Curability of Subcutaneous B16 Melanoma* *

Tumor Size at Rx** (No. Cells)	% Mice Cured
$\geq 10^9$	0
	(13% Responders)
Fragment or 10^7	4
10^5	18
10^4	33
10^3‡	70

*Modified from Griswold, 1975.

**Mice were treated with a single dose of MeCCNU, 40 mg/kg. Pooled data from six experiments, 10 mice/group in each experiment.

‡Normalized value based on 10% no-takes in the untreated controls and 78% "cures" in the drug-treated groups. There were no no-takes in any of the other control groups.

gastrointestinal cancers. In fact, such consideration has been given, and the results have been dismal.

Recently Kisner et al. (1979) reviewed the adjuvant trials in colorectal cancer and observed that no reproducible superiority of an adjuvant treatment over a concurrent control has been demonstrated. Interestingly, however, they noted in two studies, in which 5-fluorouracil was given postoperatively, a divergence in the control group and the treated group survival curves. Since that divergence was transient with no overall significant difference in survival, those authors concluded that "the divergence of the survival curves is provocative, but of questionable importance."

The same type of survival curves are often seen with surgery-chemotherapy trials of metastatic animal tumors. The data shown in Figure 1 resulted from treatment of advanced, metastatic mouse colon tumor 26. All of the mice in the untreated control died with advanced and metastatic tumors. Chemotherapy alone, single doses of BCNU (1,3-bis(2-chloroethyl)-1-nitrosourea) and 5-FU (5-fluorouracil), provided an increased survival time but no cures. Surgical removal of the SC-implanted tumors produced a 20% cure rate. But when chemotherapy was added to the surgery, a 73% cure rate was achieved. These are the results that one hopes for but often fails to see in man.

The data in Figure 2 are from another surgery-chemotherapy trial with mouse colon tumor 26. These data represent more closely the results of human colorectal surgical adjuvant trials to date. Here, one can see the divergence of the survival curves of the surgery-chemotherapy group and the surgery-only group. The divergence was not maintained, and chemotherapy added no increase in survival rate beyond that obtained by surgery alone.

Another way to look at these data is by frequency distribution analysis, in which the percentage of mice having different metastatic tumor burdens

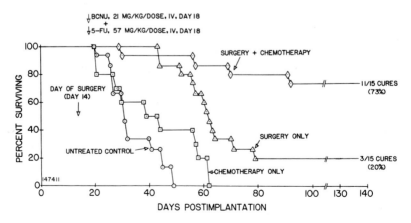

FIG. 1. Response of SC implanted colon tumor 26 to surgery with and without BCNU + 5-FU treatment. Tumors were 300 to 1,000 mg at the time of surgical removal.

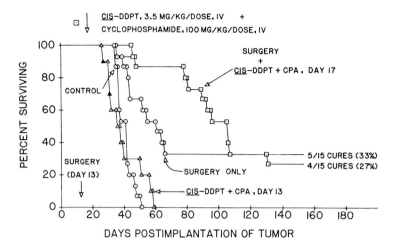

FIG. 2. Response of SC implanted colon tumor 26 to surgery with and without *Cis*-DDPt + cyclophosphamide treatment. Tumors were 400 to 1,000 mg at the time of surgical removal.

immediately following surgery or surgery plus chemotherapy are estimated. Figure 3 shows the distribution analyses for the two experiments just shown. Figure 3 (top) shows that after chemotherapy there was a shift to the left in the distribution of mice with various metastatic tumor burdens and, additionally, shows the increased percentage of cured mice. Figure 3 (bottom) shows a similar shift to the left but with a disproportionate percentage of mice left after chemotherapy with only 1–10 tumor cells. Why was the cure rate not increased? There may be several explanations. Among these would be an uneven distribution of mice or patients with various metastatic tumor burdens, coupled with the use of a relatively ineffective chemotherapy regimen. Another reason would involve the presence of tumor cell sanctuaries, which might be anatomic, pharmacologic, or kinetic in nature. A third reason, one which is becoming increasingly well recognized and of importance in chemotherapy planning, has to do with the selection of drug-resistant mutants.

Thus the divergent survival curves seen in surgical adjuvant trials may be of more than "questionable importance." They may represent the beginning of success, demanding improved chemotherapeutic strategy even through the use of the "so-called" ineffective drugs presently available.

Any possible improvement in current chemotherapeutic regimens will most likely come from a full understanding of those factors in chemotherapeutic regimen design that determine success or failure, as well as knowledge of tumor, host, and drug characteristics. Simply stated, the net tumor cell kill or reduction that may be obtained is dependent on the cell kill achieved from each single dose or course of chemotherapy, the interval in time between each dose or course, the number of doses or courses, and the doubling time and other kinetic characteristics of the tumor cell population. The regimen design

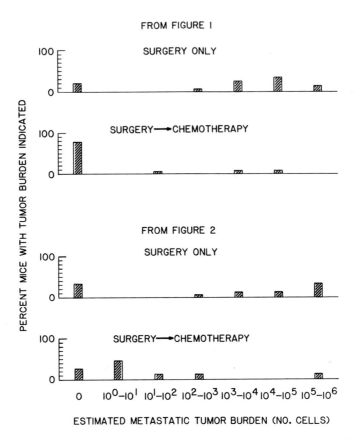

FIG. 3. Frequency distributions of mice with different metastatic tumor burdens after surgical removal of SC implanted colon tumor 26 or after surgery → chemotherapy. *Top*—Analysis of data shown in Figure 1. *Bottom*—Analysis of data shown in Figure 2.

is of course always constrained by the limitations of host toxicity. The variable frequently overlooked is that degree of cell kill that may be obtained from the individual doses or courses of a planned treatment regimen. The dosage of a drug that determines the amount of cell kill (recognizing that tumor cell populations are dose-responsive) is customarily expressed as mg/kg of body weight or as mg/M² of surface area. But since serum and tissue levels of drug following pulse treatment are dynamic (Figure 4A) rather than static, it is more realistic to determine serum concentration as a product of the duration (time) of the concentration or, for certain classes of agents, concentration with time. In Figures 4B and 4C are shown the idealized survival curves of log-phase L1210 leukemia cells in culture to various concentrations of methotrexate or BCNU. It can be seen that methotrexate produces a biphasic curve since the cell killing is not concentration-dependent at high concentrations. With drugs of this nature, e.g., cell-cycle-phase specific drugs, time (T) becomes the important parameter so long as a minimal effective concentration has been maintained. The cell killing by BCNU, on the other hand, is concentration-dependent, and in this case, as with most alkylating agents and drugs that bind tightly to or intercalate with DNA, e.g., Adriamycin, $C \times T = K$ (constant value). Again, the T in the $C \times T$ calculation must represent only the duration (T) of the minimal effective concentration (C).

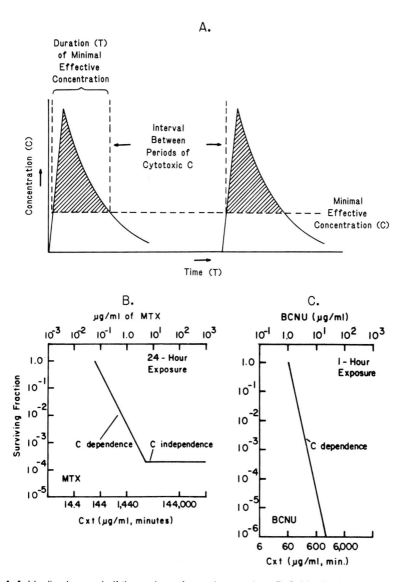

FIG. 4. A. Idealized serum half-time values of an anticancer drug. **B, C.** Idealized response of log-phase L1210 cells in culture to varying doses of methotrexate or BCNU.

Determination of minimal effective concentrations of drugs for tumors of man is no simple matter. But translation can be made from experimental tumor systems, at least for identification of baseline values, below which no antitumor activity should be expected in animals or man. Unfortunately the dosage range over which antitumor activity is observed, even in very sensitive animal tumors, is quite narrow. In Table 2 there are listed the therapeutic indices [TI = LD_{10} (mg/kg)/minimum effective dose (mg/kg)] and LD_{90}/LD_{10} ratios at the optimal schedule for each of 12 agents that were used to treat IP-L1210 leukemia. The median TI value is 3.2 and the median LD_{90}/LD_{10} value is 2.0. Using those median values a plot (Figure 5) was made showing the composite dosage-mortality curve in relationship to the minimal effective dose and the nonlethal dosage range in which a minimal (40% ILS) antitumor effect can be seen against L1210 leukemia. One can easily see what would result from a 50% dosage reduction.

Cyclophosphamide is a widely used anticancer agent. It has a broad spectrum of activity and is used in a number of clinical protocols, although it is considered inactive against colorectal cancer of man due to the short duration of response. Shown in Table 3 are the results of treating IP-L1210 leukemia in mice with single doses at various fractions of the single dose LD_{10}. Here it can be seen that a single dose of 230 mg/kg, about 80% of the LD_{10}, when used to treat mice implanted IP with 10^5 L1210 cells, cured 82% of those mice and increased the lifespan of those not cured by 70% above the untreated control. In other groups the lifespan and cure rate decreased with decreasing dose. None of the mice treated with a single dose of 25 mg/kg were cured, and the

Table 2. Therapeutic Indices (TI)* from Optimal Drug Treatment of Mice with 10^5 L1210 Cells, IP and LD_{90}/LD_{10} Ratios from Dosage-Mortality Studies in Nontumor-Bearing BDF1 (C57/BL6xDBA/2) Mice

	TI	LD_{90}/LD_{10} Ratio
5-Fluorouracil	5.6	1.1
Methotrexate	3.5	6.8
Ara-C	>2.8	2.0
Cyclophosphamide	3.0	2.1
MeCCNU	10.5	2.4
BCNU	8.0	2.0
CCNU	3.2	2.1
Mitomycin C	2.0	1.7
Melphalan	5.8	2.0
DTIC	3.1	2.4
Hexamethylmelamine	<1.0	1.7
Adriamycin	1.0	1.7
Median:	3.2	2.0

$$*TI = \frac{LD_{10} \text{ (mg/kg)}}{\text{Minimum Effective Dose (ILS}_{40} - \text{mg/kg)}}$$

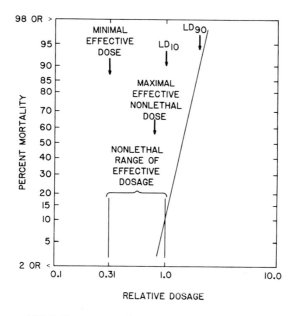

FIG. 5. Dosage-mortality curve from data in Table 2.

lifespan was increased by only 10%—inactive by any standards. But it is important to recognize that when that dosage, 25 mg/kg/dose, is given daily for 15 days (qd 1–15) it has no significantly greater antitumor effect but is lethal to 10% of mice so treated.

Three points can be made from these data: (1) Treatment to toxicity will not insure that an optimal antitumor effect has been achieved, if an inappropriate treatment schedule has been used; (2) because of the steepness of cytotoxic

Table 3. *Response of IP L1210 Leukemia in Mice to Fractions of Single-Dose LD_{10} of Cyclophosphamide*

Single Dose		C × T Mg/ml (Min.)	No. L1210 Cells	% ILS Excluding Cures	% Cures
Mg/kg	Fraction of LD_{10}				
300	1.0	10,440	10^7	200	40
		10,440	10^6	—	80
230	0.77	7,920	10^5	70	82
173	0.58	5,869	10^5	80	42
115	0.38	3,780	10^5	60	20
58	0.19	1,728	10^5	21	5
25	0.08	540	10^5	10	0
12.5	0.04	90	10^5	0	0
6.3	0.02	"0"	10^5	0	0
3.2	0.01	"0"	10^5	0	0

agent dose-response curves, dose-reduction can drastically reduce any anti-cancer effect seen in higher doses; and (3) selection of less than an optimal drug dose-regimen for initial evaluation of a new agent may provide unwarranted condemnation of that agent to the inactive status.

No one will argue with the need to obtain from each single agent as well as from combinations of agents the optimal anticancer effect with minimal host toxicity. But such endeavors demand an interdisciplinary approach and the application of biochemical and pharmacologic knowledge to dose-regimen selection and design. At the same time the search for new, more efficacious drugs must continue. One important aspect of this search points to the requirement for more relevant models and appropriate use of those models for identification and mimicry of those characteristics of human cancers that are associated with failure to respond positively to chemotherapy.

More Predictive Models

A great variety of models has been developed within the last half century for use by organic chemists, biochemists, pharmacologists, experimental oncologists, and others in attempts to provide research tools that might be used to improve the treatment for cancer in man. These include computerized mathematical models, in vitro models of animal or human tumor origin, and a great variety of in vivo animal tumor models, including those that are spontaneous in origin, chemically induced, viral associated, autochthonous, and serially transplanted. More recently, human tumor xenografts in athymic or immunologically deprived mice have been used. But today there is no model of any type that is a perfect and precise predictor for the response to drug treatment for any cancer of man; nor is any cancer of man a perfect predictor for any other cancer of man, even when of the same histologic type. The basic reason behind this problem is heterogeneity—the heterogeneity that exists from mouse to mouse or patient to patient, the heterogeneity that exists from tumor to tumor, and even that heterogeneity existing within an individual tumor cell population.

Such heterogeneity, as mentioned previously, has been well documented. Fidler (1978) demonstrated the variability in invasiveness and metastasis that is evident among subpopulations of cells within a single tumor. We (Schabel et al. 1980a, b) and many others have shown the differences in response to chemotherapy of subgroups of cells from single tumors and the variability that exists in the drug response of mice that are genetically and otherwise supposedly identical. If there were no variability, we would not need terms like LD_{50} or percent responders. Patient or mouse variability simply reflects the differences in capability and rate of drug metabolism, transport, binding, and excretion. Tumor cell populations, characterized by similar variables, also have the propensity to mutate, then presenting different biochemical and drug response characteristics. Making the matter even worse, it was shown first by

Luria and Delbrück (1943) and later by Law (1952) that such mutations are random events. Is it then any wonder that no single tumor model has ever been developed that would precisely predict for cancer of man? The recognized existence of many variables forces the use of multiple observations, with consideration of all known variables, and application of probability theory.

We believe that it is most probable that a model will be most representative if it encompasses as many variables as possible that are known to characterize the target disease. Within the past six years and with the support and encouragement of the National Large Bowel Cancer Project and the National Cancer Institute we have developed 10 distinctly different, transplantable, colon tumors of mice. These tumors were all chemically induced initially and represent a spectrum of biological and drug-response characteristics. We consider these 10 tumors, collectively, to be more representative of colorectal cancer than any one of the 10.

One of these tumors is a moderately well-differentiated mucinous adenocarcinoma. Another is a rapidly growing, undifferentiated carcinoma. The remainder are modestly to moderately well-differentiated adenocarcinomas. Following SC implantation, invasiveness ranges from very low to very high, and metastasis, which is predominantly to the lungs, is found in less than 3% of mice with one tumor and more than 90% of mice with another. Metastasis from SC implants of the other tumors varies between those two figures. Tumor growth within the liver is seen in varying percentages of mice following IP injection of tumor cells. The average doubling times of the tumors in SC sites range from about two days for the undifferentiated tumor to about seven days for one of the well-differentiated tumors.

These tumors also vary considerably in their response to drug treatment. Shown in Table 4 is the spectrum of response of the 10 mouse colon tumor lines to each of a selected group of well-known chemotherapeutic agents. Our goal was to look not only for degree of antitumor activity but also for spectrum of response, i.e., the fraction of different tumor lines that showed significant response to treatment. Tumor fragments were implanted SC and treatment was begun early, two or three days after implant or when the tumors reached a more advanced stage of growth, i.e., 300 mg or greater. In a few instances tumors were implanted by the IP route.

Although testing is not complete against all 10 tumor lines, the largest number to respond markedly to any single agent was five. One of the tumors, colon tumor 51, did not respond markedly to any of the agents listed. Furthermore, there appears to be no particular pattern in the response of the different tumor lines to these agents, and the basis for response or failure to respond is not known. But the variability of response appears to be similar to that seen in man.

It is hoped that this model tumor system may serve as a research tool that will allow the selection of new chemotherapeutic agents that will have both a

Table 4. *Spectrum of Response of 10 SC Implanted Mouse Colon Tumors to Selected Chemotherapeutic Agents*

	Fraction of Tumor Lines Responding Markedly*	
	Early Tumor	Advanced Tumor
5-Fluorouracil (or 5-fluorodeoxy-uridine)	2/10	1/6
Methotrexate	0/5	—
Arabinosylcytosine	1/4	1/1
PalmO-ara-C	5/10	4/8
Vincristine	1/9	1/1
MeCCNU (1-(2-Chloroethyl)-3-(*trans*-4-methylcyclohexyl)-1-nitrosourea)	3/10	2/5
DTIC (Imidazole carboxamide, dimethyltriazene)	5/10	3/4
Cyclophosphamide	5/9	5/7
Melphalan (L-sarcolysin)	3/7	1/2
Mitomycin C	3/8	1/4
Cis-DDPt II (*Cis*-Diamminedichloro-platinum)	2/9	0/3
M-AMSA (Cain's "Acridine")	1/7	0/4
Adriamycin	3/9	2/4

Nine of the 10 tumor lines responded markedly to at least one agent listed above.
*Marked response indicates significant reduction in tumor cell burden at the end of treatment.

significant degree of anticancer activity and a broad spectrum of activity. Certainly it would be advantageous to eliminate those false positives going into clinical trial as well as to select for clinical trial those agents that may have been false negatives by other screening criteria.

CONCLUSION

In the chemotherapy of gastrointestinal cancer today there is no magic bullet; not is there likely to be. There is, however, reason to hope that more efficacious chemotherapeutic agents will be found through congener synthesis and through the use of more predictive models. There is also reason to hope that presently available agents, either singly or in combination, will be put to better use. Further progress will depend on the coordination of effort at all levels of research and on implementation of those therapeutic concepts and principles, so derived, that offer hope, however dim that hope may be.

ACKNOWLEDGMENTS

Work from Southern Research Institute reported herein was supported by Contracts N01-CM-43756 and N01-CM-97309 from the Division of Cancer Treatment, and by Grant CA 17303 from the National Large Bowel Cancer

Project, National Cancer Institute, National Institutes of Health, Department of Health and Human Services, U.S.A.

REFERENCES

Burchenal, J. H. 1969. Success and failure in present chemotherapy and the implications of asparaginase. Cancer Res. 29:2262–2269.

DeVita, V. T., and L. M. Kershner. 1980. Cancer, the curable diseases. Am. Pharm. NS20 4:16–22.

Fidler, I. J. 1978. Tumor heterogeneity and the biology of cancer invasion and metastasis. Cancer Res. 38:2651–2660.

Griswold, D. P., Jr. 1975. The potential for murine tumor models in surgical adjuvant chemotherapy. Cancer Chem. Rep. 5:187–204.

Kisner, D. L., H. L. Davis, Jr., and F. M. Muggia. 1979. Current adjuvant trials in colorectal cancer, *in* Frontiers of Gastrointestinal Research, L. vander Reis, ed. S. Karger, Basel, pp. 102–115.

Klaassen, P. J. 1978. Chemotherapy of colorectal cancer. Can. J. Surg. 21:218–220.

Law, L. W. 1952. Origin of the resistance of leukemic cells to folic acid antagonists. Nature 169:628–629.

Luria, S. E., and M. Delbrück. 1943. Mutations of bacteria from virus sensitivity to virus resistance. Genetics 28:491–511.

Moertel, C. G. 1978. Chemotherapy of gastrointestinal cancer. New Engl. J. Med. 299:1049–1052.

Santoro, A., G. Bonadonna, V. Bonfante, and P. Valagussa. 1980. Non cross-resistant regimens (MOPP and ABVD) vs. MOPP alone in Stage IV Hodgkin's disease (Abstract). Proc. Amer. Soc. Clin. Oncol. 21:470.

Schabel, F. M., Jr., D. P. Griswold, Jr., T. H. Corbett, W. R. Laster, H. H. Lloyd, and W. C. Rose. 1980a. Variable responses of advanced solid tumors of mice to treatment with anticancer drugs, *in* Design of Models for Screening of Therapeutic Agents, I. J. Fidler and R. J. White, eds. Van Nostrand Reinhold Co., New York (in press).

Schabel, F. M., Jr., H. E. Skipper, M. W. Trader, W. R. Laster, T. H. Corbett, and D. P. Griswold, Jr. 1980b. Concepts for controlling drug-resistant tumor cells, *in* Breast Cancer, Experimental and Clinical Aspects, H. T. Mouridsen and T. Palshof, eds. Pergamon Press, Ltd., Oxford, pp. 199–211.

Silverberg, E. 1980. Cancer statistics, 1980. CA 30:23–38.

Uren, J. R., and R. E. Handschumacher. 1977. Enzyme therapy, *in* Cancer: A Comprehensive Treatise, F. F. Becker, ed. Plenum Publishing Corp., New York, pp. 457–487.

Weiss, R. B., and V. T. DeVita. 1979. Multimodal primary cancer treatment (adjuvant chemotherapy): Current results and future prospects. Ann. Intern. Med. 91:251–260.

Gastrointestinal Cancer, edited by
John R. Stroehlein and
Marvin M. Romsdahl.
Raven Press, New York © 1981.

Inhibition of Neoplasia of the Large Bowel

Lee W. Wattenberg, M.D.

*Department of Laboratory Medicine and Pathology,
University of Minnesota, Minneapolis, Minnesota*

INTRODUCTION

An increasing number and diversity of compounds have been found to prevent chemical carcinogenesis (Wattenberg 1978, 1979a, b, 1981). Inhibition can occur at different time points; the earliest is inhibition of formation of carcinogens from precursor compounds. Work of this nature has focused particularly on the inhibitory capacities of ascorbic acid and α-tocopherol (Mirvish et al. 1975, Mirvish 1981a, b). A second group of inhibitors called "blocking agents" prevent already-formed carcinogens from reaching or reacting with critical target sites. Inhibition at a still later time period is brought about by other compounds. The best studied of these are the retinoids and protease inhibitors. Both will prevent or suppress neoplasia when administered subsequent to carcinogen exposure (Sporn and Newton 1979, Matsushima et al. 1976). Occasional inhibitors can act at more than one time point. This presentation will deal primarily with "blocking agents" inhibiting carcinogen-induced neoplasia of the large bowel.

EXPERIMENTAL

Inhibition of Carcinogen-Induced Neoplasia
of the Large Bowel by Blocking Agents

A wide variety of compounds exist that inhibit carcinogenesis when administered prior to and/or simultaneously with exposure to chemical carcinogens. Some of these inhibitors are synthetic but many are naturally occurring constituents of plants. Blocking agents include: phenols, indoles, flavones, aromatic isothiocyanates, coumarins, disulfiram and related chemicals, and selenium and its salts, as well as a number of other compounds (Wattenberg 1978, 1979a, b, Griffin 1979, Wattenberg 1981). Three general mechanisms of inhibition of chemical carcinogenesis by blocking agents have been identified. The first is the inhibition of enzymatic activation of carcinogens to their reactive carcinogenic forms (Wattenberg 1979). The second entails the stimulation of a coordinated detoxification response which results in increased

Table. *Inhibitors of Carcinogen-Induced Neoplasia of the Large Bowel by Blocking Agents*

Carcinogen	Species	Inhibitor	Authors
1,2-Dimethylhydrazine	mouse	disulfiram	Wattenberg 1975
	mouse	diethyldithiocarbamate	Wattenberg et al. 1977
	mouse	bis(ethylxanthogen)	Wattenberg et al. 1977
	mouse	bis(dithiocarbamate) manganese	Wattenberg et al. 1977
	mouse	carbon disulfide	Wattenberg and Fiala 1978
	mouse	vitamin E	Cook and McNamara 1980
	rat	sodium selenite	Jacobs et al. 1977
Azoxymethane	mouse	disulfiram	Wattenberg et al. 1977
	rat	butylated hydroxytoluene	Weisburger et al. 1977
	rat	sodium selenite	Jacobs et al. 1977
	rat	disulfiram	Nigro and Campbell 1978
Methylazoxymethanol	mouse	butylated hydroxyanisole	Wattenberg and Sparnins 1979
	rat	pyrazole	Zedeck and Tan 1978
Bracken fern*	rat	phenothiazine	Pamukcu et al. 1971

*Neoplasms occur in the small intestine.

activity of several different detoxifying enzymes (Wattenberg 1979, 1981). The third general mechanism of carcinogen inhibition is the direct scavenging of reactive carcinogenic species by the inhibitor. Compounds inhibiting carcinogens which induce neoplasia of the bowel are listed in the Table. The inhibitors as well as some relevant studies have been placed into four sections to facilitate presentation.

Disulfiram and Related Compounds

Disulfiram, diethyldithiocarbamate, and bis(ethylxanthogen), when added to the diet, profoundly inhibit large bowel neoplasia resulting from subcutaneous administration of symmetrical 1,2-dimethylhydrazine (DMH) (Wattenberg 1975, Wattenberg et al. 1977). In these experiments the inhibitor is added to the diet which is fed for approximately one week prior to the initial subcutaneous administration of the carcinogen. The diets are continued until one day after the last dose of the carcinogen. Similar studies have been carried out with azoxymethane (AOM), an oxidative metabolite of DMH. Under comparable experimental conditions to those used with DMH, disulfiram inhibits AOM-induced neoplasia of the large intestine, but to a lesser extent than when DMH is the carcinogen. Studies of the mechanism of inhibition of neoplasia of the large bowel by DMH and AOM have shown that disulfiram inhibits the oxidation of both of these carcinogens in vivo (Fiala et al. 1977). Disulfiram does not inhibit methylazoxymethanol (MAM)-induced neoplasia of the large bowel.

Work has been carried out on the question of whether the inhibitory function resides in the intact molecule of disulfiram or a metabolite of this compound. These investigations have demonstrated that CS_2, a metabolite of disulfiram, inhibits the oxidation of DMH and AOM. Further work also showed that CS_2 will inhibit DMH-induced neoplasia of the large intestine in the mouse (Fiala et al. 1977, Wattenberg and Fiala 1978). Investigations also have been undertaken on the effects of CS_2 on cytochrome P-450. Incubation of microsomes with CS_2 in the presence of reduced nicotinamide adenine dinucleotide phosphate (NADPH) results in covalent binding of the sulfur to the microsomes. There is an accompanying decrease in unaltered cytochrome P-450. Several thiono-sulfur-containing compounds including disulfiram and diethyldithiocarbamate produce a similar decrease in cytochrome P-450 when incubated with microsomes under comparable conditions (Hunter and Neal 1975). This raises the possibility that thiono-sulfur-containing compounds as a group may have the potential capacity to modify cytochrome P-450 and thus alter microsomal metabolism in a manner which decreases the carcinogenicity of DMH and related carcinogens.

Recent studies have been done on the effect of disulfiram on the carcinogenicity of N-2-fluorenylacetamide (2-FAA) and N-hydroxy-N-2-fluorenylacetamide (N-OH-2-FAA) for the rat breast. Disulfiram inhibited 2-FAA but not N-OH-2-FAA. Consistent with these results was the demonstration that the inhibitory effect of disulfiram was on the metabolic conversion of 2-FAA to N-OH-2-FAA (Malejka-Giganti et al. 1980). These findings are of particular interest because, as described previously, disulfiram inhibits the N-oxidation of azomethane to AOM. Since a number of nitrogenous carcinogens are activated by N-oxidation reactions, the capacity of an inhibitor to suppress such reactions could be of importance. Disulfiram has also been shown to inhibit N-n-butyl-N-(4-hydroxybutyl)-nitrosamine-induced urinary bladder cancer in the rat (Irving et al. 1979).

The carcinogen-inhibiting effects brought about by disulfiram and diethyldithiocarbamate have drawn attention to the possibility that pesticides containing a carbon disulfide moiety in their chemical structure might have similar properties. A number of such pesticides have been used in agriculture. Two of these studied thus far have been found to inhibit DMH-induced neoplasia of the large bowel in mice. The compounds are ethylene bis(dithiocarbamate) manganese (Maneb) and bis(ethylxanthogen) (Bexide) (Wattenberg et al. 1977).

Butylated Hydroxyanisole (BHA)

BHA inhibits a variety of chemical carcinogens. Studies have been carried out to determine the effect of this phenolic antioxidant on MAM acetate-induced neoplasia of the large intestine. Female CF_1 mice were fed a diet containing BHA 5 mg/g or 10 mg/g. The diets were fed for about one week prior to the first subcutaneous administration of MAM acetate and were continued until one day after the last dose of the carcinogen. Under these conditions, almost total inhibition of neoplasia of the large intestine was produced (Wattenberg and Sparnins 1979). Grab and Zedeck have suggested that MAM might be activated to a reactive form by an NAD^+-dependent dehydrogenase that also has the capacity to oxidize ethanol. The tissue distribution of the dehydrogenase activity corresponds to the target sites of MAM acetate-induced neoplasia. In addition, pyrazole, a potent inhibitor of alcohol dehydrogenase, was found to reduce the acute lethal action of MAM acetate (Grab and Zedeck 1977). Accordingly, the effects of BHA on NAD^+-dependent alcohol dehydrogenase were determined in the livers and large bowels of CF_1 mice. BHA reduced the alcohol dehydrogenase activity in crude tissue preparations of both of these tissues in vitro (Wattenberg and Sparnins 1979). The parallel finding of BHA inhibition of MAM acetate-induced carcinogenesis of the large bowel and of NAD^+-dependent dehydrogenase activity lends support to the postulated role of the dehydrogenase activity in activating MAM to an ultimate carcinogenic form. However, BHA has multiple biologic actions so that its inhibitory effect on neoplasia of the large intestine resulting from MAM acetate may entail some other mechanism.

A study has been reported in which the effects of pyrazole on MAM acetate-induced neoplasia in the rat has been determined (Zedeck and Tan 1978). Pyrazole is a potent inhibitor of NAD^+-dependent alcohol dehydrogenase. Rats injected with MAM acetate developed tumors of the colon and duodenum. Animals treated in a comparable fashion but also given pyrazole showed no intestinal tumors. However, the latter group developed tumors of the kidney, Zymbal's gland, and the skin. The authors speculated that tumors of these latter three sites might have become apparent as a result of enhanced survival of the animals receiving the pyrazole.

Other Blocking Agents

Selenium salts have been shown to inhibit DMH- and AOM-induced neoplasia of the large bowel in rats (Jacobs et al. 1977). Selenium salts are of particular interest because of their widespread presence in the environment. Epidemiological evidence exists suggesting that there may be an inverse relationship between consumption of selenium and the occurrence of neoplasia (Shamberger and Willis 1971, Shamberger et al. 1976). The role of selenium and its salts in neoplasia has been reviewed by Griffin (1979).

There has been a recent report that addition to the diet of large amounts of vitamin E, i.e., 600 mg/kg of diet, partially inhibits the occurrence of DMH-induced colon tumors in mice. Animals fed a diet containing the high vitamin E level showed a reduction in the total number of neoplasms of the large bowel. Of particular note was the marked reduction in occurrence of malignant tumors (Cook and McNamara 1980).

Butylated hydroxytoluene (BHT) has been reported to inhibit the occurrence of tumors of the large bowel resulting from subcutaneous injection of AOM. This inhibitory effect was observed when the BHT was fed concurrently with the administrations of AOM. In addition to inhibition of neoplasia of the large bowel, a reduction in the number of malignant neoplasms of the ear ducts was also observed (Weisburger et al. 1977).

Additional Inhibitory Effects

An inhibitory study is included in the Table in which bracken fern was the carcinogenic agent. Bracken fern produces cancer of the small intestine and bladder in rats. Neoplasia at both of these sites is inhibited by addition of phenothiazine to the diet (Pamukcu et al. 1971). These findings take on increased significance because of data showing that quercetin, which is present in bracken fern, causes neoplasia of the small intestine and bladder (Pamukcu et al. 1980). Quercetin is a naturally occurring flavone commonly found in plant material consumed by man. Thus any carcinogenic effects that it may have and their inhibition could have implications for the occurrence of human neoplasia.

Increasing attention is being given to the role of the intestinal microflora in producing or activating chemical carcinogens. Metronidazole and 4-nitro-4'-isothiocyanodiphenylamine can be activated to mutagenic metabolites by the intestinal microflora of rodents. Work carried out by Batzinger and co-workers (1978) showed that this activation can be inhibited by administration of antibacterial agents acting on the enteric flora. Human feces contain mutagenic compounds (Bruce et al. 1977). If in fact mutagens occurring in the intestinal contents prove to be carcinogenic, their control by antibacterial agents could provide a useful means for cancer prevention.

A study has been reported by Raicht and his colleagues (1980) in which the plant sterol, β-sitosterol, was found to inhibit carcinogen-induced neoplasia of the large bowel of the rat. In this work, N-methyl-N-nitrosourea (MNU), a direct-acting carcinogen, was given intrarectally and the β-sitosterol added to the diet. Fewer rats fed β-sitosterol had tumors of the large bowel. The number of tumors per tumor-bearing animal also was decreased. Since the β-sitosterol-containing diet was fed concurrently with the administrations of the carcinogen and also subsequent to the last dose, it is not possible to ascertain the point or points that were inhibited in the carcinogenic process.

DISCUSSION

As is evident from the material presented in previous sections, there are a wide variety of compounds which have the capacity to inhibit carcinogen-induced neoplasia. The general area of cancer research in which administration of chemical compounds is used to prevent the occurrence of neoplasia has been called by various terms: chemoprevention, chemoprophylaxis, or simply inhibition of carcinogenesis. The term chemoprevention is simple, inclusive, and the one of choice. The core achievement at the present time in this area of research is the identification of a large number of inhibitors. Some of these are naturally occurring compounds; others are synthetic. Included are compounds which have the attractive feature of very low toxicity. It is a large pool of compounds, clearly offering multiple options and strategies. Many of these compounds have been identified on the basis of empirical work, so that for the most part they can be considered as "first generation," or at least early generation. Thus, there is the likelihood that considerable improvement can be made in terms of potency, specificity, and diminished toxicity. In contrast to achievements in identification of inhibitors, there is a relative paucity of data on mechanisms of inhibition. However, as is evident from the preceding section of this paper, progress is being made in this area. Obviously the more one understands mechanisms, the better will be the possibilities for obtaining improved inhibitors and applying those we have more effectively.

At present, chemoprevention is an area of cancer research in mid-development. It is largely focused at the moment on experimental systems, but with a few early applications to man. The importance of prevention in cancer control is evident. We have a field with potential and with promise; it remains to be determined to what extent these become realities.

ACKNOWLEDGMENTS

Work reported in this manuscript was supported by U.S. Public Health Service research grant CA 15638 from the National Cancer Institute through the National Large Bowel Cancer Project.

REFERENCES

Batzinger, R. P., S. L. Ou, and E. Bueding. 1978. Antimutagenic effects of 2(3)-tert-butyl-4-hydroxyanisole and of antimicrobial agents. Cancer Res. 12:4478–4485.

Bruce, W. R., A. J. Varghese, R. Furrer, and P. C. Land. 1977. A mutagen in the feces of normal humans, *in* Origins of Human Cancer, H. H. Hiatt, J. D. Watson, and J. A. Winsten, eds. Cold Spring Harbor Laboratory Press, New York, pp. 1641–1646.

Cook, M. G., and P. McNamara. 1980. Effect of dietary vitamin E on dimethylhydrazine-induced colonic tumors in mice. Cancer Res. 40:1329–1331.

Fiala, E. S., G. Bobotas, C. Kulakis, L. W. Wattenberg, and J. H. Weisburger. 1977. The effects of disulfiram and related compounds on the in vivo metabolism of the colon carcinogen 1,2-dimethylhydrazine. Biochem. Pharmacol. 26:1763–1768.

Grab, D. J., and M. S. Zedeck. 1977. Organ-specific effects of the carcinogen methylazoxymethanol related to metabolism by nicotinamide adenine dinucleotide-dependent dehydrogenases. Cancer Res. 37:4182–4189.

Griffin, A. C. 1979. Role of selenium in the chemoprevention of cancer. Adv. Cancer Res. 29:419–442.

Hunter, A. L., and R. A. Neal. 1975. Inhibition of hepatic mixed-function oxidase activity in vitro and in vivo by various thiono-sulfur-containing compounds. Biochem. Pharmacol. 24:2199–2205.

Irving, C. C., A. J. Tice, and W. M. Murphy. 1979. Inhibition of N-n-butyl-N-(4-hydroxybutyl)nitrosamine-induced urinary bladder cancer in rats by administration of disulfiram in the diet. Cancer Res. 39:3040–3043.

Jacobs, M. M., B. Jansson, and A. C. Griffin. 1977. Inhibitory effects of selenium on 1,2-dimethylhydrazine and methylazoxymethanol acetate induction of colon tumors. Cancer Lett. 2:133–138.

Malejka-Giganti, D., R. C. McIver, and R. E. Rydell. 1980. Inhibitory effect of disulfiram on rat mammary tumor induction by N-2-fluorenylacetamide and on its metabolic conversion to N-hydroxy-N-2-fluorenylacetamide. J. Natl. Cancer Inst. 64:1471–1477.

Matsushima, T., T. Kakizoe, T. Kawachi, H. Kazuko, T. Sugimura, T. Takeuchi, and H. Umezawa. 1976. Effects of protease-inhibitors of microbial origin on experimental carcinogenesis, *in* Fundamentals of Cancer Prevention, P. N. Magee, S. Takayama, T. Sugimura, and T. Matsushima, eds. University of Tokyo Press, Tokyo, Japan, pp. 57–69.

Mirvish, S. S. 1981a. Inhibition of the formation of N-nitroso compounds by ascorbic acid and other compounds, *in* Cancer 1980: Achievements, Challenges, Prospects, J. H. Burchenal, ed. Grune and Stratton, New York, pp. 557–587.

Mirvish, S. S. 1981b. Ascorbic acid inhibition of N-nitroso compound formation in chemical, food and biological systems, *in* Inhibition of Tumor Induction and Development, M. Zedeck and M. Lipkin, eds. Plenum Publishing Corp., New York (in press).

Mirvish, S. S., A. Cardesa, L. Wallcave, and P. Shubik. 1975. Induction of mouse lung adenomas by amines and amides plus nitrite and by N-nitroso compounds: Effect of nitrite dose and of ascorbate, gallate, thiocyanate and caffeine. J. Natl. Cancer Inst. 55:633–636.

Nigro, N. D., and R. L. Campbell. 1978. Inhibition of azoxymethane-induced intestinal cancer by disulfiram. Cancer Lett. 5:91–95.

Pamukcu, A. M., L. W. Wattenberg, J. M. Price, and G. T. Bryan. 1971. Phenothiazine inhibition of intestinal and urinary bladder tumors induced in rats by bracken fern. J. Natl. Cancer Inst. 47:155–159.

Pamukcu, A. M., S. Yalciner, J. F. Hatcher, and G. T. Bryan. 1980. Quercetin, a rat intestinal and bladder carcinogen present in bracken fern (*Pteridium aquilinum*). Cancer Res. 40:3468–3472.

Raicht, R. F., B. I. Cohen, E. P. Fazzini, A. N. Sarwal, and M. Takahashi. 1980. Protective effect of plant sterols against chemically induced colon tumors in rats. Cancer Res. 40:403–405.

Shamberger, R. J., and C. E. Willis. 1971. Selenium distribution and human cancer mortality. Crit. Rev. Clin. Lab. Sci. 2:211–221.

Shamberger, R. J., S. A. Tytko, and C. E. Willis. 1976. Antioxidants and cancer: Selenium and age-adjusted human cancer mortality. Arch. Environ. Health 31:231–235.

Sporn, M. B., and D. L. Newton. 1979. Chemoprevention of cancer with retinoids. Fed. Proc. 38:84–90.

Wattenberg, L. W. 1975. Inhibition of dimethylhydrazine-induced neoplasia of the large intestine by disulfiram. J. Natl. Cancer Inst. 54:1005–1006.

Wattenberg, L. W. 1978. Inhibitors of chemical carcinogens. Adv. Cancer Res. 26:197–226.

Wattenberg, L. W. 1979a. Naturally-occurring inhibitors of chemical carcinogenesis, *in* Naturally Occurring Carcinogens-Mutagens and Modulators of Carcinogenesis (Proceedings of the Ninth International Symposium of the Princess Takamatsu Cancer Research Fund, 1979). University Park Press, Baltimore, pp. 315–329.

Wattenberg, L. W. 1979b. Inhibitors of chemical carcinogens, *in* Environmental Carcinogenesis, P. Emmelot and E. Kriek, eds. Elsevier, New York, pp. 241–264.

Wattenberg, L. W. 1981. Inhibitors of chemical carcinogens, *in* Cancer 1980: Achievements, Challenges, Prospects, J. H. Burchenal, ed. Grune and Stratton, New York, pp. 517–539.

Wattenberg, L. W., and E. S. Fiala. 1978. Inhibition of 1,2-dimethyl-hydrazine-induced neoplasia of the large intestine in female CF_1 mice by carbon disulfide. J. Natl. Cancer Inst. 60:1515–1517.

Wattenberg, L. W., L. K. T. Lam, A. Fladmoe, and P. Borchert. 1977. Inhibitors of colon carcinogenesis. Cancer 40:2432–2435.

Wattenberg, L. W., and V. L. Sparnins. 1979. Inhibitory effects of butylation hydroxyanisole on methylazoxy acetate-induced neoplasia of the large intestine and on nicotinamide adenine dinucleotide-dependent alcohol dehydrogenase activity in mice. J. Natl. Cancer Inst. 63:219–222.

Weisburger, E. K., R. P. Evarts, and M. L. Wenk. 1977. Inhibitory effect of butylated hydroxy-toluene (BHT) on intestinal carcinogenesis in rats by azoxymethane. J. Cosmet. Toxicol. 15:139–141.

Zedeck, M. S., and Q. H. Tan. 1978. Effect of pyrazole on tumor induction by methylazoxy-methanol (MAM) acetate: Relationship to metabolism of MAM (Abstract). Pharmacologist 20:174.

Author Index

Subject Index